T0226422

Reproductive Consequences of Pediatric Disease

Editors

PETER A. LEE
CHRISTOPHER P. HOUK

ENDOCRINOLOGY AND METABOLISM CLINICS OF NORTH AMERICA

www.endo.theclinics.com

Consulting Editor
DEREK LᴇROITH

December 2015 • Volume 44 • Number 4

ELSEVIER

1600 John F. Kennedy Boulevard • Suite 1800 • Philadelphia, Pennsylvania, 19103-2899

http://www.theclinics.com

ENDOCRINOLOGY AND METABOLISM CLINICS OF NORTH AMERICA Volume 44, Number 4
December 2015 ISSN 0889-8529, ISBN 13: 978-0-323-40244-6

Editor: Jessica McCool
Developmental Editor: Meredith Clinton

Endocrinology and Metabolism Clinics of North America (ISSN 0889-8529) is published quarterly by Elsevier
Inc., 360 Park Avenue South, New York, NY 10010-1710. Months of issue are March, June, September, and
December. Periodicals postage paid at New York, NY and additional mailing offices. Subscription prices are
USD 330.00 per year for US individuals, USD 581.00 per year for US institutions, USD 165.00 per year for US
students and residents, USD 415.00 per year for Canadian individuals, USD 718.00 per year for Canadian institutions, USD 480.00 per year for international individuals, USD 718.00 per year for international institutions, and
USD 245.00 per year for international and Canadian and foreign students/residents. To receive student/resident
rate, orders must be accompanied by name of affiliated institution, date of term, and the signature of program/
residency coordinator on institution letterhead. Orders will be billed at individual rate until proof of status is received. Foreign air speed delivery is included in all *Clinics* subscription prices. All prices are subject to change
without notice. **POSTMASTER:** Send address changes to *Endocrinology and Metabolism Clinics of North
America*, Elsevier Health Sciences Division, Subscription Customer Service, 3251 Riverport Lane, Maryland
Heights, MO 63043. **Customer Service: Telephone: 1-800-654-2452** (U.S. and Canada); **1-314-447-8871** (outside U.S. and Canada). **Fax: 1-314-447-8029. E-mail: journalscustomerservice-usa@elsevier.com (for print
support); journalsonlinesupport-usa@elsevier.com (for online support).**

Reprints. For copies of 100 or more, of articles in this publication, please contact the Commercial Rights
Department, Elsevier Inc., 360 Park Avenue South, New York, NY 10010-1710; phone: +1-212-633-3874;
fax: +1-212-633-3820; E-mail: reprints@elsevier.com.

Endocrinology and Metabolism Clinics of North America is covered in *MEDLINE/PubMed (Index Medicus),
EMBASE/Excerpta Medica, Current Contents/Clinical Medicine, Current Contents/Life Sciences, Science
Citation Index, ISI/BIOMED, BIOSIS*, and *Chemical Abstracts*.

Contributors

CONSULTING EDITOR

DEREK LEROITH, MD, PhD
Director of Research, Division of Endocrinology, Diabetes and Bone Diseases, Icahn School of Medicine at Mt Sinai, New York, New York

EDITORS

PETER A. LEE, MD, PhD
Pennsylvania State University, College of Medicine, Hershey Medical Center, Hershey, Pennsylvania

CHRISTOPHER P. HOUK, MD
Associate Director, Georgia Prevention Center, Georgia Regents University, Health Sciences Campus, Augusta, Georgia

AUTHORS

ZOLTAN ANTAL, MD
Assistant Professor of Pediatrics, Department of Pediatric Endocrinology, New York Presbyterian Hospital, Weill Cornell Medical College; Memorial Sloan-Kettering Cancer Center, New York, New York

ENRICO CARMINA, MD
Professor of Endocrinology; Director of Reproductive Endocrinology Unit, Department of Mother and Child Health, University of Palermo, Palermo, Italy

JESSICA T. CASEY, MS, MD
Fellow, Department of Pediatric Urology, Riley Hospital for Children, Indianapolis, Indiana

YEE-MING CHAN, MD, PhD
Assistant Professor of Pediatrics, Harvard Medical School; Division of Endocrinology, Department of Medicine, Boston Children's Hospital, Boston, Massachusetts

MARIANA COSTANZO, MD
Servicio de Endocrinología, Hospital de Pediatría "Prof Dr Juan P. Garrahan", Buenos Aires, Argentina

SHANLEE M. DAVIS, MD
Fellow, Department of Pediatrics, Section of Endocrinology, Children's Hospital Colorado, University of Colorado, Aurora, Colorado

STEPHANIE J. ESTES, MD, FACOG
Director, Donor Oocyte Program; Director, Robotic Surgical Services; Associate Professor, Division of Reproductive Endocrinology and Infertility, Department of Obstetrics and Gynecology, Pennsylvania State University, College of Medicine, Hershey Medical Center, Hershey, Pennsylvania

LISAL J. FOLSOM, MD
Division of Endocrinology and Metabolism, Department of Medicine, Indiana University School of Medicine; Section of Pediatric Endocrinology and Diabetology, Department of Pediatrics, Riley Hospital for Children, Indianapolis, Indiana

JOHN S. FUQUA, MD
Professor of Clinical Pediatrics, Section of Pediatric Endocrinology and Diabetology, Department of Pediatrics, Riley Hospital for Children, Indianapolis, Indiana

ROMINA P. GRINSPON, MD, PhD
Centro de Investigaciones Endocrinológicas "Dr César Bergadá" (CEDIE), CONICET - FEI - División de Endocrinología, Hospital de Niños Ricardo Gutiérrez, Buenos Aires, Argentina

GABRIELA GUERCIO, MD, PhD
Servicio de Endocrinología, Hospital de Pediatría "Prof Dr Juan P. Garrahan", Buenos Aires, Argentina

WIELAND KIESS, MD
Department of Women and Child Health, Hospital for Children and Adolescents, University of Leipzig; Leipzig University Medical Centre, LIFE, Leipzig Civilization Diseases Research Centre, LIFE Child, Centre for Paediatric Research, Leipzig, Germany

ANTJE KÖRNER, MD
Department of Women and Child Health, Hospital for Children and Adolescents, University of Leipzig; Leipzig University Medical Centre, LIFE, Leipzig Civilization Diseases Research Centre, LIFE Child, Centre for Paediatric Research; IFB Adiposity Diseases, University of Leipzig, Leipzig, Germany

JÜRGEN KRATZSCH, PhD
Institute of Laboratory Medicine, Clinical Chemistry and Molecular Diagnostics, University of Leipzig, Leipzig, Germany

OKSANA LEKAREV, DO
Assistant Professor of Pediatrics, Pediatric Endocrinology, Weill Cornell Medical College, New York, New York

RACHEL LEVINE, MD
Professor of Pediatrics and Psychiatry, Pennsylvania State University College of Medicine, Hershey Medical Center, Hershey, Pennsylvania

KAREN LIN-SU, MD
Clinical Associate Professor of Pediatrics, Pediatric Endocrinology, Weill Cornell Medical College, New York, New York

ROSALIA MISSERI, MD
Associate Professor, Department of Pediatric Urology, Riley Hospital for Children, Indianapolis, Indiana

RODOLFO A. REY, MD, PhD
Centro de Investigaciones Endocrinológicas "Dr César Bergadá" (CEDIE), CONICET - FEI - División de Endocrinología, Hospital de Niños Ricardo Gutiérrez; Departamento de Histología, Biología Celular, Embriología y Genética, Facultad de Medicina, Universidad de Buenos Aires, Buenos Aires, Argentina

ALAN D. ROGOL, MD, PhD
Professor Emeritus, Department of Pediatrics, University of Virginia, Charlottesville, Virginia

JUDITH L. ROSS, MD
Professor, Department of Pediatric Endocrinology, A.I. DuPont Hospital for Children, Wilmington, Delaware; Department of Pediatrics, Thomas Jefferson University, Philadelphia, Pennsylvania

LAUREN SCHMIDT, MD
Department of Psychiatry, Yale University School of Medicine, New Haven, Connecticut

CHARLES A. SKLAR, MD
Professor of Pediatrics, Memorial Sloan-Kettering Cancer Center, New York, New York

JORMA TOPPARI, MD, PhD
Professor, Department of Physiology, Institute of Biomedicine, University of Turku; Department of Pediatrics, Turku University Hospital, Turku, Finland

HELENA E. VIRTANEN, MD, PhD
University Teacher, Department of Physiology, Institute of Biomedicine, University of Turku, Turku, Finland

MARIA G. VOGIATZI, MD
Associate Professor of Pediatrics - Clinician-Educator track, Division of Endocrinology and Diabetes, Children's Hospital of Philadelphia, Philadelphia, Pennsylvania

ISABEL V. WAGNER, MD
Department of Women and Child Health, Hospital for Children and Adolescents, University of Leipzig; Leipzig University Medical Centre, LIFE, Leipzig Civilization Diseases Research Centre, LIFE Child, Centre for Paediatric Research; IFB Adiposity Diseases, University of Leipzig, Leipzig, Germany

JIA ZHU, MD
Division of Endocrinology, Department of Medicine, Boston Children's Hospital, Boston, Massachusetts

Contents

Foreword: Reproductive Endocrinology   xiii

Derek LeRoith

Preface   xvii

Peter A. Lee and Christopher P. Houk

Infertility and Reproductive Function in Patients with Congenital Adrenal Hyperplasia: Pathophysiology, Advances in Management, and Recent Outcomes   705

Oksana Lekarev, Karen Lin-Su, and Maria G. Vogiatzi

> Individuals with congenital adrenal hyperplasia have reduced fertility, but reproductive outcomes have improved over the years. This review provides an update on the multiple pathologic processes that contribute to reduced fertility in both sexes, from alterations of the hypothalamic-pituitary-gonadal axis to the direct effect on gonadal function by elevated circulating adrenal androgens. In addition, elevated serum progesterone concentrations may hinder ovulation and embryo implantation in women, whereas in men testicular adrenal rest tumors can be a major cause of infertility. Suppression of adrenal androgen secretion represents the first line of therapy toward spontaneous conception in both sexes.

Reproductive Issues in Women with Turner Syndrome   723

Lisal J. Folsom and John S. Fuqua

> Turner syndrome is one of the most common chromosomal abnormalities affecting female infants. The severity of clinical manifestations varies and it affects multiple organ systems. Women with Turner syndrome have a 3-fold increase in mortality, which becomes even more pronounced in pregnancy. Reproductive options include adoption or surrogacy, assisted reproductive techniques, and in rare cases spontaneous pregnancy. Risks for women with Turner syndrome during pregnancy include aortic disorders, hepatic disease, thyroid disease, type 2 diabetes, and cesarean section delivery. Providers must be familiar with the risks and recommendations in caring for women with Turner syndrome of reproductive age.

Gonadal Function and Fertility Among Survivors of Childhood Cancer   739

Zoltan Antal and Charles A. Sklar

> Reproductive health and fertility are of great importance to the increasing number of survivors of childhood cancer, approximately 70% of whom are estimated to be over 20 years old. This article reviews the various treatment exposures that have been associated with makers of gonadal injury and decreased fertility in childhood cancer survivors. Identifying risk factors that decrease fertility is essential in proper counseling and timely referral for interventions that may allow for future fertility in high-risk populations.

viii   Contents

Cryptorchidism and Fertility   751

Helena E. Virtanen and Jorma Toppari

Congenital cryptorchidism, also known as undescended testis, is one of the most common urogenital abnormalities observed in newborn boys. In addition to the congenital form, there is also an acquired form of cryptorchidism. Fertility potential of patients with cryptorchidism has been evaluated by testicular histology and volume, semen quality, reproductive hormone levels, time to conception, and paternity rates. Cryptorchidism is associated with abnormalities in testicular development, and early treatment is recommended to optimize the fertility potential of the patients.

Male Obesity   761

Wieland Kiess, Isabel V. Wagner, Jürgen Kratzsch, and Antje Körner

Many cross-sectional analyses and longitudinal studies have examined the association between adiposity and pubertal development. In addition, the impact of an increased fat mass on reproduction and fertility in human obese men and in male animal models of obesity has been studied. A trend toward earlier pubertal development and maturation in both sexes has been shown, and the notion that obese boys might progress to puberty at a slower pace than their nonobese peers can no longer be substantiated. Impaired fertility markers and reduced reproductive functions have been observed in obesity. Obesity affects both pubertal development and fertility in men.

Psychological Outcomes and Reproductive Issues Among Gender Dysphoric Individuals   773

Lauren Schmidt and Rachel Levine

Gender dysphoria is a condition in which a person experiences discrepancy between the natal anatomic sex and the gender he or she identifies with, resulting in internal distress and a desire to live as the preferred gender. There is increasing demand for treatment, which includes suppression of puberty, cross-sex hormone therapy, and sex reassignment surgery. This article reviews longitudinal outcome data evaluating psychological well-being and quality of life among transgender individuals who have undergone cross-sex hormone treatment or sex reassignment surgery. Proposed methodologies for diagnosis and initiation of treatment are discussed, and the effects of cross-sex hormones and sex reassignment surgery on future reproductive potential.

Reproductive System Outcome Among Patients with Polycystic Ovarian Syndrome   787

Enrico Carmina

Polycystic ovarian syndrome (PCOS) may present with different clinical patterns, and the anovulatory phenotype may not be the most common. Data suggest that anovulation in PCOS is not the consequence of increased androgen ovarian secretion, but rather of a severe derangement of early follicle development. Other mechanisms may be operative in subgroups of patients and may contribute to the arrest of follicle growth and anovulation. At least 50% of anovulatory patients with PCOS become ovulatory in their late reproductive age. There is also evidence that menopause may occur later in women with PCOS. Finally, a strategy for treatment of infertility in PCOS is presented.

Fertility Preservation in Children and Adolescents   799

Stephanie J. Estes

Fertility preservation is the process by which either oocytes (eggs) or sperm undergo an intervention to preserve their use for future attempts at conception. Consideration of fertility preservation in the pediatric and adolescent population is important, as future childbearing is usually a central life goal. For postpubertal girls, both oocyte and embryo cryopreservation are standard of care and for postpubertal boys, sperm cryopreservation continues to be recommended. Although all the risks are unknown, it appears that fertility preservation in most cases does not worsen prognosis, allows for the birth of healthy children, and does not increase the chance of recurrence.

Fertility Issues for Patients with Hypogonadotropic Causes of Delayed Puberty   821

Jia Zhu and Yee-Ming Chan

Delayed puberty presenting with low gonadotropins has multiple causes. Self-limited delay (constitutional delay) is generally considered benign, but adult height and bone mineral density may be compromised, and fertility has not been studied. Functional hypogonadotropic hypogonadism due to a stressor is thought to resolve with removal of the stressor, but reproductive endocrine dysfunction can sometimes persist. Most, but not all, patients with idiopathic hypogonadotropic hypogonadism, a typically long-lasting condition, can achieve fertility with exogenous hormone therapy. Future studies are needed to determine fertility outcomes in self-limited delayed puberty and to more clearly define prognostic factors for fertility in functional and idiopathic hypogonadotropic hypogonadism.

Adolescent Varicoceles and Infertility   835

Jessica T. Casey and Rosalia Misseri

Varicoceles are associated with testicular atrophy and abnormal spermatogenesis. Varicocele-related testicular damage is thought to be progressive in nature. Adult varicoceles are common in men with infertility, and varicocele repair in this population has demonstrated improved semen parameters and paternity outcomes. However, without solid objective endpoints (reproducible semen analyses, paternity), the indications for adolescent varicocele repair remain controversial. Given the controversy surrounding adolescent varicocele management, it is not surprising that surveys of pediatric urologists have revealed a lack of consensus on diagnostic approaches, treatment decisions, and operative approaches.

Testis Development and Fertility Potential in Boys with Klinefelter Syndrome   843

Shanlee M. Davis, Alan D. Rogol, and Judith L. Ross

Klinefelter syndrome (KS) is the leading genetic cause of primary hypogonadism and infertility in men. The clinical phenotype has expanded beyond the original description of infertility, small testes, and gynecomastia. Animal models, epidemiologic studies, and clinical research of male subjects with KS throughout the lifespan have allowed the better characterization of the variable phenotype of this condition. This review provides an overview on what is known of the epidemiology, clinical features, and pathophysiology of KS, followed by a more focused discussion of testicular development and the clinical management of hypogonadism and fertility in boys and men with KS.

Fertility Issues in Disorders of Sex Development   867

Gabriela Guercio, Mariana Costanzo, Romina P. Grinspon, and Rodolfo A. Rey

Fertility potential should be considered by the multidisciplinary team when addressing gender assignment, surgical management, and patient and family counselling of individuals with disorders of sex development. In 46,XY individuals, defects of gonadal differentiation, or androgen, or anti-Müllerian hormone synthesis, or action result in incomplete or absent masculinization. In severe forms, raised as females, motherhood is possible with oocyte donation if Müllerian ducts have developed. In milder forms, raised as males, azoospermia or oligospermia are frequently found, however paternity has been reported. Most 46,XX patients with normal ovarian organogenesis are raised as females, and fertility might be possible after treatment.

Index   883

ENDOCRINOLOGY AND METABOLISM CLINICS OF NORTH AMERICA

FORTHCOMING ISSUES

March 2016
Lipidology
Edward A. Gill, Christie M. Ballantyne,
and Kathleen L. Wyne, *Editors*

June 2016
Pediatric Endocrinology
Robert Rapaport, *Editor*

September 2016
Obesity
Caroline M. Apovian and
Nawfal Istfan, *Editors*

RECENT ISSUES

September 2015
Postmenopausal Endocrinology
Nanette Santoro and Lubna Pal, *Editors*

June 2015
Adrenal Cortical Neoplasia
Alice C. Levine, *Editor*

March 2015
Pituitary Disorders
Anat Ben-Shlomo and Maria Fleseriu,
Editors

RELATED INTEREST

Obstetrics and Gynecology Clinics, Volume 42, Issue 1 (March 2015)
Reproductive Endocrinology
Michelle L. Matthews, *Editor*
Available at: http://www.obgyn.theclinics.com/

VISIT THE CLINICS ONLINE!
Access your subscription at:
www.theclinics.com

Foreword

Reproductive Endocrinology

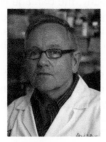

Derek LeRoith, MD, PhD
Consulting Editor

In this issue on reproductive endocrinology, a number of issues are raised: primarily, endocrine therapy and fertility assistance that reproductive and general endocrinologists are dealing with, with our patients. Given that we have more advanced investigational tools and a number of therapeutic options, we as health care providers need to be more aware of the problems and their possible therapies.

Drs Lekarev, Lin-Su, and Vogiatzi discuss, in their article, the reduced fertility rates in both males and females with congenital adrenal hyperplasia; primarily those with 21-hydroxylase deficiency, which is the most common cause. The major feature seen that affects fertility is the excess androgen secretion, secondary to the reduction in cortisol production. In women, the excess progesterone affects ovulation and implantation. Nevertheless, fertility rates are now almost 95% in well-treated patients where androgen levels are reduced. Men have an additional effect: testicular adrenal rest tumors that usually respond to glucocorticoid therapy. Finally, as the authors point out, pregnancy outcomes are excellent. The risk of an affected child is 1:1 if the other parent is a carrier.

Turner syndrome, a well-described chromosomal abnormality in female patients, is associated with impaired ovarian function, such that most cases do not undergo spontaneous puberty and pregnancy. As stressed by Drs Folsom and Fuqua, since Turners patients have numerous defects in other organs, such as aortic pathology, liver and thyroid disease, as well as diabetes, pregnancy may be an especially dangerous undertaking. Therefore, it is clearly the responsibility of the caretaker to understand and follow the recommendations with regard to preconception, and throughout pregnancy, to reduce the risk of mortality for the patients.

A serious consequence of cancer therapy in children is the subsequent infertility in both male and female patients. These effects are secondary to alkylating agents, agents used in hematopoietic stem cell transplantation, and radiation to the hypothalamus, testes, or ovaries. Drs Antal and Sklar discuss how elevations in FSH, decreases

Endocrinol Metab Clin N Am 44 (2015) xiii–xv
http://dx.doi.org/10.1016/j.ecl.2015.09.015
0889-8529/15/$ – see front matter © 2015 Published by Elsevier Inc.

endo.theclinics.com

in anti-Mullerian hormone, and inhibin B may indicate this damage and correlate with fertility capability.

Drs Virtanen and Toppari highlight the association between cryptorchidism and infertility. Cryptorchidism may be congenital, and in those cases with dysgenetic testicular development, even if the cryptorchidism is corrected early, the damage is most likely irreversible. On the other hand, acquired forms of cryptorchidism should be corrected early to avoid the changes occurring secondary to temperature effects. In cases of bilateral cryptorchidism, even early intervention may be associated with reduced fertility.

Drs Kiess, Wagner, Kratzsch, and Körner discuss the obesity epidemic and its effects on fertility. The obesity epidemic is also clearly seen in adolescents, and in male and female adolescents, obesity leads to earlier puberty, but also reduced fertility. There are numerous potential factors that could explain this relationship, including hormonal as well as some congenital factors. Furthermore, there are environmental factors that could contribute to both obesity and the infertility. One factor that is receiving attention is bisphenol-A.

There is increased interest in gender dysphoric individuals, both regarding therapeutic regimens and dealing with the psychological problems that the patients suffer from as well as appropriate diagnosis and therapy. Practicing endocrinologists are increasingly dealing with the need to suppress puberty, the use of hormonal therapy for cross-sexual results, and importantly, reassignment surgery. Successful reassignment and correct hormonal therapy have been shown to improve psychological aspects of the patients. Drs Schmidt and Levine also describe that cryopreservation of gametes and gonadal tissue banking are currently the only aspects of fertility preservation.

Dr Carmina describes in his article that polycystic ovarian syndrome is one of the most common causes of infertility in young women. It is associated with insulin resistance and hyperinsulinemia and is thought to be etiologically important. Once therapeutic interventions are successful, the hyperinsulinemia/insulin resistance is reversed, the anovulatory cycles normalize, and a percentage of women become fertile. The most commonly used interventions include lifestyle changes to reduce obesity, when present, and clomiphene citrate, metformin, and possibly thiazolidinediones.

In children or adolescents who are to be treated for cancer, an important step is the cryopreservation of oocytes and sperm. As discussed by Dr Estes, many of the chemotherapeutic regimens affect the sexual organs, and this cryopreservation allows for the surviving patients to consider fertility management later in life. A coordinated approach between pediatrician and oncologist should be very effective.

Idiopathic hypogonadotropic delayed puberty with spontaneous recovery, hypogonadotropic amenorrhea secondary to some temporary stressor, and idiopathic hypogonadotropic hypogonadism are all associated with fertility issues even after spontaneous recovery, as discussed by Drs Zhu and Chan. While many individuals become spontaneously fertile, many will require therapeutic interventions.

Varicoceles, if left untreated, are commonly associated with progressive abnormal spermatogenesis and testicular atrophy and can be reversed or halted with surgical repair. Drs Casey and Misseri discuss the situation in adolescent boys where a similar process is apparently occurring and requires immediate intervention, although the issue remains controversial among certain pediatricians. However, the recent evidence does support repair since the procedure results in improved sperm density and motility.

As discussed by Drs Davis, Rogol, and Ross, Klinefelter syndrome is the most common cause of hypogonadism and infertility in male patients. The basic cause is an extra X chromosome, and this leads to hypergonadotropic hypogonadism, due to a primary testicular abnormality that is well described. In addition, there are neurodevelopmental abnormalities and cognitive dysfunction. The primary testicular abnormality leads to infertility due to azospermia, although this may not be complete in some cases, and retrieval of sperm can be performed for later fertilization of an oocyte via intracytoplasmic sperm injection, if assisted fertility is requested. Low testosterone can be treated by standard therapy.

Disorders of sex development are very varied, and fertility issues need to be determined and treated appropriately. As discussed by Drs Guercio, Costanzo, Grinspon, and Rey, examples include 46,XY individuals and 46,XX patients. In the former, androgen defects result in reduced masculinization, and the more severe forms may be raised as females, where fertility is possible if Mullerian ducts have developed with occyte donations. In the less severe forms, raised as males, usually oligospermia or azoospermia is found, although rare cases of male fertility may occur. These and other forms require a multidisciplinary approach to diagnosis and therapy.

Drs Lee and Houk are to be praised for assembling these authors and editing these articles on some very vexing topics, and the authors are to be thanked for their efforts in writing these important topics in a clinically relevant manner.

Derek LeRoith, MD, PhD
Division of Endocrinology, Diabetes
and Bone Diseases
Icahn School of Medicine at Mt Sinai
1 Gustave Levy Place (1055)
Atran B4-35
New York, NY 10029, USA

E-mail address:
derek.leroith@mssm.edu

Preface

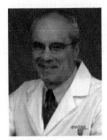 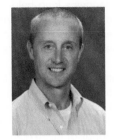

Peter A. Lee, MD, PhD   Christopher P. Houk, MD
Editors

In this issue of *Endocrinology and Metabolism Clinics of North America*: Reproductive Endocrinology, the topics were chosen because they represent conditions with reproductive consequences that are initially diagnosed or the onset of which occurs in childhood and adolescence. The reproductive topics discussed are broad, ranging from (1) classical endocrine conditions, such as Turner or Klinefelter syndrome, congenital adrenal hyperplasia, hypogonadotropic hypogonadism, constitutional delay, and polycystic ovarian syndrome, to (2) uniquely male problems like cryptorchidism, varicocele, and male obesity, to (3) conditions with significant contemporary relevance: disorders of sexual development and transgender.

Only a few decades ago, many of these conditions were strongly associated with infertility. More recently, parenthood options for these conditions have broadened significantly. Furthermore, a newer understanding of the relationship between constitutional delay and "permanent" hypogonadotropic hypogonadism instructs us that some diagnoses previously considered benign may not always be, and that some diagnoses previously considered permanent problems may in fact resolve in adulthood.

For genetic conditions associated with gonadal failure, Turner and Klinefelter syndromes, modern reproductive science has improved to the point that fertility has become a topic of discussion for all patients. Fertility options for females with congenital adrenal hyperplasia (21-hydroxylase deficiency) or polycystic ovarian syndrome have been focused on progressively intensifying traditional medical therapy to normalize the hormone imbalance in an attempt to allow normal ovulation. In recent decades, it has become obvious that such a goal is highly unlikely with traditional therapy; nonetheless, fertility is often possible among women with these diagnoses using assisted fertility techniques.

Among males with cryptorchidism and varicocele, the risk of infertility, although known, was previously not well defined. Current knowledge of factors that impact fertility in these testicular conditions is reviewed. Among those presenting with delayed puberty, the traditional understanding was that those with constitutional delay or functional delay represented an extreme variant of normal, and thus had the potential for normal fertility. Those with long-standing hypogonadotropic

Endocrinol Metab Clin N Am 44 (2015) xvii–xviii
http://dx.doi.org/10.1016/j.ecl.2015.09.014
endo.theclinics.com

hypogonadism were always permanent and were therefore infertile. Current evidence refutes this normal variant concept and suggests that future subfertility can be associated with constitutional delay and challenges a long-held understanding that long-standing hypogonadotropic hypogonadism is always permanent. The impact of current therapy upon reproductive potential of childhood cancer survivors as well as the status of fertility preservation in pediatrics, which have both changed in recent decades, is also summarized.

Two additional topics that were not primary topics relating to fertility concerns in the past include a discussion of the fertility considerations in men with obesity and individuals with disorders of sex development and transgender as fertility issues, among those with updates regarding transgender individuals and the effects of obesity on male fertility. The current fertility options for all of these diagnoses are reviewed here.

Peter A. Lee, MD, PhD
Pennsylvania State University
College of Medicine
Hershey Medical Center
500 University Drive
Hershey, PA 17033, USA

Christopher P. Houk, MD
Georgia Prevention Center
Georgia Regents University
Health Sciences Campus
1120 15th Street
Augusta, GA 30912, USA

E-mail addresses:
plee@hmc.psu.edu (P.A. Lee)
chouk@gru.edu (C.P. Houk)

Infertility and Reproductive Function in Patients with Congenital Adrenal Hyperplasia

Pathophysiology, Advances in Management, and Recent Outcomes

Oksana Lekarev, DO[a], Karen Lin-Su, MD[a], Maria G. Vogiatzi, MD[b],*

KEYWORDS

- 21-Hydroxylase deficiency • Congenital adrenal hyperplasia • Fertility • Pregnancy
- Testicular adrenal rest tumors (TART)

KEY POINTS

- Fertility data in CAH focus primarily on 21-hydroxylase deficiency.
- Fertility rates in women with CAH have improved over time. Current pregnancy rates approach 90% among those with classic disease seeking conception.
- Children born to mothers with CAH typically have no evidence of virilization.
- Fertility rates are decreased in men with classic CAH; testicular adrenal rest tumors are a common cause of infertility, require surveillance with repeated ultrasonography, and can respond to therapy with glucocorticoids.
- Suppression of adrenal androgen secretion represents the first treatment strategy toward spontaneous conception in both men and women with CAH.

INTRODUCTION

Congenital adrenal hyperplasia (CAH) refers to a group of inherited autosomal recessive disorders that lead to defective steroidogenesis. Cortisol production in the zona fasciculata of the adrenal cortex occurs in several enzyme-mediated steps. Compromised enzyme function at each step leads to a characteristic combination of elevated

The authors have nothing to disclose.
[a] Pediatric Endocrinology, Weill Cornell Medical College, New York, NY, USA; [b] Division of Endocrinology and Diabetes, Children's Hospital of Philadelphia, 3401 Civic Center Blvd, Philadelphia, PA 19104, USA
* Corresponding author. Division of Endocrinology and Diabetes, Children's Hospital of Philadelphia, 3401 Civic Center Blvd, Philadelphia, PA 19104.
E-mail address: vogiatzim@email.chop.edu

Endocrinol Metab Clin N Am 44 (2015) 705–722
http://dx.doi.org/10.1016/j.ecl.2015.07.009
0889-8529/15/$ – see front matter © 2015 Elsevier Inc. All rights reserved.

endo.theclinics.com

precursors and deficient products that is distinctive for each form of CAH. The most common form of CAH, 21-hydroxylase deficiency, accounts for approximately 95% of all cases. It is further subdivided into salt-wasting and simple-virilizing 21-hydroxylase deficiency, both of which are considered to be classic CAH, and into nonclassic CAH. In salt-wasting CAH, aldosterone and cortisol are deficient and adrenal androgens are elevated, leading to development of atypical external genitalia. In simple-virilizing CAH, aldosterone production is adequate and salt wasting does not occur; however, androgens are elevated and females are also born with atypical genitalia. In nonclassic CAH, the enzymatic deficiency is mild; although androgens are also elevated, the elevation is not significant to cause genital abnormalities in utero.[1] Thanks to life-saving glucocorticoid therapy and newborn screening programs, patients with CAH are living longer. In fact, CAH has become a life-long chronic illness with multiple complications in adulthood, including impaired fertility.

Other forms of CAH include deficiencies of 11 β-hydroxylase, 3β-hydroxysteroid dehydrogenase (HSD) or 17-α hydroxylase/17–20 lyase, congenital lipoid adrenal hyperplasia (steroidogenic acute regulatory protein), and cytochrome P450 oxidoreductase deficiency (POR). These rare forms of CAH are also associated with impaired fertility as presented in single case reports or small series of cases (**Table 1**). Most publications on

Table 1	
Various forms of CAH and summary of known effects on fertility	
Congenital lipoid hyperplasia	Severe form: • Infertility is found in both 46XX- and 46XY-affected individuals. • Spontaneous puberty and menses have been observed in 46XX-affected individuals[106]; there are anovulatory cycles with development of ovarian cysts.[107] • Successful pregnancies have been reported with reproductive assistance.[108] Partial form: There is wide variation in gonadal function in both men and women.[109,110]
17α-Hydroxylase/17,20-lyase deficiency	Severe form: There is hypergonadotropic hypogonadism and infertility (impaired spermatogenesis and folliculogenesis) in both 46XX- and 46XY-affected individuals.[111] Partial form: • Case reports of girls with spontaneous puberty and irregular or regular menses. • Single pregnancy has been reported after IVF[112]; there are several other case reports of failed IVF.
3β-HSD deficiency	Infertility is usually seen in both 46XX- and 46XY-affected individuals, with isolated reports of spontaneous puberty and conception.[113]
11β-Hydroxylase deficiency	Severe form: It resembles classic 21-hydroxylase deficiency. • Successful pregnancies of affected women have been reported.[114] • TART can develop in men.[83] Mild or nonclassic form: It resembles nonclassic 21-hydroxylase deficiency.[115]
P450 Oxidoreductase deficiency	Sexual development during puberty is disturbed in patients of both sexes, but experience is limited.[116]

Abbreviations: HSD, hydroxysteroid dehydrogenase; IVF, in vitro fertilization; TART, testicular adrenal rest tumor.

impaired fertility in CAH focus on 21-hydroxylase deficiency; unless otherwise indicated, in the authors' review the term *CAH* refers to 21-hydroxylase deficiency.

FERTILITY IN WOMEN WITH CONGENITAL ADRENAL HYPERPLASIA
Pregnancy and Fertility Rates

Estimates of spontaneous pregnancy and fertility in women with CAH correlate with the severity of the enzymatic defect, with the lowest reported rates in salt-wasting CAH and the highest reported rates in nonclassic disease. Older papers report extremely low spontaneous fertility rates (0%–10%) among women with salt-wasting CAH and moderately low rates (33%–60%) in women with the simple-virilizing type.[2–6] However, these results do not take into account whether or not patients were actively pursuing conception. Indeed, compared with the general population, adult women with classic CAH are less sexually active and less likely to engage in heterosexual relationships or actively pursue motherhood.[7,8] These facts are likely to contribute to the overall low fertility rates in this population. Reports of the pregnancy rate for women with classic disease actually trying to conceive are much more optimistic. A more recent evaluation of 106 women with classic CAH (81 with salt wasting and 25 with simple virilizing) showed that of the 23 who actively pursued conception, 91.3% achieved pregnancy. Pregnancy rates were similar in the salt-wasting (88.9%) and simple-virilizing (92.9%) groups, but those with simple-virilizing CAH were more likely to seek pregnancy.[9]

Fertility in patients with nonclassic (NC)-CAH seems to be mildly reduced. Cumulative pregnancy rates at 6 and 12 months among treated and untreated women who want pregnancy have been reported at little less than the general population at 67% and 76%, respectively.[10] Pregnancy rates may vary according to a study, from approximately 65% up to a normal rate of 95% among those seeking conception.[8,11–13] These studies involve women who came to medical attention either because of symptoms of hyperandrogenemia or infertility and, therefore, are likely to represent a more severe phenotype. The true fertility rate in nonclassic women is difficult to assess because many nonclassic patients with mild symptoms never seek medical attention and remain undiagnosed.

Proposed Factors Contributing to Reduced Fertility
Both classic and nonclassic congenital adrenal hyperplasia

Chronic anovulation and endometrial dysfunction have been described in women with CAH.[14,15] The most salient factor that can lead to these abnormalities in both classic and nonclassic CAH is adrenal androgens excess, including adrenal hypersecretion of progesterone. Elevated serum androgens can negatively affect reproductive function by several complex mechanisms that include alterations of the hypothalamic-pituitary-gonadal (HPG) axis and a direct effect on the ovary itself.[14,16]

Although the exact mechanisms by which elevated serum androgen may affect the HPG axis remain unclear, animal studies and studies in women with polycystic ovarian syndrome (PCOS) suggest that elevated androgens may alter normal central feedback pathways or interfere with the gonadotropin-releasing hormone (GnRH) pulse generator, thus, hindering ovulation.[17–19] Timing of the exposure to androgens, that is, during puberty, may also be important.[19] Estrogens produced from aromatization of excess androgens have also been proposed to suppress the HPG axis, thus, leading to anovulation and irregular menstrual cycles.[20] Regardless of the mechanism, luteinizing hormone (LH) pulsatility and secretion abnormalities have been reported in women with CAH. Compared with controls, women with nonclassic CAH have increased LH pulse amplitude but normal intervals.[21] In women with classic CAH, perinatal androgenization of the neuroendocrine function has been proposed to lead to LH hypersecretion.[22] More recently, poor adrenal control was found to be associated with reduced LH pulse frequency and amplitude.[23] Finally, elevated serum androgens have been proposed to affect folliculogenesis directly and to modulate ovarian hormone secretion by several pathways, including inhibition of follicle-stimulating hormone (FSH)–stimulated LH receptor formation in granulosa cells.[24]

Ovarian hyperandrogenism with secondary PCOS is a common finding in both classic and nonclassic CAH[22] because of chronic exposure to excess adrenal androgens, which can impair hypothalamic sensitivity to progesterone and subsequently cause LH hypersecretion. PCOS can hinder fertility through ovarian androgen production, anovulation, and irregular menstrual cycles.[16,25,26]

Another postulated factor contributing to decreased fertility is increased adrenal progesterone production in CAH. The elevated progesterone levels may potentially impede ovulation and implantation by altering GnRH pulsatility and interfering with endometrial development.[27] Other reported effects of excess progesterone are diminished sperm motility and thickening of cervical mucus, thereby acting as a form of contraception. Continuous high levels of progesterone (in contrast to the normal biphasic pattern in a healthy woman) have been documented in CAH and may adversely affect both the quality of oocytes and implantation.[10,14,16,28]

Although testicular adrenal rests are a relatively common finding in men with CAH, ovarian adrenal rests have been infrequently reported in women with CAH.[29–33] Ovarian adrenal rest tumors are difficult to identify with conventional imaging,[34] however, so it is possible that they are a more significant contributor to impaired fertility than currently estimated.

Factors unique to classic congenital adrenal hyperplasia

Women with classic CAH may face additional challenges related to their sexual and reproductive function. In these women, the excessive adrenal androgen secretion in utero affects the development of the external genitalia, including the presence of a urogenital sinus, labial fusion, and varying degrees of clitoral hypertrophy. Depending on the introital width, vaginal length, and clitoral integrity, sexual intercourse may be prohibitively uncomfortable and, thus, reduce chances for pregnancy.[14]

Women with classic CAH report being less sexually active and engaging in relationships less frequently than the general population.[7] Postsurgical difficulties may contribute to these behaviors. A study of adult women with classic CAH who had undergone genital surgery reported reduced clitoral sensation, vaginal stenosis, and painful intercourse, negatively affecting intercourse frequency.[35] Short-term results on younger patients who have undergone newer surgical techniques, such as nerve-sparing ventral clitoroplasty, have shown improved innervation and clitoral sensation.[36,37] Further studies in this cohort are needed to document if fecundity rates improve along with the evolution of surgical techniques.

Psychosexual development and psychological factors may also play a role in the reduced pregnancy rates in women with classic CAH. Prenatal exposure to high adrenal androgens seems to affect typically gender-related behavior. Girls with classic CAH have been shown to have more masculine interests in terms of sports, toys, and play behavior.[38] They also report low interest in getting married and performing a traditional child-care role, which may be an important factor.[39] Although behavior may be more masculinized, most adult women with CAH have a clearly female sex identity and gender dysphoria is rare. Most patients report a heterosexual orientation, but there is an increased rate of homosexual and bisexual orientation compared with the general population.[38]

Women with primary adrenal insufficiency also have reduced fertility[40]; therefore, cortisol deficiency itself may affect folliculogenesis and, thus, impact fertility in women with classic CAH. Glucocorticoid receptors have been shown to be present in the ovary,[14,41] and in vitro fertilization (IVF) success rates are increased with higher cortisol/cortisone ratios.[42] A direct role of cortisol on oocyte maturation or reproductive potential, however, is not clear.

Fertility Treatments

Almost all patients with classic CAH require glucocorticoid replacement in order to ovulate, and salt wasters require mineralocorticoid replacement as well. Therefore, spontaneous conception without any treatment in this patient group is exceedingly low.[14] Nonclassic patients diagnosed because of symptoms of hyperandrogenemia are also likely to benefit from therapy, although spontaneous pregnancies without any glucocorticoid replacement have been reported in rates close to 57% to 65% in this population.[10,13]

Women with CAH may conceive while on routine maintenance therapy. However, some patients may require higher doses of glucocorticoids in order to adequately suppress adrenal androgen and progesterone secretion.[14] Serum progesterone concentrations, in particular, may remain elevated despite adequate suppression of 17-hydroxyprogesterone,[43] a situation that may require treatment with higher glucocorticoid doses than routine replacement. Indeed, using a regimen of prednisolone 2 to 5 mg 3 times per day to decrease circulating progesterone levels to less than 2 nmol/L during the follicular phase, Casteras and colleagues[9] were able to attain high spontaneous pregnancy rates among women with classic disease.

For patients who remain anovulatory despite appropriate glucocorticoid and mineralocorticoid therapy and satisfactory androgen and progesterone suppression, ovulation can be induced with injectable gonadotropins or clomiphene.[44] As many adults with CAH suffer from obesity and insulin resistance,[45] an adjunct therapy with metformin can be considered, although data on its effects on androgen secretion and ovulation are limited at the moment. A decrease in circulating adrenal androgen concentrations was documented in a recent small study using metformin in diabetic women with nonclassic CAH.[46] Ovulation rates were not studied in this report.

Bilateral laparoscopic adrenalectomy is a controversial but potentially effective treatment for rare cases in which adequate adrenal androgen and progesterone suppression cannot be attained with medical therapy alone.[47] Although adrenalectomy will effectively remove the adrenal source of excess androgens, it also increases the risk for adrenal crisis, especially if patients are not completely compliant with medical therapy.[48] An increase in adrenocorticotropic hormone (ACTH) may also stimulate any adrenal rest tumors present in the ovaries.

IVF is another option if other fertility treatments are ineffective. For women with CAH whose partners are carriers, preimplantation genetic diagnosis can be performed to determine if CAH is present in embryos before they are transferred to the uterus. With this method, the parents have the option of selecting embryos unaffected by CAH for implantation.[49]

PREGNANCY AND ITS OUTCOMES

A growing body of literature reports on practice management and outcomes of women with CAH who achieve pregnancy.[5,9,15,43,50] Spontaneous miscarriages have been reported at higher rates among glucocorticoid-untreated women than in the general population. These rates reach those of the general population with steroid therapy.[9,10,13] A single report suggests that women with CAH may be at high risk for gestational diabetes.[5] This finding has not been confirmed by other studies, although it is unclear if and how patients were screened for this complication in various publications. Rates of preeclampsia or premature delivery do not seem to be affected.[9] Stress doses of glucocorticoids are recommended for labor and delivery, using similar protocols as in primary adrenal insufficiency. Finally, cesarean section is usually performed in individuals with prior genital reconstructive surgery, although vaginal deliveries have also been reported.[15,50]

Maternal use of dexamethasone to prevent virilization of the external genitalia of a female fetus affected with CAH remains a topic of heated debate, the details of which are outside the scope of this review. For women with CAH who carry an unaffected baby, hydrocortisone, prednisone, or prednisolone are the preferred steroids as these medications are inactivated by the placental 11b-hydroxysteroid dehydrogenase type 2 and, therefore, do not affect the fetus. However, there is no consensus or established guidelines on the management of glucocorticoid and/or mineralocorticoid doses during pregnancy.[43,50] One approach is to maintain prepregnancy doses and adjust them as needed based on clinical symptoms. Alternatively, therapy can be adjusted to maintain serum adrenal androgen concentrations in the upper normal range for laboratory-established pregnancy norms. Regardless, management of a pregnant woman with CAH can be challenging for multiple reasons. Symptoms of fatigue, nausea, and vomiting are common in pregnancy and overlap with those of adrenal insufficiency. Overtreatment with steroids can lead to fluid retention, excessive weight gain, and hypertension. In addition, optimal adrenal suppression during pregnancy in CAH is difficult to assess because of the multiple changes in steroidogenesis that occur during pregnancy.[4,50,51] They include a significant increase in adrenal steroid secretion along with altered steroid clearance, an increase in sex hormone–binding globulin and an increase in placenta aromatization during the third trimester. Despite all of these concerns, many pregnancies do not require an increase in prepregnancy glucocorticoid doses[9] and few obstetric problems have been reported thus far under the care of a multidisciplinary team.

Fetal outcomes are thus far reassuring. Current experience includes reports on approximately 190 babies born to mothers with classic disease.[4–7,9,52–54] No virilization was observed with the exception of 2 babies born to untreated or poorly treated mothers.[55,56] The lack of fetal masculinization is attributed to the protective effect of placental aromatase, which converts maternal androgens into estrogens. However, one should remain aware that the placental capacity for aromatization can be overcome in cases of extreme hyperandrogenemia, such as seen with maternal luteomas. Beyond this concern, fetal growth restriction and fetal distress have been linked to poorly treated adrenal insufficiency[57,58] and can be applicable to CAH pregnancies. Higher rates of babies born small for gestational age were observed in one study in CAH,[52] but the findings have not been replicated by others. Finally, long-term follow-up data remain limited at the moment[5,52] and raise no particular concerns but need to be validated by future studies.

FERTILITY IN MEN WITH CONGENITAL ADRENAL HYPERPLASIA
Fertility and Fecundity Rates

Although the subject of fertility in CAH is more frequently addressed in the literature from the female perspective, fertility remains an important topic of investigation in affected men. Earlier reports failed to show impairment in fertility.[59] However, more recent studies from Europe document significantly reduced fecundity and fertility rates in men with classic disease compared with age-matched controls or the general population.[60,61] Similar results were observed in another large study of 65 adult men with classic CAH. In this cohort, only 37% of affected men attempted fertility and 67% of them were successful, rates again significantly lower than in the general population.[8] The largest reported series to date looking at men with CAH is from a French group and includes 219 men. In those who reported cohabitation with a female partner, 51% stated that they had at least one child, a rate that is significantly lower than the French general population whereby 79% had fathered a child.[62]

Little is known about fertility rates in men with nonclassic disease. There are several case reports of men with nonclassic CAH and reduced fertility because of low sperm counts, which was reversed with glucocorticoid treatment.[63–66] However, in a recent study of 222 men who underwent a fertility evaluation because of abnormal sperm parameters, none were diagnosed with CAH.[67] Of interest, study participants were of mixed Jewish backgrounds, a population with high prevalence for nonclassic CAH. The authors do not know of any large studies directly investigating fertility in men with nonclassic CAH.

Factors Contributing to Reduced Fertility

Testicular adrenal rest tumors (TARTs) have been widely described in men with CAH and are considered to be the main culprit in reduced fertility in this population. Dysregulation of the HPG axis, Sertoli and Leydig cell dysfunction, glucocorticoid overtreatment, elevated body mass index (BMI), as well as psychological factors have also all been described as contributing factors. In addition, men with 46, XX karyotype who have CAH are unable to conceive.

Testicular adrenal rest tumors

TARTs are benign tumors, histologically resembling adrenocortical tissue and typically found in the rete testes, located at the hilum of the testicle (mediastinum testis). The rete testis consists of a network of interconnecting tubules that carry sperm from the terminal part of the seminiferous tubules to empty it into the efferent ducts. Because of their location, even small sized tumors can cause obstruction of the terminal seminiferous tubules, resulting in mechanical oligospermia or azoospermia.

Wilkins and colleagues[68] published the first case of TART in 1940. Multiple case reports followed.[66,69–72] The reported prevalence of TARTs varies widely between 0% and 94%,[8,59,60,62,73,74] depending on the age, hormonal control of the patients, and the surveillance method that was used. A limited number of studies in the pediatric population has indicated that these tumors are already present in early childhood, with a prevalence anywhere from 18% to 43%, in patients as young as few weeks of age.[69,75–79] Attempts to link the presence of TART with the CYP21A2 genotype have demonstrated no particular association, with tumors being detected in patients with salt-wasting *null* and *I2splice* mutations,[61,80,81] simple virilizing *I172N* mutation,[73,82] and even in men with nonclassic disease.[61] TARTs have also been described in men with 11-β hydroxylase deficiency[79,83] and 3-β hydroxysteroid dehydrogenase deficiency forms of CAH.[61]

The cause of TART is not completely understood, although recent studies have shed some light on the subject. It has been proposed that TARTs originate from ectopic adrenal cells that descend with the testes during fetal life and grow under ACTH stimulation; however, this hypothesis has been challenged by recent data.[84] Clinical evidence demonstrates that tumor growth is promoted in conditions whereby ACTH levels are high, such as in poorly controlled CAH and Nelson syndrome, and is reduced with high doses of glucocorticoids, suggesting the presence of ACTH receptors on tumor cells.[66,85] Recent molecular studies have supported the presence of ACTH and angiotensin II receptors as well as adrenal-specific enzymes, such as CYP11B1 and CYP11B2, directly on the tumor cells.[86] In addition, adrenal-specific steroids have been detected in blood from gonadal veins of men with TARTs[87] suggesting that these tumors have steroidogenic capacity similar to adrenals. Interestingly, some men with CAH never develop TART, despite poor adrenal control, suggesting complete regression of testicular adrenal cells prenatally. Conversely, others do not respond to intensifying glucocorticoid treatment with a reduction in tumor size.[88,89] Furthermore, Reich and colleagues[90] failed to observe an association between adrenal hormone control and TART development, again suggesting that factors other than ACTH may contribute to tumor growth. More recently, gene expression studies from TART-derived tissue revealed the presence of both adrenal cortex and Leydig cell–specific genes and expression of ACTH, angiotensin II, and LH/human chorionic gonadotropin (hCG) receptors.[84] The results provide evidence that cells in TART derive from totipotent embryonic cells that resemble fetal Leydig cells. Growth of these cells under ACTH stimulation in prenatal and postnatal life in patients with CAH and further proliferation by increased LH secretion during puberty have been proposed to lead to TART formation in men with CAH.[84]

Leydig cell dysfunction

Decreased testosterone levels have been described in several studies investigating men with CAH.[73,74,82] Although direct intratesticular mechanisms, such as TART, can cause Leydig cell damage, inadequately controlled adrenal androgens and their conversion to estrogens can suppress gonadotropins, primarily LH secretion. Cross-sectional studies as well as isolated case reports have demonstrated that men with CAH may have high androstenedione and estradiol levels along with low LH and testosterone levels, indicating an HPG axis dysregulation,[66,73,74,82,91] whereas others may have normal LH levels and low testosterone levels, indicating that TARTs may impair Leydig cell function either mechanically or by local steroid production.[74,82] In turn, impaired Leydig cell function leads to reduced semen volume and sperm number.[74,79,82] In the largest study to date, sperm analysis was performed in 71 men with classic CAH; more than 40% were found to have significant oligospermia or azoospermia, and TART was a major risk factor.[62] In one study looking at men with classic CAH, all but one patient had normal GnRH stimulation test results, indicating that HPG axis dysfunction can be overcome by stimulation and should be reversible.[82] LH suppression along with low testosterone has also been described in men with nonclassic CAH.[63–66]

Sertoli cell dysfunction

Serum inhibin B levels, which serve as a reliable marker of Sertoli cell function and number as well as seminiferous tubule damage,[92–94] have been demonstrated to be lower in men with CAH.[61,62,82,95] Inhibin B levels showed a strong positive correlation with all semen parameters, including decreased sperm count, decreased concentration, abnormal morphology, and lower motility.[82] TARTs have been shown to cause testicular parenchymal damage and seminiferous tubule obstruction in adult men with CAH, and the prevalence of TART has been shown to be significantly higher in men with low inhibin B levels than in men with normal inhibin B levels.[62] Inhibin B levels have also been shown to be lower in prepubertal boys with CAH who have no evidence of TART, implying that these patients may have had impaired Sertoli cell development independent of tumor effect.[78]

Glucocorticoid overtreatment

Overtreatment with glucocorticoids in CAH has been associated with suppression of the HPG axis[82,96] and increased BMI.[8,97,98] Obesity in itself is associated with an increased likelihood of abnormal semen parameters and reduced fertility in otherwise healthy men,[99,100] likely caused by aromatization of androgens to estrogens in the adipose tissue and subsequent dysregulation of the HPG axis.[99] Mirroring the studies in the general population, patients with CAH who have abnormal semen parameters demonstrate increased total and abdominal body fat and greater fat to lean mass ratio compared with men with CAH with normal semen.[61] Furthermore, metabolic syndrome in CAH has been linked to both high glucocorticoid replacement doses[8] and lower fertility and fecundity rates.[61]

Psychological factors and quality of life

It is unclear if psychological factors and issues contributing to quality of life have a similar impact on male fertility and fecundity rates as they do in women with CAH. The rate of marriage has been reported to be the same[61] or even higher than in healthy controls.[101] Men with CAH have been shown to have lasting employment rates comparable with healthy controls; however, they were reported to be on sick leave and receive disability pension more often than healthy controls,[101] which may play a role in their desire to have children. Anxiety and depression scores were also increased.[8] Further studies are needed to determine whether these factors influence fecundity rates in men with CAH.

Diagnostic Approach and Evaluation

The work-up of impaired fertility in a men with CAH is multifold and should include an assessment of adrenal hormone secretion and function of the HPG axis, measurement of inhibin B concentrations, as well as semen analysis. Because TART is the most common cause of infertility, men with CAH should be screened for these tumors early on in the evaluation. As the tumors are embedded within the rete testes, practitioners should not rely on palpation alone for TART detection. Typically tumors greater than 2 cm can be palpated; however, imaging techniques, such as MRI and ultrasonography, can pick up tumors only a few millimeters in diameter.[74,89] Because ultrasound is quick, noninvasive, and inexpensive, it is the study of choice for TART screening and monitoring. The age at which screening should start has not been established, but some clinics propose imaging in boys as young as 8 years of age.[96]

It is important to note that TART may be mistaken for Leydig cell tumors, and cases of unnecessary orchiectomy have been reported.[8,102] Although the tumors may be difficult to differentiate, several clinical features can aid in the differential. Up to 80% of TARTs are bilateral, whereas only 3% of Leydig cell tumors are present in both testes. Reinke crystals are found in 25% to 40% of Leydig cell tumors and are absent in TARTs. Reassuringly, malignant degeneration has never been described in TARTs; however, it occurs in 10% of Leydig cell tumors.[96]

A TART classification system has been proposed by Claahsen-van der Grinten and colleagues[96] and is summarized in **Table 2**. Beyond an effect on fertility, large TARTs can cause significant discomfort and pain.

Fertility Treatments

Because TART is the most common cause of impaired fertility in men with CAH, most of the treatment efforts aim at tumor reduction. Intensifying glucocorticoid treatment is the mainstay of medical therapy; however, there are no specific treatment protocols in place, and glucocorticoid dosing and treatment outcomes have mostly been reported

Table 2
Classification of TART

Stage 1	Adrenal rest cells present within the rete testes and are not detected on ultrasound. No treatment necessary is necessary.
Stage 2	Adrenal rest cells become visible on ultrasound as one or more small hypoechoic lesions. Optimizing glucocorticoid therapy frequently leads to tumor regression.
Stage 3	There is further growth of adrenal rest cells with compression of the rete testes. Because of obstruction of the seminiferous tubules, oligospermia and azoospermia may already be present and hormonal gonadal dysfunction is evident. Tumor size can be temporarily reduced with high glucocorticoid dosing, but tumor growth will typically resume when the dose is lowered again.
Stage 4	There is further tumor growth with progressive obstruction of the rete testes with fibrosis and focal lymphocytic infiltrates. Glucocorticoid therapy is typically not effective, and testes-sparing surgery is the treatment of choice.
Stage 5	There is irreversible damage of testicular parenchyma.

Adapted from Claahsen-van der Grinten HL, Hermus AR, Otten BJ. Testicular adrenal rest tumors in congenital adrenal hyperplasia. Int J Pediatr Endocrinol 2009;2009:624823; with permission.

Table 3
TART treatment strategies: case report summary

Case Report	Original Dosage	TART Treatment	Outcome
23-y-old man with well-controlled SV-CAH, bilateral TART, and azoospermia[117]	Hydrocortisone 30 mg divided twice daily (16 mg/m²)	Dexamethasone 0.75 mg divided 3 times daily Two 7-mo courses	• Successful pregnancy with each course of therapy • Cushingoid features
30-y-old man with poorly controlled SW-CAH, 1.5-y history of infertility, bilateral TART, and poor sperm quality[95]	Hydrocortisone 10 mg daily Fludrocortisone 0.05 mg daily	Hydrocortisone 10 mg TID Dexamethasone 0.1 mg daily	• Partial bilateral TART regression after 1.5 mo and complete regression on one side after 2 y • 6 mo on treatment semen quality significantly improved and spontaneous conception occurred • Adrenal androgens well controlled • No cushingoid features
26-y-old man with poorly controlled SW-CAH, 4-y history of infertility, bilateral TART, and azoospermia[71]	Not described	Dexamethasone 0.5 mg twice daily Fludrocortisone 0.05 mg twice daily	• Spontaneous conception approximately after 3 mo of therapy (repeat semen analysis and paternity testing not performed) • Complete regression of TART
37-y-old man with previously undiagnosed SV-CAH, infertility, unilateral TART, and azoospermia[72]	None	Dexamethasone 0.5 mg daily	• Complete regression of TART within 1 y • Normal sperm parameters

Abbreviations: SV, simple virilizing; SW, salt-wasting.

as individual cases, a selection of which is summarized in **Table 3**. High-glucocorticoid dosing has side effects and is, therefore, not acceptable to some patients. Because angiotensin II may stimulate tumor growth, mineralocorticoid therapy in patients with salt-wasting (SW)-CAH should also be optimized.[86] Surgical treatment has been reserved for more advanced TART staging, such as stage 4, whereby glucocorticoid treatment is no longer effective and testes-sparing tumor removal may prevent further testicular damage. Surgery for stage 5 tumors does not reverse testicular damage and has not been demonstrated to improve pituitary-gonadal function; therefore, surgery is primarily performed to reduce pain and discomfort.[86,96,103] Claahsen-van der Grinten and colleagues,[96] a Danish group with significant TART experience, recommends conducting a testicular biopsy before surgery to evaluate the surrounding testicular parenchyma and the extent of gonadal damage.

Traditional infertility treatments, such as clomiphene citrate,[104] combination of hCG and FSH,[102] and intracytoplasmic sperm injection,[105] have been described in men with CAH. Glucocorticoid dosing should be optimized because overtreatment with steroids can both suppress the HPG axis and lead to weight gain and metabolic syndrome, further compromising fertility. Men with CAH who have an elevated BMI should aim to lose weight. As testicular damage secondary to TART can be progressive and because there may be additional risk factors that can lead to infertility in men with CAH, perhaps the idea of semen analysis and sperm cryopreservation should be discussed with families early on in the clinical course.

REFERENCES

1. Wajnrajch MP, New MI. Defects of adrenal steroidogenesis. In: Jameson JL, DeGroot LJ, editors. Endocrinology, adult and pediatric. 6th edition. Philadelphia, PA: Saunders Elsevier; 2010. p. 1897–920.

2. Mulaikal RM, Migeon CJ, Rock JA. Fertility rates in female patients with congenital adrenal hyperplasia due to 21-hydroxylase deficiency. N Engl J Med 1987; 316:178–82.

3. Jaaskelainen J, Heppelainen M, Kiekara O, et al. Child rate, pregnancy outcome and ovarian function in females with classical 21-hydroxylase deficiency. Acta Obstet Gynecol Scand 2000;79:687–92.

4. Lo JC, Grumbach MM. Pregnancy outcome in women with congenital virilizing adrenal hyperplasia. Endocrinol Metab Clin North Am 2001;30:207–29.

5. Hagenfeldt K, Janson PO, Homdahl G, et al. Fertility and pregnancy outcome in women with congenital adrenal hyperplasia due to 21-hydroxylase deficiency. Hum Reprod 2008;23:1607–13.

6. Kulshreshtha B, Maramudi E, Khurana M, et al. Fertility among women with classical congenital adrenal hyperplasia: report of seven cases where treatment was started after 9 years of age. Gynecol Endocrinol 2008;24(5):267–72.

7. Gastaud F, Bouvattier C, Duranteau L, et al. Impaired sexual and reproductive outcomes in women with classical forms of congenital adrenal hyperplasia. J Clin Endocrinol Metab 2007;92(4):1391–6.

8. Arlt W, Willis D, Wild S, et al. Health status of adults with congenital adrenal hyperplasia: a cohort study of 203 patients. J Clin Endocrinol Metab 2010;95(11): 5110–21.

9. Casteras A, De Silva P, Rumsby G, et al. Reassessing fecundity in women with classical congenital adrenal hyperplasia (CAH): normal pregnancy rate but reduced fertility rate. Clin Endocrinol 2009;70(6):833–7.

10. Bidet M, Bellane-Chantelot C, Galand-Portier MB, et al. Fertility in women with nonclassical congenital adrenal hyperplasia due to 21-hydroxylase deficiency. J Clin Endocrinol Metab 2010;95(3):1182–90.
11. Birnbaum MD, Rose LI. Late onset adrenocortical hydroxylase deficiencies associated with menstrual dysfunction. Obset Gynecol 1984;63:445–51.
12. Feldman S, Billaud L, Thalabard JC, et al. Fertility in women with late-onset adrenal hyperplasia due to 21-hydroxylase deficiency. J Clin Endocrinol Metab 1992;74:635–9.
13. Moran C, Azziz R, Weintrob N, et al. Reproductive outcome of women with 21-hydroxylase-deficient nonclassic adrenal hyperplasia. J Clin Endocrinol Metab 2006;91:3451–6.
14. Reichman DE, White PC, New MI, et al. Fertility in patients with congenital adrenal hyperplasia. Fertil Steril 2014;101:301–9.
15. Witchel SF. Management of CAH during pregnancy: optimizing outcomes. Curr Opin Endocrinol Diabetes Obes 2012;19(6):489–96.
16. Mnif MF, Kamoun M, Kacem FH, et al. Reproductive outcomes of female patients with congenital adrenal hyperplasia due to 21-hydroxylase deficiency. Indian J Endocrinol Metab 2013;17:790–3.
17. Melrose P, Gross L. Steroid effects on the secretory modalities of gonadotropin-releasing hormone release. Endocrinology 1987;121(1):190–9.
18. Blank SK, McCartney CR, Helm KD, et al. Neuroendocrine effects of androgens in adult polycystic ovary syndrome and female puberty. Semin Reprod Med 2007;25(5):352–9.
19. McGee WK, Bishop CV, Bahar A, et al. Elevated androgens during puberty in female rhesus monkeys lead to increased neuronal drive to the reproductive axis: a possible component of polycystic ovary syndrome. Hum Reprod 2012;27(2):531–40.
20. Knobil E. Discovery of the hypothalamic gonadotropin-releasing hormone pulse generator and of its physiologic significance. Am J Obstet Gynecol 2005;193(5):1765–6.
21. Levin JH, Carmina E, Lobo RA. Is the inappropriate gonadotropin secretion of patients with polycystic ovary syndrome similar to that of patients with adult-onset congenital adrenal hyperplasia? Fertil Steril 1991;56:635–40.
22. Barnes RB, Rosenfield RL, Ehrmann DA, et al. Ovarian hyperandrogynism as a result of congenital adrenal virilizing disorders: evidence for perinatal masculinization of neuroendocrine function in women. J Clin Endocrinol Metab 1994;79(5):1328–33.
23. Bachelot A, Chakhtoura Z, Plu-Bureau G, et al. Influence of hormonal control on LH pulsatility and secretion in women with classical congenital adrenal hyperplasia. Eur J Endocrinol 2012;167:499–505.
24. Jia XC, Kessel B, Welsh TH Jr, et al. Androgen inhibition of follicle-stimulating hormone-stimulated luteinizing hormone receptor formation in cultured rat granulosa cells. Endocrinology 1985;117:13–22.
25. Forest MG. Recent advances in the diagnosis and management of congenital adrenal hyperplasia due to 21-hydroxylase deficiency. Hum Reprod Update 2004;10:469–85.
26. Robyr D, Llor J, Gaudin G, et al. Polycystic ovary syndrome and congenital adrenal hyperplasia: a different entity for comparable phenotypes? Rev Med Suisse 2007;3:1595–601.
27. Holmes-Walker DJ, Conway GS, Honour JW, et al. Menstrual disturbance and hypersecretion of progesterone in women with congenital adrenal hyperplasia due to 21-hydroxylase deficiency. Clin Endocrinol 1995;43:291–6.

28. Labarta E, Martinez-Conejero JA, Alama P, et al. Endometrial receptivity is affected in women with high circulating progesterone levels at the end of the follicular phase: a functional genomics analysis. Hum Reprod 2011;26: 1813–25.
29. Russo G, Paesano P, Taccagni G, et al. Ovarian adrenal-like tissue in congenital adrenal hyperplasia. N Engl J Med 1998;339:853–5.
30. Al-Ahmadie HA, Stanek J, Liu J, et al. Ovarian 'tumor' of the adrenogenital syndrome: the first reported case. Am J Surg Pathol 2001;25:436–42.
31. Claahsen-van der Grinten HL, Hulsbergen-van de Kaa CA, Otten BJ. Ovarian adrenal rest tissue in congenital adrenal hyperplasia: a patient report. J Pediatr Endocrinol Metab 2006;19:177–82.
32. Tiosana D, Vlodavsky E, Filmar S, et al. Ovarian adrenal rest tumor in a congenital adrenal hyperplasia patient with adrenocorticotropin hypersecretion following adrenalectomy. Horm Res Paediatr 2010;74:223–8.
33. Zaarour MG, Atallah DM, Trak-Smayra VE, et al. Bilateral ovary adrenal rest tumor in a congenital adrenal hyperplasia following adrenalectomy. Endocr Pract 2014;20:e69–74.
34. Crocker MK, Barak S, Millo CM, et al. Use of PET/CT with cosyntropin stimulation to identify and localize adrenal rest tissue following adrenalectomy in a woman with congenital adrenal hyperplasia. J Clin Endocrinol Metab 2012; 97:E2084–9.
35. Crouch NS, Liao LM, Woodhouse CR, et al. Sexual function and genital sensitivity following feminizing genitoplasty for congenital adrenal hyperplasia. J Urol 2008;179:634–8.
36. Yang J, Felsen D, Poppas DP. Nerve sparing ventral clitoroplasty: analysis of clitoral sensitivity and viability. J Urol 2007;178:1598–601.
37. Leslie JA, Cain MP, Rink RC. Feminizing genital reconstruction in congenital adrenal hyperplasia. Indian J Urol 2009;25:17–26.
38. Meyer-Bahlburg HF, Dolezal C, Baker SW, et al. Gender development in women with congenital adrenal hyperplasia as a function of disorder severity. Arch Sex Behav 2006;35:667–84.
39. Meyer-Bahlburg HFL. What causes low rate of child-bearing in congenital adrenal hyperplasia? J Clin Endocrinol Metab 1999;84:1844–7.
40. Erichson MM, Husebye ES, Michelsen TM, et al. Sexuality and fertility in women with Addison's disease. J Clin Endocrinol Metab 2010;95:4354–60.
41. Rae MT, Price D, Harlow CR, et al. Glucocorticoid receptor-mediated regulation of MMP9 gene expression in human ovarian surface epithelial cells. Fertil Steril 2009;92:703–8.
42. Keay SD, Harlow CR, Wood PJ, et al. Higher cortisol: cortisone ratios in the pre-ovulatory follicle of completely unstimulated IVF cycles indicate oocytes with increased pregnancy potential. Humanit Rep 2002;17:2410–4.
43. Ogilvie CM, Crouch NS, Rumsby G, et al. Congenital adrenal hyperplasia in adults: a review of medical, surgical and psychological issues. Clin Endocrinol (Oxf) 2006;64(1):2–11.
44. Laohaprasitiporn C, Barbieri RL, Yeh J. Induction of ovulation with the sole use of clomiphene citrate in late-onset 21-hydroxylase deficiency. Gynecol Obstet Invest 1996;41:224–6.
45. Saygili F, Oge A, Yilmaz C. Hyperinsulinemia and insulin insensitivity in women with nonclassical congenital adrenal hyperplasia due to 21-hydroxylase deficiency: the relationship between serum leptin levels and chronic hyperinsulinemia. Horm Res 2005;63:270–4.

46. Krysiak R, Okopien B. The effect of metformin on androgen production in diabetic women with non-classic congenital adrenal hyperplasia. Exp Clin Endocrinol Diabetes 2014;122:568–71.

47. Gmyrek GA, New MI, Sosa RE, et al. Bilateral laparoscopic adrenalectomy as a treatment for classic congenital adrenal hyperplasia attributable to 21-hydroxylase deficiency. Pediatrics 2002;109:E28.

48. Van Wyk JJ, Ritzen EM. The role of bilateral adrenalectomy in the treatment of congenital adrenal hyperplasia. J Clin Endocrinol Metab 2003;88:2993–8.

49. Van de Velde H, Sermon K, De Vos A, et al. Fluorescent PCR and automated fragment analysis in preimplantation genetic diagnosis for 21-hydroxylase deficiency in congenital adrenal hyperplasia. Mol Hum Reprod 1999;5:691–6.

50. Lekarev O, New MI. Adrenal disease in pregnancy. Best Pract Res Clin Endocrinol Metab 2011;25(6):959–73.

51. Suri D, Moran J, Hibbard JU, et al. Assessment of adrenal reserve in pregnancy: defining the normal response to the adrenocorticotropin stimulation test. J Clin Endocrinol Metab 2006;91(10):3866–72.

52. Krone N, Wachter I, Stefanidou M, et al. Mothers with congenital adrenal hyperplasia and their children: outcome of pregnancy, birth and childhood. Clin Endocrinol (Oxf) 2001;55(4):523–9.

53. Dumic M, Janjanin N, Ille J, et al. Pregnancy outcomes in women with classical congenital adrenal hyperplasia due to 21-hydroxylase deficiency. J Pediatr Endocrinol Metab 2005;18(9):887–95.

54. Hoepffner W, Schulze E, Bennek J, et al. Pregnancies in patients with congenital adrenal hyperplasia with complete or almost complete impairment of 21-hydroxylase activity. Fertil Steril 2004;81(5):1314–21.

55. Kai H, Nose O, Iida Y, et al. Female pseudohermaphroditism caused by maternal congenital adrenal hyperplasia. J Pediatr 1979;95(3):418–20.

56. Zacharin M. Fertility and its complications in a patient with salt losing congenital adrenal hyperplasia. J Pediatr Endocrinol Metab 1999;12(1):89–94.

57. Albert E, Dalaker K, Jorde R, et al. Addison's disease and pregnancy. Acta Obstet Gynecol Scand 1989;68:185–7.

58. Björnsdottir S, Cnattingius S, Brandt L, et al. Addison's disease in women is a risk factor for an adverse pregnancy outcome. J Clin Endocrinol Metab 2010; 95:5249–57.

59. Urban MD, Lee PA, Migeon CJ. Adult height and fertility in men with congenital virilizing adrenal hyperplasia. N Engl J Med 1978;299(25):1392–6.

60. Jaaskelainen J, Kiekara O, Hippeläinen M, et al. Pituitary gonadal axis and child rate in males with classical 21-hydroxylase deficiency. J Endocrinol Invest 2000; 23(1):23–7.

61. Falhammar H, Nyström HF, Ekström U, et al. Fertility, sexuality and testicular adrenal rest tumors in adult males with congenital adrenal hyperplasia. Eur J Endocrinol 2012;166(3):441–9.

62. Bouvattier C, Esterle L, Renoult-pierre P, et al. Clinical outcome, hormonal status, gonadotrope axis and testicular function in 219 adult men born with classic 21-hydroxylase deficiency. A French national survey. J Clin Endocrinol Metab 2015;100(6):2303–13.

63. Augarten A, Weissenberg R, Pariente C, et al. Reversible make infertility in late onset congenital adrenal hyperplasia. J Endocrinol Invest 1991;14(3): 237–40.

64. Mirsky HA, Hines JH. Infertility in a man with 21-hydroxylase deficient congenital adrenal hyperplasia. J Urol 1989;142(1):111–3.

65. Kalachanis I, Rousso D, Kourtis A, et al. Reversible infertility, pharmaceutical and spontaneous, in a male with late onset congenital adrenal hyperplasia, due to 21-hydroxylase deficiency. Arch Androl 2002;48(1):37–41.

66. Bonaccorsi AC, Adler I, Figueiredo JG. Male infertility due to congenital adrenal hyperplasia: testicular biopsy findings, hormonal evaluation, and therapeutic results in three patients. Fertil Steril 1987;47(4):664–70.

67. Pinkas H, Fuchs S, Klipper-Aurbach Y, et al. Non-classical 21-hydroxylase deficiency: prevalence in males with unexplained abnormal sperm analysis. Fertil Steril 2010;93(6):1887–91.

68. Wilkins L, Fleiscmann W, Howard JE. Macrogenitosomia precox associated with hyperplasia of the androgenic tissue and death from corticoadrenal insufficiency. Endocrinology 1940;26:385–95.

69. Shanklin MA, Keating MA, Levin HS, et al. Testicular hilar nodules in adrenogenital syndrome. The nature of the nodules. Am J Dis Child 1963;106:243–50.

70. Rutgers JL, Young RH, Scully RE. The testicular "tumor" of the adrenogenital syndrome. A report of six cases and review of the literature on testicular masses in patients with adrenogenital disorders. Am J Surg Pathol 1988;12(7):503–13.

71. Collet TH, Pralong F. Reversal of primary male infertility and testicular adrenal rest tumors in salt-wasting congenital adrenal hyperplasia. J Clin Endocrinol Metab 2010;95(5):2013–4.

72. Sumida C, Kondoh N, Kurajoh M, et al. 21-hydroxylase deficiency associated with male infertility: report of 2 cases with gene analyses. Intern Med 2011;50:1317–21.

73. Cabrera M, Vogiatzi M, New M. Long term outcomes in adult males with classic congenital adrenal hyperplasia. J Clin Endocrinol Metab 2001;86:3070–8.

74. Stikkelbroeck N, Otten B, Pasic A, et al. High prevalence of testicular adrenal rest tumors, impaired spermatogenesis, and Leydig cell failure in adolescent and adult males with congenital adrenal hyperplasia. J Clin Endocrinol Metab 2001;86(12):5721–8.

75. Avila NA, Premkunar A, Shawker TH, et al. Testicular adrenal rest tissue in congenital adrenal hyperplasia: findings at gray-scale and color Doppler US. Radiology 1996;198(1):99–104.

76. Vanzulli A, DelMaschio A, Paesano P, et al. Testicular masses in association with adrenogenital syndrome: US findings. Radiology 1992;183(2):425–9.

77. Claahsen-van der Grinten HL, Sweep FC, Blickman JG, et al. Prevalence of testicular adrenal rest tumours in male children with congenital adrenal hyperplasia due to 21-hydroxylase deficiency. Eur J Endocrinol 2007;157(3):339–44.

78. Martinez-Aguayo A, Rocha A, Rojas N, et al. Testicular adrenal res tumors and Leydig and Sertoli cell function in boys with classical congenital adrenal hyperplasia. J Clin Endocrinol Metab 2007;92:4583–9.

79. Aycan Z, Bas VN, Cestinkaya S, et al. Prevalence and long-term outcomes of testicular adrenal rest tumors in children and adolescent males with congenital adrenal hyperplasia. Clin Endoctinol (Oxf) 2013;78(5):667–72.

80. Mouritsen A, Jorgensen N, Main KM, et al. Testicular adrenal rest tumors in boys, adolescents and adult men with congenital adrenal hyperplasia may be associated with the CYP21A2 mutation. Int J Androl 2010;33:521–7.

81. Nermoen I, Rorvik J, Holmedal SH, et al. High frequency of adrenal myelolipomas and testicular adrenal rest tumours in adult Norwegian patients with classical congenital adrenal hyperplasia because of 21-hydroxylase deficiency. Clin Endocrinol (Oxf) 2011;75(6):753–9.

82. Reisch N, Flade L, Scherr M, et al. High prevalence of reduced fecundity in men with congenital adrenal hyperplasia. J Clin Endocrinol Metab 2009;94:1665–70.
83. Kaynar M, Sonmez MG, Unlü Y, et al. Testicular adrenal rest tumor in 11-beta-hydroxylase deficiency driven congenital adrenal hyperplasia. Korean J Urol 2014; 55(4):292–4.
84. Smeets E, Span P, van Herwaarden A, et al. Molecular characterization of testicular adrenal rest tumors in congenital adrenal hyperplasia; lesions with both adrenocortical and Leydig cell features. J Clin Endocrinol Metab 2015;100(3):E524–30.
85. Cunnah D, Perry L, Dacie JL, et al. Bilateral testicular tumours in congenital adrenal hyperplasia: a continuing diagnostic and therapeutic dilemma. Clin Endocrinol (Oxf) 1989;30(2):141–7.
86. Claahsen-van der Grinten HL, Otten BJ, Sweep F, et al. Testicular tumors in patients with congenital adrenal hyperplasia due to 21-hydroxylase deficiency show functional features of adrenocortical tissue. J Clin Endocrinol Metab 2007;92(9):3674–80.
87. Blumberg-Tick J, Boudou P, Nahoul K, et al. Testicular tumors in congenital adrenal hyperplasia: steroid measurements from adrenal and spermatic veins. Clin Endocrinol Metab 1991;73(5):1129–33.
88. Walker BR, Skoog SJ, Winslow BH, et al. Testis sparing surgery for steroid unresponsive testicular tumors of the adrenogenital syndrome. J Urol 1997; 157(4):1460–3.
89. Stikkelbroeck NM, Hermus AR, Suliman HM, et al. Asymptomatic testicular adrenal rest tumours in adolescent and adult males with congenital adrenal hyperplasia: basal and follow-up investigation after 2.6 years. J Pediatr Endocrinol Metab 2004;17(4):645–53.
90. Reisch N, Rottenkolber M, Greifenstein A, et al. Testicular adrenal rest tumors develop independently of long-term disease control: a longitudinal analysis of 50 adult men with congenital adrenal hyperplasia due to classic 21-hydroxylase deficiency. J Clin Endocrinol Metab 2013;98(11):E1820–6.
91. Radfar N, Bartter FC, Easley R, et al. Evidence of endogenous LH suppression in a man with bilateral testicular tumors and congenital adrenal hyperplasia. J Clin Endocrinol Metab 1977;45:1194–204.
92. Andersson AM, Petersen JH, Jorgensen N, et al. Serum inhibin B and follicle-stimulating hormone levels as tools in the evaluation of infertile men: significance of adequate reference values from proven fertile men. J Clin Endocrinol Metab 2004;89:2873–9.
93. Ramaswamy S, Mashall GR, McNeilly AS, et al. Evidence that in a physiological setting Sertoli cell number is the major determinant of circulating concentration of inhibin B in the adult male rhesus monkey. J Androl 1999;20:430–4.
94. Suescun MO, Lustig L, Calandras RS, et al. Correlation between inhibin secretion and damage of seminiferous tubules in a model of experimental autoimmune orchitis. J Endocrinol 2001;170:113–20.
95. Mouritsen A, Juul A, Jørgensen N. Improvement of semen quality in an infertile man with 21-hydroxylase deficiency, suppressed serum gonadotropins and testicular adrenal rest tumours. Int J Androl 2010;33(3):518–20.
96. Claahsen-van der Grinten HL, Hermus AR, Otten BJ. Testicular adrenal rest tumors in congenital adrenal hyperplasia. Int J Pediatr Endocrinol 2009;2009: 624823.
97. Mooji CF, Kroese JM, Claahsen-van der Grinten HL, et al. Unfavourable trends in cardiovascular and metabolic risk in paediatric and adult patients with a congenital adrenal hyperplasia. Clin Endocrinol 2010;73:137–46.

98. Falhammar H, Filipsson H, Holmdahl G, et al. Metabolic profile and body composition in adult women with congenital adrenal hyperplasia due to 21-hydroxylase deficiency. J Clin Endocrinol Metab 2007;92:110–6.

99. Du Plessis SS, Cabler S, McAlister DA, et al. The effect of obesity on sperm disorders and male infertility. Nature Reviews. Urology 2010;7:153–61.

100. Hammoud AO, Wilde N, Gibson M, et al. Male obesity and alterations in sperm parameters. Fertil Steril 2008;90:2222–5.

101. Strandqvist A, Falhammar H, Lichtenstein P, et al. Suboptimal psychosocial outcomes in patients with congenital adrenal hyperplasia: epidemiological studies in a non-biased national cohort in Sweden. J Clin Endocrinol Metab 2014;99(4):1425–32.

102. Rohayem J, Tüttelmann F, Mallidis C, et al. Restoration of fertility by gonadotropin replacement in a man with hypogonadotropic azoospermia and testicular adrenal rest tumors due to untreated simple virilizing congenital adrenal hyperplasia. Eur J Endocrinol 2014;170(4):K11–7.

103. Claahsen-van der grinten HL, Otten BJ, Takahashi S, et al. Testicular adrenal rest tumors in adult males with congenital adrenal hyperplasia: evaluation of pituitary-gonadal function before and after successful testis-sparing surgery in eight patients. J Clin Endocrinol Metab 2007;92(2):612–5.

104. Yang RM, Fefferman RA, Shapiro CE. Reversible infertility in a man with 21-hydroxylase deficiency congenital adrenal hyperplasia. Fertil Steril 2005;83(1):223–5.

105. Murphy H, George C, de Kretser D, et al. Successful treatment with ICSI of infertility caused by azoospermia associated with adrenal rests in testes. Hum Reprod 2001;16(2):263–7.

106. Bose HS, Pescovitz OH, Miller WL. Spontaneous feminization in a 46, XX female patient with congenital lipoid adrenal hyperplasia due to a homozygous frameshift mutation in the steroidogenic acute regulatory protein. J Clin Endocrinol Metab 1997;82(5):1511–5.

107. Kim CJ. Congenital lipoid adrenal hyperplasia. Ann Pediatr Endocrinol Metab 2014;19(4):179–83.

108. Khoury K, Barbar E, Ainmelk Y, et al. Gonadal function, first cases of pregnancy, and child delivery in a woman with lipoid congenital adrenal hyperplasia. J Clin Endocrinol Metab 2009;94(4):1333–7.

109. Flück CE, Pandey AV, Dick B, et al. Characterization of novel StAR (steroidogenic acute regulatory protein) mutations causing non-classic lipoid adrenal hyperplasia. PLoS One 2011;6(5):e20178.

110. Sahakitrungruang T, Tee MK, Blackett PR, et al. Partial defect in the cholesterol side-chain cleavage enzyme P450scc (CYP11A1) resembling nonclassic congenital lipoid adrenal hyperplasia. J Clin Endocrinol Metab 2011;96(3):792–8.

111. Marsh CA, Auchus RJ. Fertility in patients with genetic deficiencies of cytochrome P450c17 (CYP17A1): combined 17-hydroxylase/17,20-lyase deficiency and isolated 17,20-lyase deficiency. Fertil Steril 2014;101(2):317–22.

112. Levran D, Ben-Shlomo I, Pariente C, et al. Familial partial 17,20-desmolase and 17alpha-hydroxylase deficiency presenting as infertility. J Assist Reprod Genet 2003;20(1):21–8.

113. Simard J, Ricketts ML, Gingras S, et al. Molecular biology of the 3beta-hydroxysteroid dehydrogenase/delta5-delta4 isomerase gene family. Endocr Rev 2005;26(4):525–82.

114. Simm PJ, Zacharin MR. Successful pregnancy in a patient with severe 11-beta-hydroxylase deficiency and novel mutations in CYP11B1 gene. Horm Res 2007;68(6):294–7.

115. Reisch N, Högler W, Parajes S, et al. A diagnosis not to be missed: nonclassic steroid 11β-hydroxylase deficiency presenting with premature adrenarche and hirsutism. J Clin Endocrinol Metab 2013;98(10):E1620–5.
116. Fukami M, Ogata T. Cytochrome P450 oxidoreductase deficiency: rare congenital disorder leading to skeletal malformations and steroidogenic defects. Pediatr Int 2014;56(6):805–8.
117. Claahsen-van der Grinten HL, Otten BJ, Sweep F, et al. Repeated successful induction of fertility after replacing hydrocortisone with dexamethasone in a patient with congenital adrenal hyperplasia and testicular adrenal rest tumors. Fertil Steril 2007;88(3):705.e5–8.

Reproductive Issues in Women with Turner Syndrome

Lisal J. Folsom, MD[a,b,*], John S. Fuqua, MD[b]

KEYWORDS

- Turner syndrome • Fertility • Reproduction • Pregnancy risks
- Society recommendations • Prepregnancy counseling

KEY POINTS

- Turner syndrome is one of the most common chromosomal abnormalities in female infants.
- Clinical manifestations of Turner syndrome include abnormalities of the skeletal, cardiovascular and lymphatic, endocrine, gastrointestinal, renal, and central nervous systems.
- Ovarian function sufficient to result in puberty is uncommon, and subsequent fertility is even less common in women with Turner syndrome; however, there are several options for women who desire to expand their families.
- Because of the unique pregnancy risks and complications in women with Turner syndrome it is important to be familiar with the current guidelines for preconception counseling and monitoring during gestation.

INTRODUCTION

Turner syndrome, defined as typical features in a phenotypic female with partial or complete loss of the second sex chromosome, is one of the most common chromosomal abnormalities, with an annual incidence of 1:2500 live-born female infants.[1,2] Approximately 50% of affected women are missing an entire X chromosome and have a karyotype of 45,X. About 25% have a partial deletion of 1 X chromosome, whereas about 20% have varying degrees of mosaicism, most commonly a 45,X/46,XX karyotype.[3] A small group of affected women carries an XY cell line.

In general, the phenotypic severity of Turner syndrome varies with the extent of X chromosome loss. Clinical manifestations of Turner syndrome (**Fig. 1**) may be categorized as

Disclosures: The authors have nothing to disclose.
[a] Division of Endocrinology and Metabolism, Department of Medicine, Indiana University School of Medicine, 541 N. Clinical Drive CL 365, Indianapolis, IN 46202, USA; [b] Section of Pediatric Endocrinology and Diabetology, Department of Pediatrics, Riley Hospital for Children, 705 Riley Hospital Drive, Room 5960, Indianapolis, IN 46202, USA
* Corresponding author. 705 Riley Hospital Drive, Room 5960, Indianapolis, IN 46202.
E-mail address: FolsomL@iupui.edu

Endocrinol Metab Clin N Am 44 (2015) 723–737
http://dx.doi.org/10.1016/j.ecl.2015.07.004
0889-8529/15/$ – see front matter © 2015 Elsevier Inc. All rights reserved.

endo.theclinics.com

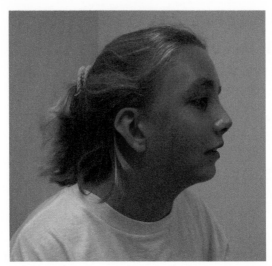

Fig. 1. Adolescent with Turner syndrome. Note the phenotypic features, including ptosis, downslanting palpebral fissures, micrognathia, low-set and posteriorly rotated ears, low posterior hairline, and pigmented nevi. (*Courtesy of* Erica Eugster, MD, Indianapolis, IN.)

abnormalities affecting multiple organ systems, including the skeletal, cardiovascular and lymphatic, endocrine, gastrointestinal, renal, and the central nervous systems (**Box 1**). Major morbidities may occur during adult life, and these result in a 3-fold increase in mortality.[4] Particularly relevant to the discussion of reproductive function is the increased prevalence of aortic root dilatation and aortic dissection, which occur in 32% and 1% to 2% of affected women, respectively.[5,6] Dissection occurs at an average age of 31.5 years, making it particularly relevant to women in their reproductive years.[7]

OVARIAN DEVELOPMENT IN WOMEN WITH TURNER SYNDROME

In normal developing women, the number of nongrowing ovarian follicles increases through the first half of gestation, reaching an average maximum of 300,000 per ovary at 18 to 22 weeks of gestation.[8] Oogonia enter meiosis, which is arrested at prophase I, forming oocytes. Oocytes are incorporated into primordial follicles starting at 14 to 20 weeks of gestation. Throughout the second half of gestation, the number of nongrowing follicles remains fairly constant, and by birth the number of follicles averages 295,000 per ovary. This number then decreases over prepubertal life, reaching about 180,000 per ovary by the age at menarche, and then declines further in an accelerating fashion until menopause (**Fig. 2**).

During the first trimester, ovarian development in fetuses with Turner syndrome is initially normal. Examination of ovaries at 14 to 18 weeks' gestation has revealed normal gonadal development.[9] Shortly thereafter, oocyte loss is accelerated in many girls with Turner syndrome, with oocyte depletion being nearly complete prenatally or by the first few months after birth. In fetuses with 46,XX karyotypes, oogonia were seen as early as 18 weeks, ovaries from 20 weeks onward were found to have primordial follicles, and preantral and antral follicles were seen at 26 weeks. In contrast, some ovaries from fetuses with 45,X karyotypes had oogonia, but no follicles were visualized.[10] There is evidence that some girls with Turner syndrome continue to

Box 1
Phenotypic features of Turner syndrome

Skeletal system
  Short stature
  Broad chest
  Scoliosis
  Cubitus valgum
  Short fourth metacarpal
  Madelung deformity of the wrist
  Genu valgum

Cardiovascular and lymphatic systems
  Bicuspid aortic valve
  Coarctation of the aorta
  Hypertension
  Aortic root dilatation
  Aortic dissection
  Lymphedema of hands and feet
  Pterygium colli
  Low posterior hairline
  Low-set and posteriorly rotated ears
  Downslanting palpebral fissures

Endocrine system
  Primary ovarian failure
  Hashimoto thyroiditis
  Glucose intolerance
  Type 2 diabetes mellitus

Gastrointestinal system
  Celiac disease

Central nervous system
  Sensorineural hearing loss
  Attention-deficit/hyperactivity disorder
  Learning disability
  Decreased visuospatial skills and executive function

Renal system
  Duplicated renal collecting system
  Horseshoe kidney

Other
  Arched palate
  Micrognathia
  Otitis media
  Conductive hearing loss
  Pigmented nevi
  Hyperconvex fingernails

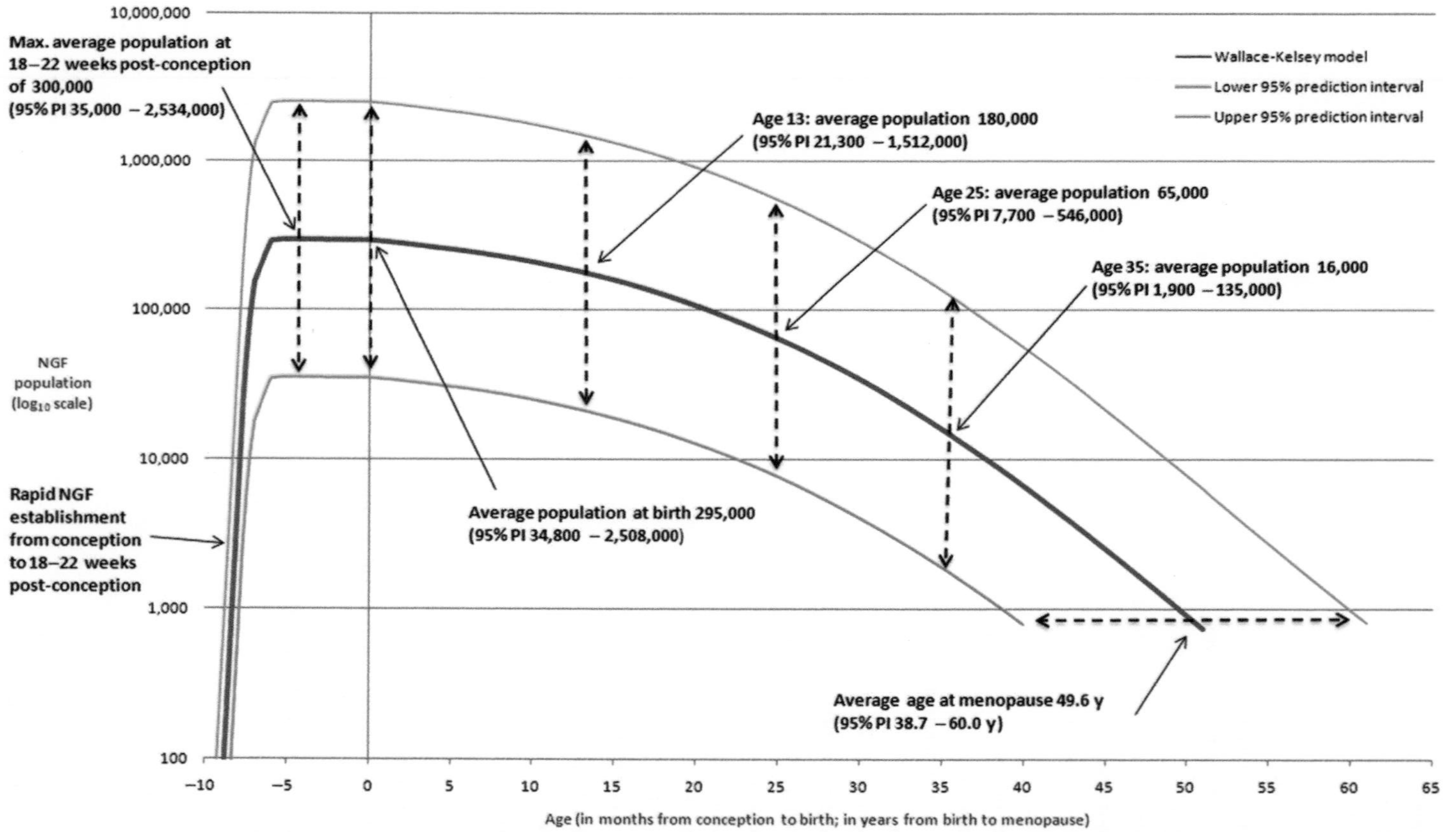

Fig. 2. Changes in ovarian follicle number across the life span in normal women. These data were derived from 8 histologic studies of ovaries from women ranging from 7 weeks postconception to 51 years. Note the rapid proliferation up to 18 to 22 weeks postconception and the gradually increasing rate of decline until menopause. NGF, nongrowing follicles; PI, prediction interval. (*From* Wallace WH, Kelsey TW. Human ovarian reserve from conception to the menopause. PLoS One 2010;5(1):e8772, 4.)

have oocytes and functional follicles after birth. In a study to assess for the presence of ovarian follicles in adolescents with Turner syndrome, one-quarter to one whole ovary was removed laparoscopically from 9 adolescent girls with Turner syndrome and histologically analyzed. Eight of the 9 ovaries had follicles, with higher numbers of follicles in younger adolescents and girls with mosaicism. Follicular density inversely correlated with follicle-stimulating hormone (FSH) level.[11]

PUBERTAL MATURATION IN TURNER SYNDROME
Gonadotropins and Ovarian Hormone Production

In 46,XX fetal development, the hypothalamic-pituitary-gonadal axis becomes active in late gestation. At birth, there is a surge of luteinizing hormone (LH) and FSH.[9] In newborns with Turner syndrome, an exaggerated FSH surge has been documented, suggesting the onset of ovarian failure. Increased FSH levels during infancy decline between the ages of 4 and 11 years, as they do in normal girls, although average FSH concentrations in children with Turner syndrome are generally higher than normal.[9] After the age of 11 years, FSH concentrations in girls with Turner syndrome again increase sharply to levels much higher than those typically seen in normal puberty.[12] Using an ultrasensitive assay, prepubertal girls with Turner syndrome were found to have lower estradiol levels compared with age-matched girls without Turner syndrome.

Chromosomal analysis was performed on a group of 40 patients diagnosed with Turner syndrome with variable degrees of mosaicism. Six of these patients had spontaneous menarche, with the remainder having primary amenorrhea. Cytogenetic analyses showed that, in those with mosaicism, the presence of at least 10% euploid cells is predictive of spontaneous pubertal development.[13]

Ovarian and Uterine Growth

Uterine development is altered in girls with Turner syndrome. A cohort of 38 patients with Turner syndrome was followed longitudinally, and serial pelvic ultrasonography was performed to document ovarian and uterine size before and during the expected time of puberty. Between 27% and 46% of patients had ultrasonographically detectable ovaries; in these patients, the investigators documented an initial increase in ovarian size at a skeletal age of approximately 9 years, and this increase became more pronounced after 14 years of age, suggesting continued estrogen production in these patients. Seventy-six percent of the patients with mosaic Turner syndrome had 2 detectable ovaries and larger ovarian volumes, compared with girls with 45,X karyotypes, of whom only 26% had ovaries detected by ultrasonography. Girls with mosaicism more frequently had spontaneous thelarche (50%) and menarche (38.5%) than those with 45,X karyotypes. Uterine size was only assessed in patients who were not prescribed estrogen therapy, and increased in all patients with Turner syndrome; however, girls with mosaicism had larger increases in uterine size than girls with 45,X karyotypes. Even though all patients with Turner syndrome had increased uterine size, these measurements were still significantly lower than those from the control group.[14]

Menstrual Function

Menarche is infrequent in girls with Turner syndrome. However, one recent report noted that as many as 40% to 50% of girls with Turner syndrome may have some observed pubertal development. Rates are higher in girls with mosaic karyotypes, but up to 25% of girls with 45,X karyotypes have some signs of spontaneous puberty. Up to 10% of girls with Turner syndrome achieve menarche.[15] In another study, 522 subjects with Turner syndrome were observed for spontaneous puberty, and spontaneous menarche occurred in 84 (16.1%) subjects.[16] During follow-up, 30 patients were found to have regular menses 9 years after the onset of menarche, 12 patients developed secondary amenorrhea 1 to 3 years after the onset of menarche, and 19 patients developed oligomenorrhea. Of the remaining patients, long-term data were not available in 10, and 13 were lost to follow-up. Spontaneous menarche was more common in patients with mosaicism than in those with 45,X karyotypes, leading the investigators to conclude that the additional X chromosome likely has a significant influence on the progression of puberty. In addition, a serum FSH level less than 10 mIU/mL at age 12 years is predictive of the onset of spontaneous menarche and regular cycles.[17]

Because most patients with Turner syndrome (>80%) do not undergo spontaneous puberty or menarche, estrogen therapy is typically required to initiate pubertal development.[16] The age at which estrogen is initiated varies but is generally around 12 years. Estrogen is initiated in very low doses, generally one-tenth to one-eighth of the adult dose, and slowly increased to full replacement doses over a period of 2 years to promote normal breast and uterine growth. After 2 years of treatment or once breakthrough bleeding occurs, a progestin is typically added to allow for regular menstrual cycles. With the assistance of hormone therapy, girls with Turner syndrome may have regular monthly menses throughout life until hormone therapy is discontinued at the typical time of menopause.[2]

PREGNANCY IN TURNER SYNDROME

Spontaneous pregnancy can be seen in a small percentage of individuals with Turner syndrome and generally is more likely in women with mosaicism and those who report spontaneous puberty and regular menses.[18,19] However, there are reports of individuals with 45,X karyotypes spontaneously conceiving and delivering healthy infants, indicating that although women with mosaicism are more likely to conceive spontaneously, women with monosomy may also be fertile. More than 90% of women with Turner syndrome who have spontaneous pregnancies have a mosaic karyotype.[18–21] In a study of 482 women with Turner syndrome, 57 women (12%) reported a total number of 124 pregnancies, occurring either spontaneously or through in vitro fertilization (IVF). Twenty-seven women (47%) became pregnant using their own oocytes; of these, 23 women (85%) conceived spontaneously, and 4 (15%) conceived with the use of either IVF or insemination. Thirty women (53%) became pregnant as a result of oocyte donation. Ninety-two percent of the women who achieved pregnancy via autologous oocyte transfer had a mosaic karyotype.[19]

Assisted Reproductive Technology

In rare incidences, individuals with Turner syndrome are able to conceive spontaneously and deliver. However, for most women with Turner syndrome, infertility is inevitable. In the past, all women with Turner syndrome were advised to avoid pregnancy because of risks of complications. However, recent studies have shown that in selected cases women with Turner syndrome are able to become pregnant successfully and deliver healthy infants. There are several options for women with Turner syndrome who desire to have children: adoption and surrogate gestational carriers have been the traditionally recommended options, although more recently additional alternatives have been developed that allow women with Turner syndrome to carry and deliver children themselves.

The most commonly sought fertility option is IVF with donor oocytes.[22] In this option, a donor oocyte is obtained and fertilized, with the resulting embryo being transferred into the uterus of the individual with Turner syndrome (donor IVF). Oocyte donation programs cite pregnancy success rates of 24% to 47%, which are consistent with pregnancy rates in women undergoing IVF who do not have Turner syndrome.[23] Khastgir and colleagues[24] cite an implantation rate of 17.1% per embryo transferred at a facility in London. Miscarriages are most often caused by the presence of a hypoplastic or bicornuate uterus and a thinner endometrial lining than that typically seen in pregnant women without Turner syndrome.[24] Because of the small uterine size of women with Turner syndrome, even after hormonal preparation to ensure adequate uterine growth, is it recommended that only 1 embryo be transferred per IVF cycle to prevent undue complications, many of which are discussed later in this article. Hormone replacement therapy is continued during the IVF process for up to 12 weeks, until the placenta is able to produce sufficient amounts of estrogens and progestins to maintain the pregnancy.[25]

More recently, there have been reports of women with Turner syndrome who have functional ovaries undergoing IVF using their own oocytes (autologous IVF). In this option, if a woman with Turner syndrome is thought to be a good candidate, she undergoes FSH stimulation to promote follicle growth. Her own individual follicles are then removed and cryopreserved, later undergoing IVF and implantation. Predictors for successful autologous IVF include a mosaic peripheral blood karyotype, normal serum FSH and antimüllerian hormone (AMH) levels, and spontaneous puberty. Negative predictors for successful autologous IVF are monosomy or a structurally anomalous X chromosome, increased FSH levels, low AMH levels, and lack of spontaneous puberty.[15,22,26]

Timing for oocyte retrieval is controversial. Although some girls do have spontaneous puberty, most do not, and those who start puberty spontaneously often do not complete puberty or have premature ovarian failure in the teenage years. It may be better to obtain oocytes for cryopreservation before ovarian failure begins. In addition, there have been several case reports of adolescents and adults with Turner syndrome undergoing ovarian stimulation followed by both oocyte and ovarian tissue cryopreservation for later IVF.[27–29] However, there is currently no evidence regarding the safety of ovarian stimulation regimens in prepubertal girls, and it is unknown what effect these treatments may have on overall pubertal development or adult height. An alternative is laparoscopic ovarian wedge resection with subsequent cryopreservation. This approach has succeeded in a 16-year-old girl with mosaic Turner syndrome.[30]

Pregnancy Outcomes

Pregnancy outcomes in women with Turner syndrome have been studied closely. In 2011 Bryman and colleagues[19] reported an overall delivery rate of live babies of 54%, with a rate of 44% in pregnancies that resulted from autologous oocytes, either spontaneous pregnancies or with IVF assistance, and a rate of 74% in pregnancies resulting from oocyte donation. In the 68 live births, only 5 infants (7.4%) had complications or birth defects, including cerebral palsy, neuropsychological disorder, coarctation of the aorta, cleft lip and palate, and congenital tumor. The infants were nondysmorphic and without chromosomal anomalies. Tarani and colleagues[31] cited a 20% rate of birth defects in children born to women with Turner syndrome, and a higher incidence of chromosomal abnormalities, including trisomy 21. In a Belgian study, 24 women with Turner syndrome were followed from conception to delivery. Pregnancies were monitored for complications in both mothers and infants, and the investigators documented a miscarriage rate of 23%. However, when considering loss of biochemical pregnancies as well, the rate of early pregnancy losses approached 44%.[32] A recent study of 103 women with Turner syndrome who underwent oocyte donation with IVF reported reassuring neonatal outcomes with live birth per embryo transfer rates ranging from 30.5% to 33.3%, preterm birth rate of 8%, low birth weight in 8.8%, and major birth defects in 3.8%, with overall perinatal mortality of 2.3%. These numbers are reassuring because of their similarity to neonatal complication rates in normal pregnancies.[6]

RISKS AND COMPLICATIONS OF PREGNANCY
Cardiovascular Disorders

Despite improved expectations for fertility in individuals with Turner syndrome, pregnancy-related mortality remains higher than in the general population: approximately 2% compared with 0.013% in normal women.[33] One of the most significant risks is worsening of cardiovascular disease during pregnancy. Coarctation of the aorta and bicuspid aortic valve are the two most common cardiovascular manifestations in Turner syndrome, with prevalence rates of 11% and 16%, respectively.[2] Other cardiovascular abnormalities include elongated transverse aortic arch, partial anomalous pulmonary connection, and persistent left superior vena cava.[34] In addition, women with Turner syndrome also have dilated vasculature compared with those with 46,XX karyotypes, particularly dilatation of the aortic root.[2] Women with Turner syndrome are at increased risk for aortic dissection or rupture related to the increased cardiovascular stress that occurs during pregnancy. Another reason that single oocyte transfer is recommended for women undergoing IVF (see earlier) is that the stress on the cardiovascular system increases with multiple gestations. There is also some evidence that the changes to the aorta persist even after pregnancy and can be exacerbated by subsequent pregnancies.[35] Because of these risks, it is imperative to perform careful preconception counseling and screening in all women with Turner syndrome who are considering pregnancy. Specific factors that increase the risk of aortic dissection or rupture during pregnancy include aortic size index of greater than 2.0 cm/m^2, history of surgery to repair cardiovascular defects, bicuspid aortic valve, current aortic dilatation, and systemic hypertension.[2,36] Despite careful screening and intrapregnancy monitoring, aortic dissection and rupture can still occur, and the risk for this is highest in the third trimester of pregnancy or postpartum.[37] Women with any of these risk factors should be offered alternatives to pregnancy, including adoption and surrogacy.

Hypertension and its sequelae, including preeclampsia and eclampsia, are major risks for cardiovascular complications during pregnancy. Pregnancy-induced hypertension is defined as 2 increased blood pressure readings of greater than or equal to 140/90 mm Hg occurring after 20 weeks of gestation, measured at least 4 hours apart or on 2 separate occasions, and preeclampsia is defined as increased blood pressure in combination with proteinuria. The incidence of any pregnancy-associated hypertensive disorder in women with Turner syndrome is variable and has been reported to range from 35% to 67%.[6,38] Severe hypertensive syndromes, such as preeclampsia, eclampsia, and HELLP (hemolysis, elevated liver enzyme levels, and low platelets) syndrome, have been documented in 50% of women with Turner syndrome and hypertension during pregnancy. In a study of 21 women with Turner syndrome, Bodri and colleagues[38] documented pregnancy-associated hypertensive disorders in 5 patients: 2 with pregnancy-induced hypertension, 2 with preeclampsia, and 1 with HELLP syndrome. One hypothesis for the increased incidence of preeclampsia is endothelial dysfunction resulting from a mismatch between proangiogenic factors, such as vascular endothelial growth factor, and antiangiogenic factors, including soluble *fms*-like tyrosine kinase 1 (FLT-1).[39] There is some thought that the higher incidence of intrauterine growth restriction and pre-term births seen in the infants of women with Turner syndrome could be related to pregnancy-associated hypertension. Therefore, careful blood pressure screening both before and during pregnancy is indicated.

Hepatic Disease

Nonpregnant women with Turner syndrome are more likely to have abnormal liver function tests, including increased concentrations of transaminases and alkaline phosphatase, as well as an increased incidence of regenerative nodular hyperplasia and portal hypertension.[2] In 1998, a review of the Danish Cytogenetic Central Register revealed a relative risk of 5.69 for cirrhosis in women with Turner syndrome compared with the general population.[40] A more recent study of 218 women with Turner syndrome in Sweden noted increased concentrations of liver enzymes in 36% of patients at baseline, with an additional 23% developing abnormalities at the 5-year follow-up evaluation.[41] Six percent of the original cohort of women normalized their transaminase levels at follow-up. Six of the women with abnormal liver enzyme concentrations underwent liver biopsy, and pathology was consistent with cholangitis and hepatitis C in 1 subject each, with steatosis and normal biopsies in 2 patients each.

With an increased incidence at baseline, there is concern that pregnancy may contribute to worsening liver disease. A retrospective cohort study of 106 European women with Turner syndrome revealed that 2 women (1.9%) had increased liver enzyme concentrations at baseline.[6] During pregnancy, 6 women were found to have intrahepatic cholestasis, and 1 woman developed HELLP syndrome, requiring early cesarean section (C-section) delivery. Although it is clear that hepatic disease is more common in women with Turner syndrome than in the general population, further studies are required before the magnitude of risk during pregnancy can be determined.

Thyroid Disease

Thyroid dysfunction is common in women with Turner syndrome, with a prevalence approaching 24%. However, the incidence of hypothyroidism seems to increase during pregnancy,[2] with reported rates ranging from 7.7% to 43.8%,[6,42] whereas in normal women the incidence of thyroid dysfunction in pregnancy is around 1% to 2%.[43] To prevent complications from uncontrolled or undiagnosed maternal hypothyroidism, all women with Turner syndrome should have annual thyroid function testing, including thyroid-stimulating hormone, either total or free thyroxine, and antithyroid antibodies.[6]

Diabetes and Glucose Metabolism

Women with Turner syndrome are at a higher risk of glucose intolerance and diabetes compared with normal women. Fifty percent of adult women with Turner syndrome who undergo an oral glucose tolerance test are diagnosed with either abnormal glucose tolerance or type 2 diabetes mellitus.[2] In one study of 26 adult women with Turner syndrome who underwent oral glucose tolerance testing, 38.4% had abnormal glucose tolerance, and 7.7% were diagnosed with type 2 diabetes.[44] In a study of 57 pregnancies in Swedish women with Turner syndrome with previously normal glucose tolerance, 5% were found to have gestational diabetes.[19] One-hundred and ten women with Turner syndrome who became pregnant via oocyte donation were followed for nearly 20 years, and 9.4% of pregnancies were complicated by gestational diabetes.[6] The increased incidence of diabetes in women with Turner syndrome is thought to be related to impaired first-phase insulin secretion caused by pancreatic beta-cell dysfunction, and this effect seems to be amplified during sex hormone administration. Gravholt and colleagues[40] reported 26 women with Turner syndrome who underwent oral glucose tolerance testing before and after receiving 6 months of sex hormone replacement therapy. Most of the women had impaired first-phase insulin secretion at baseline as well as lower basal insulin levels; these effects were intensified after 6 months of sex hormone therapy. Because pregnancy is a condition in which sex hormone levels are significantly increased, pregnant women with Turner syndrome are more likely to develop diabetes. Hence, these women should be screened diligently before and during pregnancy to ensure that gestational diabetes is promptly diagnosed.

Cesarean Section Delivery

Because of their short stature and narrow pelvic diameter, women with Turner syndrome have a higher rate of C-section deliveries than normal women.[2] Bryman and colleagues[19] evaluated 124 pregnancies in 57 Swedish women with Turner syndrome and documented C-section rates of 63% in women who became pregnant using their own oocytes and 80% after oocyte donation, compared with a C-section rate of 16% in the general population. Hagman and colleagues[6] evaluated 117 pregnancies in 106 women with Turner syndrome. C-sections, either planned or emergent, were performed in 82% of all deliveries; 34.4% of these were emergent. The most common reasons for nonemergent C-sections were cephalopelvic disproportion and breech presentation. Induction of labor was attempted in 34% of the women. However, 72.2% of these attempts required unplanned C-section because of slow labor or failure to progress. Only 21% of women were able to deliver via spontaneous vaginal delivery. Risks of C-section delivery include pelvic fetal head impaction, hemorrhage, uterine atony, damage to bladder or bowel, and complications from anesthesia.[45] Because women with Turner syndrome have a significantly higher rate of C-section delivery than those without Turner syndrome, the risks of C-section delivery should be discussed thoroughly during prepregnancy counseling.

Prepregnancy Counseling

Because of the pregnancy risks specific to women with Turner syndrome, all women of reproductive age who have been diagnosed with Turner syndrome should be provided with comprehensive prepregnancy counseling. Although uncommon, women with Turner syndrome have been reported to spontaneously conceive. Therefore, all women should be provided with adequate information regarding the importance of contraception.[18,20] The risks of increased overall mortality, cardiovascular disease (including aortic dissection, hypertension, preeclampsia, and eclampsia), liver disease, hypothyroidism, diabetes, and the increased chance of cesarean delivery should all be discussed as part of the prepregnancy visit. Because of the risks of pregnancy, all women with Turner syndrome should be informed of alternative methods to expand their families, including adoption or surrogacy. These options should be especially stressed in women who have relative contraindications for pregnancy.[2]

PROFESSIONAL SOCIETY RECOMMENDATIONS

Several professional organizations and expert groups have developed consensus guidelines and position statements regarding pregnancy in women with Turner syndrome, with similar recommendations[2,36,46] (**Table 1**), and many other

Table 1
Position and consensus statements on pregnancy in women with Turner syndrome

Organization	Contraindication to Pregnancy	Preconception	ART	Monitoring During Gestation	Delivery
American Society for Reproductive Medicine,[36] 2012	Pregnancy is absolutely contraindicated if any cardiac defects on MRI, including ASI>2 cm/m^2 Pregnancy is relatively contraindicated, even if there are no cardiovascular defects	Maternal counseling, including cardiology and high-risk OB Encourage other options for children Cardiac MRI	Single embryo transfer	Careful observation Periodic echocardiography or MRI Treat HTN Monitor for gestational diabetes, HTN, hepatic failure	ASI<2 cm/m^2: vaginal delivery possible ASI>2 cm/m^2: C-section with epidural anesthesia before labor
French Joint Practice Committee,[46] 2010	Contraindicated if any past or current aortic disease, uncontrolled HTN, or portal HTN with esophageal varices Not contraindicated if isolated BAV	Maternal counseling, including cardiology and endocrinology Blood pressure Echocardiography Cardiac/aortic MRA	Single embryo transfer	Echocardiography at end of first and second trimesters and monthly during third trimester, confirm suspected aortic dilatation with MRI Treat HTN with beta-blockade Echocardiography 5–8 d postpartum	ASI<2.5 cm/m^2: assisted vaginal delivery possible ASI>2.5 cm/m^2: hospitalize, accelerate fetal lung maturity, C-section
Turner Syndrome Consensus Study Group,[2] 2007	Relatively contraindicated if: surgically repaired cardiovascular disease, BAV, aortic dilatation, HTN. Counsel against pregnancy if these conditions present	Maternal counseling Echocardiography ECG Cardiac MRI	Single embryo transfer	Care by cardiology and high-risk OB at a tertiary care facility Monitor for gestational diabetes, hypothyroidism, HTN	Vaginal delivery allowable under optimal conditions

Abbreviations: ART, assisted reproductive technology; ASI, aortic size index; BAV, bicuspid aortic valve; ECG, electrocardiogram; HTN, hypertension; MRA, magnetic resonance angiography; OB, obstetrics.

investigators have put forward additional suggestions.[22,33,47] All women carrying the diagnosis of Turner syndrome are at risk during pregnancy, and there is no distinction between those with 45,X karyotypes and those with partial X chromosome deletions or mosaic karyotypes. A careful, complete prepregnancy medical evaluation is mandated, including meticulous cardiovascular assessment with cardiac imaging using echocardiography and cardiac MRI. Consultation with specialists in cardiovascular disease, endocrinology, and high-risk obstetrics is required to ensure the best chance for a successful pregnancy and delivery of a healthy infant. Pregnancy is considered contraindicated in the presence of significant hypertension or structural cardiac disease, including bicuspid aortic valve, aortic coarctation, and aortic dilatation at baseline. Mothers require detailed prepregnancy counseling about the increased risk for aortic dilatation and aortic dissection and the increased risk for C-section. If assisted reproductive technology is required, a single embryo should be transferred to avoid the increased risks of multiple gestation. Throughout pregnancy, close follow-up with subspecialty care is needed, including periodic echocardiography or MRI, and monitoring of thyroid dysfunction, glucose metabolism, hepatic function, and blood pressure. At delivery, if there is no evidence of aortic dilatation, vaginal delivery may be attempted. However, if the aortic size index or absolute aortic diameter is increased, the infant should be delivered by C-section, without allowing the mother to labor.

SUMMARY

Turner syndrome is one of the most common chromosomal abnormalities, with clinical manifestations affecting multiple organ systems. As children with Turner syndrome transition into adulthood it is important for practitioners to be familiar with screening guidelines and health concerns, particularly with regard to fertility and pregnancy. There are unique health issues to consider in women with Turner syndrome who desire fertility, including stature, cardiovascular risk, and disorders of the endocrine system, including thyroid disease and type 2 diabetes. It is imperative that providers who care for women with Turner syndrome be familiar with the current guidelines in order to provide the highest level of care.

REFERENCES

1. Nielsen J, Sillesen I, Hansen KB. Fertility in women with Turner's syndrome. Case report and review of literature. Br J Obstet Gynaecol 1979;86(11):833–5.
2. Bondy CA, Turner Syndrome Study Group. Care of girls and women with Turner syndrome: a guideline of the Turner Syndrome Study Group. J Clin Endocrinol Metab 2007;92(1):10–25.
3. Stochholm K, Juul S, Juel K, et al. Prevalence, incidence, diagnostic delay, and mortality in Turner syndrome. J Clin Endocrinol Metab 2006;91(10):3897–902.
4. Schoemaker MJ, Swerdlow AJ, Higgins CD, et al, United Kingdom Clinical Cytogenetics Group. Mortality in women with turner syndrome in Great Britain: a national cohort study. J Clin Endocrinol Metab 2008;93(12):4735–42.
5. Matura LA, Ho VB, Rosing DR, et al. Aortic dilatation and dissection in Turner syndrome. Circulation 2007;116(15):1663–70.
6. Hagman A, Loft A, Wennerholm UB, et al. Obstetric and neonatal outcome after oocyte donation in 106 women with Turner syndrome: a Nordic cohort study. Hum Reprod 2013;28(6):1598–609.
7. Carlson M, Airhart N, Lopez L, et al. Moderate aortic enlargement and bicuspid aortic valve are associated with aortic dissection in Turner syndrome: report of

the International Turner Syndrome Aortic Dissection Registry. Circulation 2012; 126(18):2220–6.

8. Wallace WH, Kelsey TW. Human ovarian reserve from conception to the menopause. PLoS One 2010;5(1):e8772.

9. Saenger P. Turner syndrome. In: Sperling M, editor. Pediatric endocrinology. 3rd edition. Philadelphia: Saunders; 2008. p. 610–61.

10. Reynaud K, Cortvrindt R, Verlinde F, et al. Number of ovarian follicles in human fetuses with the 45,X karyotype. Fertil steril 2004;81(4):1112–9.

11. Hreinsson JG, Otala M, Fridstrom M, et al. Follicles are found in the ovaries of adolescent girls with Turner's syndrome. J Clin Endocrinol Metab 2002;87(8): 3618–23.

12. Hagen CP, Main KM, Kjaergaard S, et al. FSH, LH, inhibin B and estradiol levels in Turner syndrome depend on age and karyotype: longitudinal study of 70 Turner girls with or without spontaneous puberty. Hum Reprod 2010;25(12): 3134–41.

13. Castronovo C, Rossetti R, Rusconi D, et al. Gene dosage as a relevant mechanism contributing to the determination of ovarian function in Turner syndrome. Hum Reprod 2014;29(2):368–79.

14. Mazzanti L, Cacciari E, Bergamaschi R, et al. Pelvic ultrasonography in patients with Turner syndrome: age-related findings in different karyotypes. J Pediatr 1997;131(1 Pt 1):135–40.

15. Hovatta O. Ovarian function and in vitro fertilization (IVF) in Turner syndrome. Pediatr Endocrinol Rev 2012;9(Suppl 2):713–7.

16. Pasquino AM, Passeri F, Pucarelli I, et al. Spontaneous pubertal development in Turner's syndrome. Italian Study Group for Turner's Syndrome. J Clin Endocrinol Metab 1997;82(6):1810–3.

17. Aso K, Koto S, Higuchi A, et al. Serum FSH level below 10 mIU/mL at twelve years old is an index of spontaneous and cyclical menstruation in Turner syndrome. Endocr J 2010;57(10):909–13.

18. Hadnott TN, Gould HN, Gharib AM, et al. Outcomes of spontaneous and assisted pregnancies in Turner syndrome: the U.S. National Institutes of Health experience. Fertil steril 2011;95(7):2251–6.

19. Bryman I, Sylven L, Berntorp K, et al. Pregnancy rate and outcome in Swedish women with Turner syndrome. Fertil steril 2011;95(8):2507–10.

20. El-Shawarby SA, Steer CV. Spontaneous monozygotic monochorionic twin pregnancy in non-mosaic Turner's syndrome. Int J Gynaecol Obstet 2007; 97(2):155.

21. Baudier MM, Chihal HJ, Dickey RP. Pregnancy and reproductive function in a patient with non-mosaic Turner syndrome. Obstet Gynecol 1985;65(3 Suppl): 60S–4S.

22. Hewitt JK, Jayasinghe Y, Amor DJ, et al. Fertility in Turner syndrome. Clin Endocrinol 2013;79(5):606–14.

23. Abir R, Fisch B, Nahum R, et al. Turner's syndrome and fertility: current status and possible putative prospects. Hum Reprod Update 2001;7(6):603–10.

24. Khastgir G, Abdalla H, Thomas A, et al. Oocyte donation in Turner's syndrome: an analysis of the factors affecting the outcome. Hum Reprod 1997;12(2):279–85.

25. Foudila T, Soderstrom-Anttila V, Hovatta O. Turner's syndrome and pregnancies after oocyte donation. Hum Reprod 1999;14(2):532–5.

26. Borgstrom B, Hreinsson J, Rasmussen C, et al. Fertility preservation in girls with turner syndrome: prognostic signs of the presence of ovarian follicles. J Clin Endocrinol Metab 2009;94(1):74–80.

27. Balen AH, Harris SE, Chambers EL, et al. Conservation of fertility and oocyte genetics in a young woman with mosaic Turner syndrome. BJOG 2010;117(2):238–42.

28. Oktay K, Rodriguez-Wallberg KA, Sahin G. Fertility preservation by ovarian stimulation and oocyte cryopreservation in a 14-year-old adolescent with Turner syndrome mosaicism and impending premature ovarian failure. Fertil steril 2010;94(2):753.e715–59.

29. Lau NM, Huang JY, MacDonald S, et al. Feasibility of fertility preservation in young females with Turner syndrome. Reprod Biomed Online 2009;18(2):290–5.

30. Huang JY, Tulandi T, Holzer H, et al. Cryopreservation of ovarian tissue and in vitro matured oocytes in a female with mosaic Turner syndrome: case report. Hum Reprod 2008;23(2):336–9.

31. Tarani L, Lampariello S, Raguso G, et al. Pregnancy in patients with Turner's syndrome: six new cases and review of literature. Gynecol Endocrinol 1998; 12(2):83–7.

32. Alvaro Mercadal B, Imbert R, Demeestere I, et al. Pregnancy outcome after oocyte donation in patients with Turner's syndrome and partial X monosomy. Hum Reprod 2011;26(8):2061–8.

33. Karnis MF. Fertility, pregnancy, and medical management of Turner syndrome in the reproductive years. Fertil steril 2012;98(4):787–91.

34. Ho VB, Bakalov VK, Cooley M, et al. Major vascular anomalies in Turner syndrome: prevalence and magnetic resonance angiographic features. Circulation 2004; 110(12):1694–700.

35. Bondy CA. Heart disease in Turner syndrome. Minerva Endocrinol 2007;32(4): 245–61.

36. Practice Committee of American Society for Reproductive Medicine. Increased maternal cardiovascular mortality associated with pregnancy in women with Turner syndrome. Fertil Steril 2012;97(2):282–4.

37. Karnis MF, Zimon AE, Lalwani SI, et al. Risk of death in pregnancy achieved through oocyte donation in patients with Turner syndrome: a national survey. Fertil steril 2003;80(3):498–501.

38. Bodri D, Vernaeve V, Figueras F, et al. Oocyte donation in patients with Turner's syndrome: a successful technique but with an accompanying high risk of hypertensive disorders during pregnancy. Hum Reprod 2006;21(3):829–32.

39. Levine RJ, Maynard SE, Qian C, et al. Circulating angiogenic factors and the risk of preeclampsia. N Engl J Med 2004;350(7):672–83.

40. Gravholt CH, Juul S, Naeraa RW, et al. Morbidity in Turner syndrome. J Clin Epidemiol 1998;51(2):147–58.

41. El-Mansoury M, Berntorp K, Bryman I, et al. Elevated liver enzymes in Turner syndrome during a 5-year follow-up study. Clin Endocrinol (Oxf) 2008;68(3): 485–90.

42. El-Mansoury M, Bryman I, Berntorp K, et al. Hypothyroidism is common in Turner syndrome: results of a five-year follow-up. J Clin Endocrinol Metab 2005;90(4): 2131–5.

43. Glinoer D. Management of hypo- and hyperthyroidism during pregnancy. Growth Horm IGF Res 2003;13(Suppl A):S45–54.

44. Gravholt CH, Naeraa RW, Nyholm B, et al. Glucose metabolism, lipid metabolism, and cardiovascular risk factors in adult Turner's syndrome. The impact of sex hormone replacement. Diabetes Care 1998;21(7):1062–70.

45. Kulas T, Bursac D, Zegarac Z, et al. New views on cesarean section, its possible complications and long-term consequences for children's health. Med Arch 2013; 67(6):460–3.

46. Cabanes L, Chalas C, Christin-Maitre S, et al. Turner syndrome and pregnancy: clinical practice. Recommendations for the management of patients with Turner syndrome before and during pregnancy. Eur J Obstet Gynecol Reprod Biol 2010;152(1):18–24.
47. Reindollar RH. Turner syndrome: contemporary thoughts and reproductive issues. Semin Reprod Med 2011;29(4):342–52.

Gonadal Function and Fertility Among Survivors of Childhood Cancer

Zoltan Antal, MD[a,b], Charles A. Sklar, MD[b,*]

KEYWORDS

- Childhood cancer survivor • Infertility • Fertility • Pregnancy • Chemotherapy
- Radiation • Gonadal injury

KEY POINTS

- Exposure to increasing doses of alkylating agents is associated with decreased rates of fertility in both male and female survivors of childhood cancer.
- Testicular radiation doses greater than 4 Gy, ovarian/uterine radiation doses greater than 5 Gy, and hypothalamic radiation doses greater than 22 to 30 Gy in girls is associated with reduced rates of fertility.
- Many survivors of childhood cancer report a pregnancy or siring a pregnancy despite meeting criteria for clinical infertility.
- Markers of gonadal toxicity, including elevated serum follicle-stimulating hormone (FSH) levels and decreased antimüllerian hormone (AMH) or inhibin B levels, may not ultimately correlate with decreased fertility.

INTRODUCTION

Overall 5-year survival rates for pediatric cancers are currently greater than 80%.[1] As of 2010, it is estimated that 70% of the approximately 380,000 survivors of childhood cancer living in the United States are over 20 years old. Reproductive health and fertility are of great importance to adolescent and young adult survivors of childhood cancer and their parents.[2] Identifying risk factors that decrease fertility is essential for proper counseling and timely referral for interventions (eg, oocyte retrieval) that may allow for future fertility in high-risk populations.

For most pediatric cancers, treatment is multimodal and includes various combinations of surgery, chemotherapy, radiation therapy (RT), and in certain cases

The authors have nothing to disclose.
[a] Department of Pediatric Endocrinology, New York Presbyterian Hospital, Weill Cornell Medical College, 505 East 70 Street, New York, NY 10021, USA; [b] Department of Pediatrics, Memorial Sloan-Kettering Cancer Center, 1275 York Avenue, New York, NY 10065, USA
* Corresponding author.
E-mail address: sklarc@mskcc.org

Endocrinol Metab Clin N Am 44 (2015) 739–749
http://dx.doi.org/10.1016/j.ecl.2015.08.002
0889-8529/15/$ – see front matter © 2015 Elsevier Inc. All rights reserved.

endo.theclinics.com

hematopoietic stem cell transplantation (SCT). The decreased rates of fertility seen in survivors are directly related to the adverse effects of these treatments and are reviewed in this article.

Although the most direct assessment of fertility is to assess an individual's ability to sire a pregnancy or become pregnant, many studies of childhood cancer survivors assess surrogate measures of gonadal injury, such as levels of gonadotropins, inhibin B, and AMH. Although these indirect measures provide important information on treatment-related adverse effects, they may not ultimately correlate with proved fertility.

FERTILITY IN MALE LONG-TERM SURVIVORS

Impaired fertility in male cancer survivors results from treatment-induced toxicity to male germ stem cells, tubular epithelium, or sperm at various stages of maturity. Serum concentrations of FSH are elevated whereas plasma levels of inhibin B tend to be low in men with germ cell damage/reduced sperm counts.

Chemotherapy

Alkylating agents are used in a variety of childhood and adolescent cancers and are the chemotherapeutic agents most often implicated in gonadal damage. Examples of such agents include cyclophosphamide, ifosfamide, procarbazine, and busulfan. Quantifying exposure to alkylating agents has been done by assigning either an alkylating agent dose (AAD) score or a cyclophosphamide equivalent dose (CED) score. An AAD score, derived by summing the total dose of alkylating agents received by every patient, dividing the resulting value into tertiles, and summing the tertile scores, is useful within an individual study but cannot be generalized to other studies. The CED score, recently described by Green and colleagues,[3] can be used to compare total alkylating agent exposure across multiple study populations exposed to different types of alkylating agents.

Gonadal damage and alkylating agents

In boys treated for Hodgkin lymphoma (HL) during childhood with combination chemotherapy that included cyclophosphamide and procarbazine, elevated FSH levels have been reported in approximately 50% of subjects a median of 6 years after completion of therapy.[4,5] A significant number of survivors in these studies had azoospermia[3] or decreased testicular volumes as surrogates for germ cell damage.[4]

Larger studies of adult male survivors of various childhood cancers have reported elevated FSH levels in one-third of patients,[6,7] with exposure to alkylating agents a significant risk factor. Casteren and colleagues[7] found that compared with age-matched controls, adult male survivors had decreased inhibin B levels, with a significant negative correlation seen between inhibin B levels and total cumulative cyclophosphamide dose ($r = -0.531$, $P<.001$).

Green and colleagues[8] used the CED score to explore the relationship between cumulative exposure to alkylating agents and sperm production. Among 214 survivors, 53 (25%) had azoospermia, 59 (28%) had oligospermia, and the remaining 102 (48%) were normospermic. Although there were significant overlaps between CED scores and sperm counts, the corresponding mean CED scores showed a negative correlation with sperm concentration ($r = -0.37$). Interestingly, 89% of men with a CED score under 4000 mg/m^2 had normospermia.

Gonadal damage and stem cell transplantation with high-dose chemotherapy

High-dose chemotherapy with busulfan and cyclophosphamide is associated with high rates of gonadal injury. Treatment with cyclophosphamide 120 to 200 mg/kg and busulfan 16 mg/kg preceding SCT in childhood is associated with gonadal damage, evidenced by elevated serum FSH levels and delayed puberty or decreased testosterone levels, in 50% to 68% of adult male survivors.[9–11]

Fertility and alkylating agents in the Childhood Cancer Survivor Study

The Childhood Cancer Survivor Study (CCSS) is a large cohort study of long-term survivors of childhood cancer who were diagnosed between 1970 and 1986 and treated at 26 institutions in North America.[12] Two studies from the CCSS provide valuable information on the prevalence of and risk factors for impaired fertility among long-term survivors.[13,14]

Green and colleagues[13] evaluated fertility, defined as ability to sire a pregnancy, in 6224 male survivors in the CCSS, ages 15 to 44, and 1292 male siblings. Overall, survivors were almost half as likely to ever sire a pregnancy compared with their siblings (hazard ratio 0.56, $P<.001$). Among survivors, a lower likelihood of siring a pregnancy was associated with a summed AAD of 2 or greater compared with an AAD score of 0 (no exposure to alkylating agents) (**Fig. 1**) and with exposure to higher cumulative doses of the individual chemotherapy agents procarbazine or cyclophosphamide.

In a subsequent study from the CCSS, Wasilewski-Masker and colleagues[14] assessed infertility, defined as "failure to achieve a pregnancy after 12 months or more of regular unprotected sex" as opposed to fertility, which does not take into account an individual's intention to sire a pregnancy. Compared with siblings, survivors within the CCSS cohort were more likely to report infertility (47% vs 17.5%) and more often cited male infertility as the cause (63.5% vs 14.8%). Among survivors, an AAD score of 3 or greater was associated with a significantly higher relative risk of infertility compared with an AAD score less than 3 (RR 2.13). Interestingly, 45% of survivors classified as having infertility reported siring at least one pregnancy, supporting the possibility of survivors siring pregnancies despite meeting criteria for infertility.

Fertility and stem cell transplantation

Fertility rates after SCT are low, as noted by Salooja and colleagues,[15] who found that among 19,412 allogeneic and 17,950 autologous transplant recipients, only 232 patients (0.6%) overall reported a pregnancy, with 119 of these pregnancies sired by

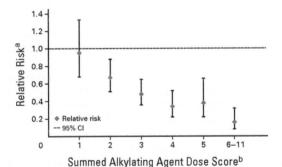

Fig. 1. Decreased relative risk of fertility with increasing AAD scores. (*From* Green DM. Fertility of male survivors of childhood cancer: a report from the Childhood Cancer Survivor Study. J Clin Oncol 2010;28(2):337; with permission.) [a], Relative risk is adjusted for age at diagnosis, race/ethnicity, marital status, educational attainment, nonalkylating chemotherapy drugs, hypothalamic/pituitary radiation dose, and testicular radiation dose; [b], Referent group = 0 score.

male survivors. Despite the low rates of fertility, there is evidence of recovery of gonadal function and fertility potential in men after SCT with a chemotherapy-only regimen.[15,16]

A few studies suggest that younger age at treatment in boys is protective against infertility.[13,17] In the CCSS cohort, survivors who were 0 to 4 years of age at diagnosis were more likely to sire a pregnancy than those who were 15 to 20 years of age at diagnosis.[13] The study was unable to demonstrate a significant difference in fertility between those who were ages 5 to 14 years at diagnosis and those 15 to 20 years at diagnosis.

Radiation Therapy

RT results in dose-dependent injury to seminiferous tubule epithelium, potentially impairing spermatogenesis. The radiation may be targeted specifically to testicular or pelvic tumors or it may arise from scatter from spinal or abdominal fields or from total body irradiation (TBI), the latter commonly used in preparation for SCT.

Immature spermatogonia are more radiosensitive than the more mature spermatocytes and spermatids, with recovery of spermatogenesis dependent on surviving spermatogonial stem cells.[18]

Gonadal damage and radiation exposure

Sklar and colleagues[19] noted germ cell dysfunction in 17% (10 of 60) long-term survivors of childhood acute leukemia and found a significant association between germ cell dysfunction and inclusion of the testes in the radiation field. Similar findings of elevated FSH levels[5,6] and small testicular volumes[5] were noted by other studies of survivors exposed to abdominal and pelvic radiation.

Gonadal dysfunction is common in boys after TBI, with elevated FSH levels reported in 81% of boys treated with a single fraction TBI dose of 10 Gy[9] and in 58%[9] and 64%[20] of those exposed to 12 to 15.75 Gy fractionated TBI doses. Mertens and colleagues,[21] in a study of 270 patients undergoing SCT, found that 92% of boys had evidence of elevated gonadotropins, with an increased likelihood among those exposed to fractionated TBI.

Fertility and gonadal radiation

Among 595 male survivors of childhood cancer, survivors exposed to RT below the diaphragm had a 25% lower risk of fertility compared with controls.[22] In the CCSS cohort, survivors exposed to testicular radiation doses above 7.5 Gy had significantly reduced fertility compared with siblings and compared with survivors who did not receive any testicular radiation.[13] Survivors exposed to testicular radiation doses greater than 4 Gy were twice as likely to report infertility compared with survivors who were not exposed to testicular radiation[14] (**Box 1**).

Fertility is significantly decreased among male survivors treated with TBI. Among boys who underwent SCT after TBI at a mean dose of 12.3 Gy, 76 of 91 (84%) met criteria for infertility, significantly less than the 56% not treated with TBI ($P<.001$).[11] Sanders and colleagues[16] found that among 463 adult men exposed to TBI doses of 10 to 15 Gy prior to SCT, only 6 (1.3%) reported siring a pregnancy. Nonetheless, Salooja and colleagues[15] found that 29% of men who reported siring a pregnancy after SCT were exposed to a mean TBI dose of 10 Gy, demonstrating the potential of siring a pregnancy after TBI.

Fertility and cranial radiation

In a study of survivors of acute leukemia treated with cranial RT, Byrne and colleagues[23] reported that although overall fertility between survivors and controls did not differ, boys treated with 24 Gy cranial RT before age 9 years had significantly

---

Box 1
Risk factors for impaired fertility of male survivors in the Childhood Cancer Survivor Study

Chemotherapy

- Increasing dose of alkylating agents (AAD score $\geq$2)
- Exposure to high doses of cyclophosphamide ($\geq$9360 mg/m^2) or procarbazine ($\geq$4201 mg/m^2)
- Age at diagnosis greater than 4 years

Radiation

- Testicular radiation greater than 4–7.5 Gy

Data from Green DM, Kawashiwa T, Stovall M, et al. Fertility of male survivors of childhood cancer: a report from the childhood cancer survivor study. J Clin Oncol 2010;28(2):332–9; and Wasilewski-Masker K, Seidel KD, Leisenrig W, et al. Male infertility in long-term survivors of pediatric cancer: a report from the childhood cancer survivor study. J Cancer Surviv 2014;8:437–47.

---

depressed fertility. By contrast, the 2 larger CCSS cohort studies[13,14] were unable to demonstrate a statistically significant effect of hypothalamic/pituitary radiation on fertility, regardless of the dose.

FERTILITY IN FEMALE LONG-TERM SURVIVORS

Because women are born with a finite number of oocytes that naturally decline over time, cancer treatment at an older age, even within the pediatric age group, carries a higher risk for decreased fertility due to a decreased ovarian reserve.[24]

Ovarian injury may manifest as acute ovarian failure (AOF), defined as loss of ovarian function during or shortly after treatment with chemotherapy and RT. Fortunately, the ovaries of young women are often resistant to acute injury and only a small percentage experience permanent ovarian failure requiring lifelong hormone replacement therapy.[25] More commonly, cancer treatments in young women result in decreased follicular reserve and the development of premature menopause after years of reasonably normal ovarian function.

Acute injury to the ovaries can result in loss of hormone production, which can manifest clinically as amenorrhea or, in a prepubertal girl, lack of pubertal development. Depletion of the primordial follicular pool is associated with elevated serum FSH levels and decreased serum estradiol levels. Serum concentrations of AMH, secreted by granulosa cells of growing follicles, correlate directly with the number of primordial follicles in adult women[26] and have been used to assess ovarian reserve and potential response to stimulation in adult women prior to undergoing in vitro fertilization.[27] Because serum concentrations of AMH are measurable even in prepubertal girls, interest has grown in its utility as a measure of ovarian reserve and future fertility in female survivors of childhood cancer.[28]

Chemotherapy

Gonadal damage and alkylating agents

Exposure to alkylating agents is associated with gonadal toxicity in female cancer survivors. After exposure to alkylating agents during treatment of HL during childhood, elevated serum FSH levels indicating gonadal injury have been reported in up to 53% of female survivors.[5,29] Among 100 adult female survivors of childhood cancer, Larsen and colleagues[30] found evidence of acute ovarian injury, indicated by elevated FSH levels and requirement for hormone replacement therapy, in 17%. Survivors with

AOF in this study had a significantly smaller number of antral follicles, an ultrasound measure associated with decreased ovarian reserve.[31] Exposure to alkylating agents was a predictor of lower antral follicle count. In a large study of 3390 female survivors from the CCSS, AOF, defined as spontaneous cessation of menses within 5 years after completion of therapy, was noted in 215 survivors (6.3%). Independent risk factors for AOF included exposure to procarbazine at any age and cyclophosphamide at ages 13 to 20 years.[32]

Sklar and colleagues[33] assessed the incidence of premature menopause (ie, onset of menopause prior to age 40 years in survivors who continued to menstruate for at least 5 years after their cancer diagnosis) in 2819 survivors from the CCSS cohort and 1065 female sibling comparators. Risk factors for nonsurgical premature menopause, which occurred significantly more often in survivors compared with sibling controls (8% vs 0.8%), included increasing AAD score compared with no alkylating agent use.

Gonadal damage and stem cell transplantation with high-dose chemotherapy

High-dose chemotherapy using 120 to 200 mg/kg of cyclophosphamide with or without busulfan, 8 to 16 mg/kg, prior to SCT is associated with elevated FSH levels in 55% to 80% of female survivors,[11,34] with a significantly higher risk among those treated with busulfan.[11] Balachandar and colleagues,[35] in a study of young medulloblastoma survivors, noted that 5 of 5 (100%) of those treated with high-dose chemotherapy and autologous stem cell rescue developed primary ovarian dysfunction.

Antimüllerian hormone

Recent studies have noted lower serum AMH levels in female survivors of childhood cancer compared with healthy controls,[36–38] with a significant association between treatment with higher AAD and lower AMH levels.[36,38] A significant decrease in AMH levels during chemotherapy, followed by recovery 12 months after completion of therapy, has also been reported in a prospective study of largely prepubertal girls.[39] As expected, FSH levels showed no significant changes in the mostly prepubertal subjects. Despite these findings, the prognostic value of AMH levels in female childhood cancer survivors remains unknown; studies to date have not found an association between markers of ovarian reserve (serum FSH and AMH levels) and impaired fertility in this population.[37]

Fertility and alkylating agents in the Childhood Cancer Survivor Study

Two key studies[40,41] directly assessed fertility and infertility in the large CCSS cohort. Fertility, defined as any pregnancy 5 or more years after the date of primary cancer diagnosis, was assessed in 5149 female participants from the CCSS and 1441 female sibling controls.[40] Survivors were overall less likely to become pregnant relative to their female siblings (relative risk [RR] 0.81). Among survivors, summed AAD scores of 3 or 4 were associated with a lower risk of pregnancy compared with an AAD score of 0.

Barton and colleagues[41] investigated treatment factors associated with infertility, defined as the inability of a woman to become pregnant after trying for 12 months or more, in 3531 female survivors in the CCSS and 1366 female sibling controls. Compared with their siblings, survivors had a higher risk of infertility (RR 1.48), which was more pronounced in those who were younger (ie, ≤24 years old) at time of study participation. Exposure to a cumulative AAD score of 3 significantly raised the risk of infertility compared with an AAD score of 0 (RR 1.48) and survivors with AAD scores of 2 (RR 0.59) or 3 (RR 0.77) were less likely to become pregnant than those with no exposure to alkylating agents.

Radiation Therapy

Radiation to the abdomen, pelvis, and spine is associated with an increased risk of ovarian damage, particularly when the ovaries are directly in the radiation field.[42]

Gonadal damage and radiation exposure

Hamre and colleagues[43] evaluated 97 female survivors of acute lymphoblastic leukemia treated with chemotherapy plus either 18 or 24 Gy cranial RT or craniospinal irradiation (CSI) or CSI plus 12 Gy abdominal RT. Elevated gonadotropins were more commonly seen among those treated with CSI plus abdominal RT (93%) or CSI (49%) compared with those treated with cranial RT alone (9%). Additionally, survivors exposed to 24 Gy CSI had a greater risk of gonadal dysfunction compared with those exposed to 18 Gy CSI. By contrast, Balachandar and colleagues[35] did not note a significantly higher rate of primary ovarian dysfunction in medulloblastoma survivors exposed to 36 Gy CSI compared with those exposed to 24 Gy CSI.

In the CCSS cohort, exposure to higher doses of pelvic radiation was associated with increasing risk of AOF[32] and nonsurgical premature menopause[33]; 75% of survivors exposed to abdominal/pelvic radiation developed AOF compared with 21% of those not so exposed ($P<.001$); 54% of all cases of AOF received at least 10 Gy to the ovaries, and 70% of patients exposed to 20 Gy RT or greater developed AOF. Survivors exposed to ovarian RT doses as low as 0.1 to 0.9 Gy had a higher risk of nonsurgical premature menopause compared with those not exposed to ovarian RT, with the highest risk seen in those exposed to the highest RT doses (>10 Gy). The cumulative incidence of nonsurgical premature menopause approached 30% in survivors treated with both alkylating agents and ovarian radiation.

TBI is associated with gonadal insufficiency and elevated gonadotropin levels in a majority of women undergoing SCT during childhood. Among 44 women conditioned with TBI (range 6–12 Gy) in preparation for SCT, Bresters and colleagues[34] found that 68% developed ovarian insufficiency after a median of 7.2 years. Other investigators have reported similarly high rates of gonadal insufficiency in female survivors exposed to TBI doses ranging from 7.5 to 15 Gy,[11,20,21] with older age and more advanced pubertal stage at the time of exposure significant risk factors.[11,20,21,34]

Fertility and gonadal radiation

Green and colleagues[40] found significantly reduced fertility in survivors exposed to ovarian/uterine radiation doses greater than 5 Gy compared with those exposed to radiation doses less than 2.5 Gy. Similarly, the risk of infertility was significantly higher among female survivors in the CCSS exposed to uterine RT doses greater than 5 Gy compared with no uterine RT.[41]

Fertility is significantly decreased among female survivors treated with TBI. Carter and colleagues[44] found that only 8 of 292 women (3%) reported a pregnancy after SCT, and a TBI-containing regimen was associated with a significantly decreased likelihood of reporting a pregnancy. Sanders and colleagues[16] found that among 532 adult women exposed to TBI doses of 10 to 15 Gy prior to SCT, only 7 (1.3%) reported a pregnancy, with a significantly higher rate of spontaneous abortions in survivors treated with TBI compared with survivors not so treated. Despite these decreased rates, Salooja and colleagues[15] found that 20% of female survivors who reported a pregnancy after SCT were exposed to a mean TBI dose of 10 Gy, demonstrating a potential for pregnancy after TBI.

In addition to causing direct damage to the ovaries, pelvic RT is associated with uterine damage that may have an impact on both fertility and pregnancy outcomes.

Box 2
Risk factors for impaired fertility of female survivors in the Childhood Cancer Survivor Study

Chemotherapy

- High doses of alkylating agents
- Exposure to cyclophosphamide or CCNU lomustine
- Age at diagnosis greater than 4 years

Radiation

- Ovarian/uterine radiation greater than 5 Gy
- Hypothalamic/pituitary radiation greater than 22–30 Gy

Data from Refs.[40,41,49]

Uterine RT is associated with decreased uterine size and absence of blood flow,[45–48] particularly in those exposed at a younger age.[46]

Fertility and cranial radiation

Although the CCSS cohort studies were unable to demonstrate a statistically significant effect of hypothalamic/pituitary RT on fertility in men, 2 separate analyses from the CCSS found a lower likelihood of pregnancy in female survivors exposed to hypothalamic/pituitary RT doses greater 22 to 30 Gy[40,49] (**Box 2**).

SUMMARY

In summary, male and female survivors of childhood cancer are at increased risk for impaired fertility after exposure to alkylating agents in a dose-dependent fashion and high-dose chemotherapy preparatory to hematopoietic SCT. Radiation-related risks for impaired fertility include exposure of the testes to testicular radiation doses greater than 4 Gy, ovarian/uterine radiation doses greater than 5 Gy, hypothalamic pituitary radiation greater than 22 to 30 Gy in girls, and TBI in both boys and girls.

REFERENCES

1. Ward E, DeSantis C, Robbins A, et al. Childhood and adolescent cancer statistics, 2014. CA Cancer J Clin 2014;64:83–103.
2. Lee SJ, Schover LR, Partridge AH, et al. American society of clinical oncology recommendations on fertility preservation in cancer patients. J Clin Oncol 2006;24:2917–31.
3. Green DM, Nolan VG, Goodman PJ, et al. The cyclophosphamide equivalent dose as an approach for quantifying alkylating agent exposure: a report from the childhood cancer survivor study. Pediatr Blood Cancer 2014;61:53–67.
4. Dhabhar BN, Malhotra H, Joseph R, et al. Gonadal function in prepubertal boys following treatment for Hodgkins disease. Am J Pediatr Hematol Oncol 1993; 15(3):306–10.
5. Papadakis V, Vlachopapadopoulou E, Syckle KV, et al. Gonadal function in young patents successfully treated for Hodgkin disease. Med Pediatr Oncol 1999;32: 366–72.
6. Tromp K, Claessens JJ, Knijnenburg SL, et al. Reproductive status in adult male long-term survivors of childhood cancer. Hum Reprod 2011;26(7):1775–83.

7. Casteren NJ, van der Linden GH, Hakvoort-Cammel GA, et al. Effect of childhood cancer treatment on fertility markers in adult male long-term survivors. Pediatr Blood Cancer 2009;52:108–12.

8. Green DM, Liu W, Kutteh WH, et al. Cumulative alkylating agent exposure and semen parameters in adult survivors or childhood cancer: a report from the St. Jude Lifetime Cohort Study. Lancet Oncol 2014;15(11):1215–23.

9. Sanders JE. Endocrine complications of high-dose therapy with stem cell transplantation. Pediatr Transplant 2004;8(Suppl 5):39–50.

10. Afify Z, Shaw PJ, Clavano-Harding A, et al. Growth and endocrine function in children with acute myeloid leukaemia after bone marrow transplantation using busulfan/cyclophosphamide. Bone Marrow Transplant 2000;25:1087–92.

11. Borgmann-Staudt A, Rendtorff R, Reinmuth S, et al. Fertility after allogeneic hematopoietic stem cell transplantation in childhood and adolescence. Bone Marrow Transplant 2010;47:271–6.

12. Robinson LL, Mertens AC, Boice JD, et al. Study design and cohort characteristics of the childhood cancer survivor study: a multi-institutional collaborative project. Med Pediatr Oncol 2002;38:229–39.

13. Green DM, Kawashiwa T, Stovall M, et al. Fertility of male survivors of childhood cancer: a report from the childhood cancer survivor study. J Clin Oncol 2010; 28(2):332–9.

14. Wasilewski-Masker K, Seidel KD, Leisenrig W, et al. Male infertility in long-term survivors of pediatric cancer: a report from the childhood cancer survivor study. J Cancer Surviv 2014;8:437–47.

15. Salooja N, Szydlo RM, Socie G, et al. Pregnancy outcomes after peripheral blood or bone marrow transplantation: a retrospective survey. Lancet 2001;358: 271–6.

16. Sanders JE, Hawley J, Levy W, et al. Pregnancies following high-dose cyclophosphamide with or without high-dose busulfan or total-body irradiation and bone marrow transplantation. Blood 1996;87:3045–52.

17. Rivkees SA, Crawford JD. The relationship of gonadal activity and chemotherapy-induced gonadal damage. JAMA 1988;259:2123–5.

18. Howell SJ, Shalet SM. Spermatogenesis after cancer treatment: damage and recovery. J Natl Cancer Monogr Inst 2005;34:12–7.

19. Sklar CA, Robison LL, Nesbit ME, et al. Effect of radiation on testicular function in long-term survivors of childhood acute lymphoblastic leukemia: a report from the children's cancer study group. J Clin Oncol 1990;8(12):1981–7.

20. Sarafoglu K, Boulad F, Gillio A, et al. Gonadal function after bone marrow transplantation for acute leukemia during childhood. J Pediatr 1997;130:210–6.

21. Mertens AC, Ramsay NKC, Kouris S, et al. Patterns of gonadal dysfunction following bone marrow transplantation. Bone Marrow Transplant 1998;22:345–50.

22. Byrne J, Mulvihill JJ, Myers MH, et al. Effects of Treatment on fertility in Long-Term Survivors of Childhood or Adolescent Cancer. N Engl J Med 1987;371:1315–21.

23. Byrne J, Fears TR, Mills JL, et al. Fertility of Long-term male survivors of acute lymphoblastic leukemia diagnosed during childhood. Pediatr Blood Cancer 2004;42:364–72.

24. Metzger ML, Meachan LR, Patterson B, et al. Female reproductive health after childhood, adolescent, and young adult cancers: guidelines for the assessment and management of female reproductive complications. J Clin Oncol 2013;31: 1239–47.

25. Sklar C. Maintenance of ovarian function and risk of premature menopause related to cancer treatment. J Natl Cancer Inst Monogr 2005;34:25–7.

26. Hansen KR, Hodnett GM, Knowlton N, et al. Correlation of ovarian reserve tests with histologically determined primordial follicle number. Fertil Steril 2011;95: 170–5.

27. Nelson SM, Yates RW, Fleming R. Serum anti-Mullerian hormone and FSH: prediction of live birth and extremes of response in stimulated cycles – implications for individualization of therapy. Hum Reprod 2007;22:2414–21.

28. Anderson RA, Wallace WHB. Antiulerrian hormone, the assessment of the ovarian reserve, and the reproductive outcome of the young patient with cancer. Fertil Steril 2013;99:1469–75.

29. Mackie EJ, Radford M, Shalet SM. Gonadal function following chemotherapy for childhood hodgkin's disease. Med Pediatr Oncol 1996;27:74–8.

30. Larsen EC, Muller J, Schmiegelow K, et al. Reduced ovarian function in long-term survivors of radiation and chemotherapy-treated childhood cancer. J Clin Endocrinol Metab 2003;88:5307–14.

31. Chang MY, Chiang CH, Hsieh TT, et al. Use of the antral follicle count to predict the outcome of assisted reproductive technologies. Fertil Steril 1998;69: 505–10.

32. Chemaitilly W, Mertens AC, Mitby P, et al. Acute ovarian failure in the childhood cancer survivor study. J Clin Endocrinol Metab 2006;91:1723–8.

33. Sklar CA, Mertens AC, Mitby P, et al. Premature menopause in survivors of childhood cancer: a report from the Childhood Cancer Survivor Study. J Natl Cancer Inst 2006;98:890–6.

34. Bresters D, Emons JA, Nuri N, et al. Ovarian insufficiency and pubertal development after hematopoietic stem cell transplantation in childhood. Pediatr Blood Cancer 2014;61:2048–53.

35. Balachandar S, Dunkel IJ, Khakoo Y, et al. Ovarian function in survivors of childhood medulloblastoma: Impact of reduced dose craniospinal irradiation and high-dose chemotherapy with autologous stem cell rescue. Pediatr Blood Cancer 2015;62:317–21.

36. Garcia CR, Samme MD, Freeman E, et al. Impact of cancer therapies on ovarian reserve. Fertil Steril 2012;97:134–40.

37. Dillon KE, Sammel MD, Ginsberg JP, et al. Pregnancy after cancer: results from a prospective cohort study of cancer survivors. Pediatr Blood Cancer 2013;60: 2001–6.

38. Charpentier AM, Chong AL, Gingras-Hill G, et al. Anti-Mullerian hormone screening to assess ovarian reserve among female survivors of childhood cancer. J Cancer Surviv 2014;8:548–54.

39. Brougham MFH, Crofton PM, Johnson EJ, et al. Anti-Mullerian Hormone is a marker of gonadotoxicity in pre- and postpubertal girls treated for cancer: a prospective study. J Clin Endocrinol Metab 2012;97:2059–67.

40. Green DM, Kawashima T, Stovall M, et al. Fertility of female survivors of childhood cancer: A report from the childhood cancer survivor study. J Clin Oncol 2009;27: 2677–85.

41. Barton S, Najita JS, Ginsburg ES, et al. Infertility, infertility treatment, and achievement of pregnancy in female survivors of childhood cancer: a report from the Childhood Cancer Survivor Study cohort. Lancet Oncol 2013;14:873–81.

42. Sklar C. Reproductive physiology and treatment-related loss of sex hormone production. Med Pediatr Oncol 1999;33:2–8.

43. Hamre MR, Robinson LL, Nesbit ME, et al. Effects of radiation on ovarian function in long-term survivors of childhood acute lymphoblastic leukemia: a report from the children's cancer study group. J Clin Oncol 1987;5:1759–65.

44. Carter A, Robison LL, Francisco L, et al. Prevalence of conception and pregnancy outcomes after hematopoietic cell transplantation: report from the bone marrow transplant survivor study. Bone Marrow Transplant 2006; 37:1023–9.

45. Critchley HO, Wallace WH, Shalet SM, et al. Abdominal irradiation in childhood: the potential for pregnancy. Br J Obstet Gynaecol 1992;99(5):392–4.

46. Larsen EC, Schmiegelow K, Rechnitzer C, et al. Radiotherapy at a young age reduces uterine volume of childhood cancer survivors. Acta Obstet Gynecol Scand 2004;83:96–102.

47. Signorello LB, Cohen SS, Bosetti C, et al. Female survivors of childhood cancer: preterm birth and low birth weight among their children. J Natl Cancer Inst 2006; 98:1453–61.

48. Signorello LB, Mulvihill JJ, Green DM, et al. Stillbirth and neonatal death in relation to radiation exposure before conception: a retrospective cohort study. Lancet 2010;376:624–30.

49. Green DM, Nolan VG, Kawashima T, et al. Decreased fertility among female childhood cancer survivors who received 22-27 Gy hypothalamic/pituitary irradiation: a report from the childhood cancer survivor study. Fertil Steril 2011;95:1922–7.

Cryptorchidism and Fertility

Helena E. Virtanen, MD, PhD[a],*, Jorma Toppari, MD, PhD[a,b]

KEYWORDS

- Congenital cryptorchidism • Acquired cryptorchidism • Germ cell
- Sperm concentration • Testicular size • Paternity • Testis

KEY POINTS

- Germ cell loss can be observed early in congenital cryptorchid testes, and the longer the testes remain undescended the more the testicular structure deteriorates. Therefore, orchiopexy at the age of 6 to 12 months is recommended to sustain as good spermatogenesis as possible.
- Orchiopexy corrects the inappropriate temperature of the testis, but it may not reverse the damage that underlies cryptorchidism in the first place.
- History of surgery for bilateral cryptorchidism has been associated with reduced paternity rate. However, currently very early operation of congenital cryptorchidism is recommended and thus further studies on paternity rates are needed.
- Acquired cryptorchidism has also been associated with reduced number of germ cells and possibly reduced testicular size, and thus operation at diagnosis is recommended in many countries.

GERM CELL PROLIFERATION DURING CHILDHOOD

Quantitative data on germ cell populations in fetal and childhood testes have been analyzed in rather few studies.[1–4] After migration of primordial germ cells to gonadal ridges, testicular cords are forming at 8 weeks of gestation, and germ cells inside the cords are called gonocytes. They normally move from the central part of the testicular cords to the basement membrane and form the spermatogonial layer by the age of 3 months. At that time, Adark and Apale spermatogonia start to appear. The former cell group is considered to include a stem cell pool, whereas the latter are

Funding Sources: This work was supported by the Academy of Finland, the Turku University Hospital, and Sigrid Jusélius Foundation.
Conflict of Interest: The authors have nothing to disclose.
a Department of Physiology, Institute of Biomedicine, University of Turku, Kiinamyllynkatu 4-8, Turku FI-20520, Finland; b Department of Pediatrics, Turku University Hospital, Kiinamyllynkatu 10, Turku FI-20520, Finland
* Corresponding author.
E-mail address: helena.virtanen@utu.fi

differentiating germ cells.[5] Occasional primary spermatocytes can be observed in the testis during early childhood, but only at puberty full spermatogenesis is established. The number of spermatogonia declines from 6 months to 3 years and then starts slowly to increase again.[2]

GERM CELL LOSS IN CRYPTORCHIDISM

In cryptorchid testis, germ cell development is not normal, and even in the contralateral descended testis, abnormalities are common.[6] The number of germ cells declines faster during the first 3 years after birth in the undescended testes than in the contralateral or normal testis.[7,8] This decline is also reflected by testicular size that lags behind in the undescended testis as compared with the normal one.[9,10] Timing of the treatment is an important determinant of testicular growth. Comparison of orchiopexy at 9 months and 36 months clearly demonstrated that earlier time of surgery was beneficial for growth of the testis.[9,11] Similar findings were reported in Korea.[12] In the histologic structure of the testes, this correlated to the number of germ cells that was dramatically reduced in the testes operated on at 36 months as compared with those operated on at 9 months.[7] Similar results have been reported in several other studies.[8,13] However, orchiopexy cannot fix all the problems that may be related to cryptorchidism: the loss of spermatogonial stem cells leads to azoospermia or oligozoospermia (sperm concentration $<5 \times 10^6$/mL). The absence of type Adark spermatogonia in testicular biopsies has been suggested to indicate the loss of spermatogenic stem cells and predict infertility in adulthood.[14] The number of germ cells per seminiferous cord at the time of orchiopexy did not correlate with adult sperm concentrations, whereas the number of Adark spermatogonia did.[15]

EFFECT OF TREATMENT ON GERM CELLS—HUMAN CHORIONIC GONADOTROPIN, GONADOTROPIN-RELEASING HORMONE

Treatment with either human chorionic gonadotropin (hCG) or gonadotropin-releasing hormone (GnRH) stimulates testicular growth and initiation of spermatogenesis both in the cryptorchid and descended testes. Part of the growth after hCG treatment is related to inflammatory reaction where vascular permeability in the testis increases and both erythrocytes and leukocytes leak into the interstitial tissue.[16,17] Apoptosis of germ cells can be observed after cessation of hCG treatment in a time-dependent manner,[18] and this may lead to permanently reduced size of the testes in adult age.[19] The efficacy of hormonal treatments in randomized controlled trials has been only around 20%, and relapses have been common.[20,21] Hormonal treatment has been reported to cause potential harm to germ cells.[22] Because of these reasons, most guidelines do not recommend hormonal treatment of cryptorchidism.[23–25]

On the other hand, Hadzicelimovic and Herzog[14,26] have advocated GnRH therapy as an adjuvant treatment after orchiopexy, because they observed improved sperm production in patients who have type Adark spermatogonia in testicular biopsy and following GnRH treatment in patients with paucity of germ cells. It was suggested that additional hormonal treatment may be beneficial for a special subgroup of cryptorchid patients, but further studies were recommended to identify such a group.[27]

PATERNITY RATES

Paternity rates among men who had undergone orchiopexy because of unilateral or bilateral cryptorchidism were compared with a control group of men who had been operated on for another reason (the controls were matched for age at operation).[28,29] When including only men who had attempted to father a child (and who had attempted at least 12 months, if they were unsuccessful), the paternity rates were significantly reduced among formerly bilaterally cryptorchid men (success rate 65% of 49 men), whereas there was no significant difference between formerly unilaterally cryptorchid men and the controls (success rates 90% of 359 men and 93% of 443 men, respectively).[28,29] Men with a history of surgery for bilateral cryptorchidism also had significantly lower sperm concentrations and inhibin B levels and significantly higher luteinizing hormone (LH) and follicle-stimulating hormone (FSH) levels than the control group or men with a history of surgery for unilateral cryptorchidism (only subgroups of each group were analyzed [n = 8, n = 53, and n = 109, respectively]).[28] Men with a history of bilateral cryptorchidism also had significantly longer time to pregnancy than men with a history of unilateral cryptorchidism or control men (n = 32, n = 215, and n = 224, respectively).[30] Formerly unilaterally cryptorchid men had significantly lower inhibin B levels than control men (n = 106 and n = 53, respectively), whereas no significant differences were observed in gonadotropin levels, in sperm concentrations (although there was a high variation among cryptorchid men n = 95, n = 48 for controls), or in time to pregnancy (n = 322 for cryptorchid men and n = 413 for control men).[29] The men included in these studies underwent surgery between the years 1955 and 1975, and they were younger than one year to older than 10.9 years at the time of operation.[28,29] Thus, both cases with congenital and acquired cryptorchidism were likely included. No significant association between the age at orchiopexy and successful paternity rate or sperm concentration was observed among the formerly unilaterally cryptorchid men.[29,31] However, inhibin B levels correlated negatively and FSH levels correlated positively with age at operation among these men (n = 84), and men who underwent surgery by the age of 2 years (n = 10) had the highest inhibin B levels,[31] which suggests positive effect of early orchiopexy. Among 103 formerly cryptorchid men, inhibin B levels correlated positively with sperm concentration, but no significant association was observed among 48 control men.[32] Inhibin B levels lower than 150 pmol/L have been shown to reflect sperm concentrations well, whereas concentrations between 150 and 300 pmol/L do not show a good correlation.[33] Furthermore, early orchiopexy has also been suggested to be beneficial for adult-age Leydig cell function, because weak negative association was observed between age at orchiopexy and adult testosterone levels among men with a history of surgery for unilateral cryptorchidism (n = 105).[34]

Men with a single testis (due to absent testis or orchiectomy) have also been reported to have similar success rates in attempted paternity as men who have been treated surgically for unilateral cryptorchidism during childhood or control men.[35]

Calleja Aguayo and colleagues[36] evaluated men with a history of surgery for unilateral or bilateral cryptorchidism during childhood and attempting to impregnate their partner.[36,37] All the men were evaluated as one group. About 64% of 53 men succeeded within 12 months, 19% succeeded after a longer period or after fertility treatments, and 17% were not able to impregnate their partner even during a period longer than 12 months. The response rate in the study was 34%, and only 56% of the respondents attempted to induce pregnancy.

SPERM CONCENTRATION AND ADULT TESTICULAR SIZE AFTER CRYPTORCHIDISM

Approximately half of men with persistent unilateral cryptorchidism and 0% of men with untreated bilateral cryptorchidism have normal sperm concentration.[38,39] According to an older review, based on studies in which orchiopexy was usually performed between the ages of 4 and 14 years, 57% and 25% of men treated (with orchiopexy and possible hormonal treatment) for unilateral or bilateral cryptorchidism, respectively, had normal sperm concentration in adulthood.[38] In the study by Taskinen and colleagues,[40] semen quality and reproductive hormone levels of men who had been treated during childhood for unilateral or bilateral cryptorchidism (n = 39 and n = 12, respectively) were analyzed. All the men had been operated on for cryptorchidism, except for 2 men with unilateral cryptorchidism, who had been treated only with hormonal therapy (hCG). All men who were treated for bilateral cryptorchidism before the age of 4 years had normal sperm concentration, whereas almost all men who were treated for bilateral cryptorchidism at an older age had sperm concentration less than 20 million/mL.[40] In the group of men treated for unilateral cryptorchidism, 90% had normal sperm concentration ($\geq$20 million/mL), and all the men with abnormal sperm concentration had been treated after the age of 3 years. Azoospermia and severe oligozoospermia were associated with increased FSH levels in men who were treated for bilateral cryptorchidism.[40] Gracia and colleagues[41] observed significantly higher sperm concentrations among men operated on for unilateral cryptorchidism than in men operated on for bilateral cryptorchidism during childhood.

In a recently published small follow-up study, men who were operated on for unilateral or bilateral cryptorchidism before the age of 1 year (n = 27) were compared with men who had orchiopexy during the second year of their life (n = 24).[42] Some of the patients were also treated with luteinizing hormone-releasing hormone and hCG before the orchiopexy. Men who were operated on during the first year of life had significantly more often normal sperm concentration (96% of men vs 75% of men) and normal sperm motility (96% of men vs 67% of men) than men who were operated on for cryptorchidism during the second year of life. No significant difference between unilateral and bilateral cases or testicular position classes or boys with or without hormonal treatment was observed in sperm concentration.[42] However, the study size was small.

In a review based on older studies, abnormal size at adult-age follow-up was reported in 28% of former cryptorchid testes.[38] Taskinen and Wikström[43] compared adult testicular size of men treated for unilateral or bilateral cryptorchidism (n = 58 and n = 15, respectively) and observed that surgically treated former cryptorchid testes were smaller than spontaneously descended testes. Operation age varied between 10 months and 13 years. In a study comparing adult men operated on for cryptorchidism between the ages of 2 and 12 years, men with a history of bilateral cryptorchidism (n = 19) had poorer semen quality, smaller testes, and lower inhibin B levels than men with a history of unilateral cryptorchidism (n = 49).[44] In the group of men operated on for unilateral cryptorchidism, higher inhibin B levels, larger testicular size, and lower FSH levels were observed among subjects operated on before the age of 8 years than among subjects who were older during the operation. Among men with a history of bilateral cryptorchidism, sperm concentrations correlated positively with inhibin B levels and negatively with FSH levels.[44]

Engeler and colleagues[45] observed that the number of germ cells in testicular biopsy taken during orchiopexy correlated positively with sperm concentration in adulthood among men operated on for bilateral cryptorchidism (n = 24). Median operation age was 6.2 years, and operation age correlated negatively with sperm concentration and testicular size in adulthood. Sperm concentration correlated positively with testicular size in adulthood.[45] Vinardi and colleagues[46] observed positive correlation between sperm concentration and testicular volume in adulthood among men who had been treated for cryptorchidism during childhood (n = 47 unilateral cases and n = 10 bilateral cases). van Brakel and colleagues[47] observed compromised fertility potential among men with a history of congenital cryptorchidism, but no significant association between operation age and testicular size or sperm concentration was observed. However, the number of patients who underwent surgery during the first year of life was limited.[47]

Lee and colleagues[48] studied adult men with a history of unilateral cryptorchidism who underwent surgery during childhood. They observed no association between testicular size at orchiopexy and paternity rates, hormone levels, sperm counts, or testicular size in adulthood. Taken together, operation age has been negatively associated with sperm concentration and testicular volume in adulthood in some studies. Bilateral cryptorchidism has been associated with poorer prognosis than unilateral cryptorchidism. However, evaluation of the association between history of cryptorchidism and sperm concentration and other predictors of fertility potential is challenged by possible combination of unilateral and bilateral cases and acquired and congenital cases (in studies with wide range of operation age), by possible combination of different testicular position classes, and by higher operation age in older studies than currently recommended (optimally between 6 and 12 months).

ACQUIRED CRYPTORCHIDISM AND FERTILITY

In addition to congenital cryptorchidism, there is also acquired form of cryptorchidism. Testicular ascent may be seen in boys with a retractile testis or in boys who have previously had ipsilateral inguinal operation (entrapment of the testis into the scar).[49,50] In addition, improper elongation of the spermatic cord due to fibrous remnant of the processus vaginalis and spasticity of the cremaster muscle have been proposed as possible causes for testicular ascent.[51,52] Acquired cryptorchidism is considered to be the main reason for high prevalence of late orchiopexies.[53,54] Spontaneously descended congenitally undescended testis may show reascent during childhood.[55,56]

According to Dutch longitudinal studies, most boys with acquired cryptorchidism show spontaneous testicular descent during puberty,[57,58] and thus, wait-and-see policy in the treatment of acquired cryptorchidism has been followed in the Netherlands.[59] In a Dutch study, men with a history of unilateral (n = 50) or bilateral (n = 15) acquired cryptorchidism were compared with healthy control men (n = 53) and with men who had been treated for unilateral or bilateral congenital cryptorchidism (n = 55 and n = 7, respectively) in terms of semen quality, testicular size and consistency, reproductive hormone levels, and paternity rates.[60] Men with a history of unilateral acquired cryptorchidism had smaller testes, lower sperm concentration and progressive sperm motility, and more often soft testicular consistency than control men. When comparing men with a history of unilateral acquired cryptorchidism with those with a history of unilateral congenital cryptorchidism, the congenital form was more often associated with soft testicular consistency, but no significant differences in other studied parameters were observed. Men with a history of bilateral acquired cryptorchidism had smaller mean testicular volume, more often soft testicular consistency, lower successful paternity rate, higher LH and FSH levels, and lower inhibin B levels, sperm concentration, and progressive motility than control men. When comparing men with a history of bilateral acquired cryptorchidism with those with a history of bilateral congenital cryptorchidism, no differences between the groups were observed in semen quality, reproductive hormones, testicular size, or successful paternity rates.[60] Thus, men with a history of acquired cryptorchidism differed from control men but were similar to men with a history of congenital cryptorchidism. Accordingly, it has been suggested that men with congenital and acquired cryptorchidism represent the same continuum.[53,60]

The study by van Brakel and colleagues[60] included men with acquired cryptorchidism for whom orchiopexy was performed after follow-up until Tanner stage G2P2 (n = 26) and men who showed spontaneous testicular descent during puberty (n = 24). No differences between these 2 groups were observed in testicular volume, reproductive hormones, semen quality, and successful paternity rates. Unilateral acquired cryptorchidism was associated with higher sperm concentration and motility than bilateral acquired cryptorchidism. However, further studies are needed to evaluate fertility potential in men with a history of acquired cryptorchidism with immediate surgery at diagnosis. Testicular volumes smaller than normal for age in ultrasonography were observed at follow-up after operation in boys and men who had previously been treated with orchiopexy at diagnosis of unilateral or bilateral acquired cryptorchidism (n = 155).[61] The age of the subjects at follow-up was 5 to 27 years. Furthermore, in unilateral cases, the treated testis was smaller than its counterpart.[61] Small testicular size for age in most ascending testes (80% of 30 testes) was also reported in another study, in which testicular size was evaluated visually at pubertal operation.[62] Hack and colleagues[63] evaluated testicular size of acquired undescended testes with orchidometer after spontaneous descent at puberty (measurement n = 494) or after pubertal orchiopexy (measurement n = 85). They observed that, although testicular size was within normal limits in most (>90%) of the measurements, in more than 50% of unilateral cases the affected testes were smaller at follow-up than the other testis that had always been descended.[63]

Rusnack and colleagues[64] reported histologic findings of bilateral testicular biopsies of 91 cases with unilateral ascended testis and compared them with histologic findings of 209 age- and position-matched controls with unilateral congenital cryptorchidism. Reduced number of germ cells per tubule was reported in the ascended testis and in its normally descended counterpart, which is similar to the situation observed in cases with congenital cryptorchidism. The investigators suggested that testicular ascent is likely to be due to endocrine defect, because the histologic changes were observed also in the testis that had always been normally descended. Processus vaginalis was more often closed among cases with ascending testis when compared with cases with congenital cryptorchidism.[64] Mayr and colleagues[65] reported in a small study (biopsy n = 13) similar type of alterations in germ and Sertoli cells in acquired cryptorchidism and in congenital cryptorchidism.

SUMMARY

Different types of evidence support the current recommendation of treatment of cryptorchidism during the first year of life or later on immediately at diagnosis to optimize the fertility potential of cryptorchid patients.

REFERENCES

1. Muller J, Skakkebaek NE. Fluctuations in the number of germ cells during the late foetal and early postnatal periods in boys. Acta Endocrinol (Copenh) 1984; 105(2):271–4.
2. Paniagua R, Nistal M. Morphological and histometric study of human spermatogonia from birth to the onset of puberty. J Anat 1984;139(Pt 3):535–52.

3. Hadziselimovic F, Thommen L, Girard J, et al. The significance of postnatal gonadotropin surge for testicular development in normal and cryptorchid testes. J Urol 1986;136(1 Pt 2):274–6.
4. Cortes D, Thorup JM, Beck BL. Quantitative histology of germ cells in the undescended testes of human fetuses, neonates and infants. J Urol 1995;154(3): 1188–92.
5. Clermont Y. Renewal of spermatogonia in man. Am J Anat 1966;118(2):509–24.
6. Cortes D. Cryptorchidism–aspects of pathogenesis, histology and treatment. Scand J Urol Nephrol Suppl 1998;196:1–54.
7. Kollin C, Stukenborg JB, Nurmio M, et al. Boys with undescended testes: endocrine, volumetric and morphometric studies on testicular function before and after orchidopexy at nine months or three years of age. J Clin Endocrinol Metab 2012; 97(12):4588–95.
8. Cortes D, Petersen BL, Thorup J. Testicular histology in cryptorchid boys - aspects of fertility. J Ped Surg Special 2007;1:32–5.
9. Kollin C, Karpe B, Hesser U, et al. Surgical treatment of unilaterally undescended testes: testicular growth after randomization to orchiopexy at age 9 months or 3 years. J Urol 2007;178(4 Pt 2):1589–93 [discussion: 1593].
10. Kollin C, Granholm T, Nordenskjöld A, et al. Growth of spontaneously descended and surgically treated testes during early childhood. Pediatrics 2013;131(4): e1174–80.
11. Kollin C, Hesser U, Ritzen EM, et al. Testicular growth from birth to two years of age, and the effect of orchidopexy at age nine months: a randomized, controlled study. Acta Paediatr 2006;95(3):318–24.
12. Kim SO, Hwang EC, Hwang IS, et al. Testicular catch up growth: the impact of orchiopexy age. Urology 2011;78(4):886–9.
13. Park KH, Lee JH, Han JJ, et al. Histological evidences suggest recommending orchiopexy within the first year of life for children with unilateral inguinal cryptorchid testis. Int J Urol 2007;14(7):616–21.
14. Hadziselimovic F, Herzog B. The importance of both an early orchidopexy and germ cell maturation for fertility. Lancet 2001;358(9288):1156–7.
15. Kraft KH, Canning DA, Snyder HM, et al. Undescended testis histology correlation with adult hormone levels and semen analysis. J Urol 2012;188(4 Suppl):1429–35.
16. Hjertkvist M, Lackgren G, Ploen L, et al. Does HCG treatment induce inflammation-like changes in undescended testes in boys? J Pediatr Surg 1993;28(2):254–8.
17. Kaleva M, Arsalo A, Louhimo I, et al. Treatment with human chorionic gonadotropin for cryptorchidism: clinical and histological effects. Int J Androl 1996; 19(5):293–8.
18. Heiskanen P, Billig H, Toppari J, et al. Apoptotic cell death in the normal and cryptorchid human testis: the effect of human chorionic gonadotropin on testicular cell survival. Pediatr Res 1996;40(2):351–6.
19. Dunkel L, Taskinen S, Hovatta O, et al. Germ cell apoptosis after treatment of cryptorchidism with human chorionic gonadotropin is associated with impaired reproductive function in the adult. J Clin Invest 1997;100(9):2341–6.
20. Pyörälä S, Huttunen NP, Uhari M. A review and meta-analysis of hormonal treatment of cryptorchidism. J Clin Endocrinol Metab 1995;80(9):2795–9.
21. Henna MR, Del Nero RG, Sampaio CZ, et al. Hormonal cryptorchidism therapy: systematic review with meta-analysis of randomized clinical trials. Pediatr Surg Int 2004;20(5):357–9.
22. Cortes D, Thorup J, Visfeldt J. Hormonal treatment may harm the germ cells in 1 to 3-year-old boys with cryptorchidism. J Urol 2000;163(4):1290–2.

23. Ritzen EM, Bergh A, Bjerknes R, et al. Nordic consensus on treatment of undescended testes. Acta Paediatr 2007;96(5):638–43.

24. Gapany C, Frey P, Cachat F, et al. Management of cryptorchidism in children: guidelines. Swiss Med Wkly 2008;138(33–34):492–8.

25. Kolon TF, Herndon CD, Baker LA, et al. Evaluation and treatment of cryptorchidism: AUA guideline. J Urol 2014;192(2):337–45.

26. Hadziselimovic F, Herzog B. Treatment with a luteinizing hormone-releasing hormone analogue after successful orchiopexy markedly improves the chance of fertility later in life. J Urol 1997;158(3 Pt 2):1193–5.

27. Chua ME, Mendoza JS, Gaston MJ, et al. Hormonal therapy using gonadotropin releasing hormone for improvement of fertility index among children with cryptorchidism: a meta-analysis and systematic review. J Pediatr Surg 2014;49(11): 1659–67.

28. Lee PA, Coughlin MT. Fertility after bilateral cryptorchidism. Evaluation by paternity, hormone, and semen data. Horm Res 2001;55(1):28–32.

29. Miller KD, Coughlin MT, Lee PA. Fertility after unilateral cryptorchidism. Paternity, time to conception, pretreatment testicular location and size, hormone and sperm parameters. Horm Res 2001;55(5):249–53.

30. Coughlin MT, O'Leary LA, Songer NJ, et al. Time to conception after orchidopexy: evidence for subfertility? Fertil Steril 1997;67(4):742–6.

31. Coughlin MT, Bellinger MF, Lee PA. Age at unilateral orchiopexy: effect on hormone levels and sperm count in adulthood. J Urol 1999;162(3 Pt 2):986–8 [discussion: 989].

32. Lee PA, Coughlin MT, Bellinger MF. Inhibin B: comparison with indexes of fertility among formerly cryptorchid and control men. J Clin Endocrinol Metab 2001; 86(6):2576–84.

33. Jørgensen N, Liu F, Andersson AM, et al. Serum inhibin-B in fertile men is strongly correlated with low but not high sperm counts: a coordinated study of 1,797 European and US men. Fertil Steril 2010;94(6):2128–34.

34. Lee PA, Coughlin MT. Leydig cell function after cryptorchidism: evidence of the beneficial result of early surgery. J Urol 2002;167(4):1824–7.

35. Lee PA, Coughlin MT. The single testis: paternity after presentation as unilateral cryptorchidism. J Urol 2002;168(4 Pt 2):1680–2 [discussion: 1682–3].

36. Calleja Aguayo E, Delgado Alvira R, Estors Sastre B, et al. Fertility survey of patients operated on of cryptorchidism in the pediatric age. Cir Pediatr 2012; 25(2):78–81 [in Spanish].

37. Lee PA, Houk CP. Cryptorchidism. Curr Opin Endocrinol Diabetes Obes 2013; 20(3):210–6.

38. Chilvers C, Dudley NE, Gough MH, et al. Undescended testis: the effect of treatment on subsequent risk of subfertility and malignancy. J Pediatr Surg 1986; 21(8):691–6.

39. Virtanen HE, Bjerknes R, Cortes D, et al. Cryptorchidism: classification, prevalence and long-term consequences. Acta Paediatr 2007;96(5):611–6.

40. Taskinen S, Hovatta O, Wikstrom S. Early treatment of cryptorchidism, semen quality and testicular endocrinology. J Urol 1996;156(1):82–4.

41. Gracia J, Sánchez Zalabardo J, Sánchez García J, et al. Clinical, physical, sperm and hormonal data in 251 adults operated on for cryptorchidism in childhood. BJU Int 2000;85(9):1100–3.

42. Feyles F, Peiretti V, Mussa A, et al. Improved sperm count and motility in young men surgically treated for cryptorchidism in the first year of life. Eur J Pediatr Surg 2014;24(5):376–80.

43. Taskinen S, Wikström S. Effect of age at operation, location of testis and preoperative hormonal treatment on testicular growth after cryptorchidism. J Urol 1997;158(2):471–3.
44. Trsinar B, Muravec UR. Fertility potential after unilateral and bilateral orchidopexy for cryptorchidism. World J Urol 2009;27(4):513–9.
45. Engeler DS, Hosli PO, John H, et al. Early orchiopexy: prepubertal intratubular germ cell neoplasia and fertility outcome. Urology 2000;56(1):144–8.
46. Vinardi S, Magro P, Manenti M, et al. Testicular function in men treated in childhood for undescended testes. J Pediatr Surg 2001;36(2):385–8.
47. van Brakel J, Kranse R, de Muinck Keizer-Schrama SM, et al. Fertility potential in men with a history of congenital undescended testes: a long-term follow-up study. Andrology 2013;1(1):100–8.
48. Lee PA, Coughlin MT, Bellinger MF. No relationship of testicular size at orchiopexy with fertility in men who previously had unilateral cryptorchidism. J Urol 2001; 166(1):236–9.
49. Lamah M, McCaughey ES, Finlay FO, et al. The ascending testis: is late orchidopexy due to failure of screening or late ascent? Pediatr Surg Int 2001;17(5–6): 421–3.
50. Eardley I, Saw KC, Whitaker RH. Surgical outcome of orchidopexy. II. Trapped and ascending testes. Br J Urol 1994;73(2):204–6.
51. Clarnette TD, Rowe D, Hasthorpe S, et al. Incomplete disappearance of the processus vaginalis as a cause of ascending testis. J Urol 1997;157(5):1889–91.
52. Smith JA, Hutson JM, Beasley SW, et al. The relationship between cerebral palsy and cryptorchidism. J Pediatr Surg 1989;24(12):1303–5.
53. Hack WW, Goede J, van der Voort-Doedens LM, et al. Acquired undescended testis: putting the pieces together. Int J Androl 2012;35(1):41–5.
54. Hack WW, Meijer RW, Van Der Voort-Doedens LM, et al. Previous testicular position in boys referred for an undescended testis: further explanation of the late orchidopexy enigma? BJU Int 2003;92(3):293–6.
55. Cryptorchidism: a prospective study of 7500 consecutive male births, 1984-8. John Radcliffe Hospital Cryptorchidism Study Group. Arch Dis Child 1992; 67(7):892–9.
56. Wohlfahrt-Veje C, Boisen KA, Boas M, et al. Acquired cryptorchidism is frequent in infancy and childhood. Int J Androl 2009;32(4):423–8.
57. Hack WW, Meijer RW, van der Voort-Doedens LM, et al. Natural course of acquired undescended testis in boys. Br J Surg 2003;90(6):728–31.
58. Sijstermans K, Hack WW, van der Voort-Doedens LM, et al. Puberty stage and spontaneous descent of acquired undescended testis: implications for therapy? Int J Androl 2006;29(6):597–602.
59. Hack WW, van der Voort-Doedens LM, Sijstermans K, et al. Reduction in the number of orchidopexies for cryptorchidism after recognition of acquired undescended testis and implementation of expectative policy. Acta Paediatr 2007;96(6):915–8.
60. van Brakel J, Kranse R, de Muinck Keizer-Schrama SM, et al. Fertility potential in a cohort of 65 men with previously acquired undescended testes. J Pediatr Surg 2014;49(4):599–605.
61. van der Plas EM, Zijp GW, Froeling FM, et al. Long-term testicular volume after orchiopexy at diagnosis of acquired undescended testis. J Urol 2013;190(1): 257–62.
62. Meij-de Vries A, Hack WW, Heij HA, et al. Perioperative surgical findings in congenital and acquired undescended testis. J Pediatr Surg 2010;45(9): 1874–81.

63. Hack WW, van der Voort-Doedens LM, Goede J, et al. Natural history and long-term testicular growth of acquired undescended testis after spontaneous descent or pubertal orchidopexy. BJU Int 2010;106(7):1052–9.
64. Rusnack SL, Wu HY, Huff DS, et al. The ascending testis and the testis undescended since birth share the same histopathology. J Urol 2002;168(6):2590–1.
65. Mayr J, Rune GM, Holas A, et al. Ascent of the testis in children. Eur J Pediatr 1995;154(11):893–5.

Male Obesity

Wieland Kiess, MD[a,b,*], Isabel V. Wagner, MD[a,b,c],
Jürgen Kratzsch, PhD[d], Antje Körner, MD[a,b,c]

KEYWORDS

- Obesity • Male puberty • Male fertility • Reproduction • Testis • Adipocytokines

KEY POINTS

- Being overweight, and being obese, are highly prevalent in men, even at a young age.
- Obesity affects the timing and progress of puberty in both sexes, and may reduce fertility in men.
- Mechanisms that may lead to reduced fertility in obese men include intrinsic (ie, genetic), endocrine, and paracrine factors, as well as extrinsic factors.
- Endocrine-disrupting chemicals such as bisphenol-A may be a link between obesity and infertility in men.

INTRODUCTION

It is hypothesized that the emergence of a pandemic of childhood obesity may have been a major driving force for earlier maturation in both genders.[1-4] This hypothesis has, for example, been suggested using data from Flanders, Belgium,[5] where a positive trend both in height and weight was observed over the years in a large population of normal children more than 5 years of age. Adult median height and weight had increased by 1.2 cm and 0.9 kg/decade, respectively, in boys and the weight distribution had become more skewed. Despite this secular trend in growth parameters, the timing of puberty had not advanced over the previous 50 years and the onset of pubertal stages of G2 (enlargement of scrotum and testes) in boys was comparable with that reported from other Western European countries.[5] These data point to the

The authors have nothing to disclose.
[a] Department of Women & Child Health, Hospital for Children and Adolescents, University of Leipzig, Liebigstr. 20a, Leipzig D 04103, Germany; [b] Leipzig University Medical Centre, LIFE, Leipzig Civilization Diseases Research Centre, LIFE Child, Centre for Paediatric Research, Leipzig, Germany; [c] IFB Adiposity Diseases, University of Leipzig, Liebigstr. 20a, Leipzig D 04103, Germany; [d] Institute of Laboratory Medicine, Clinical Chemistry and Molecular Diagnostics, University of Leipzig, Paul-List-Street 13-15, Leipzig 04103, Germany
* Corresponding author. Department of Women & Child Health, Hospital for Children and Adolescents, University of Leipzig, Liebigstr. 20a, Leipzig D 04103, Germany.
E-mail address: Wieland.kiess@medizin.uni-leipzig.de

Endocrinol Metab Clin N Am 44 (2015) 761–772
http://dx.doi.org/10.1016/j.ecl.2015.07.010
0889-8529/15/$ – see front matter © 2015 Elsevier Inc. All rights reserved.

endo.theclinics.com

need for further investigation into the association between secular trends in growth, obesity, and puberty. In addition, there is now evidence that fat mass and adipocytokines released from adipose tissue have profound effects on fertility in men. This finding has been shown in observational studies both in human adult men and in animal models of obesity.[6–11]

For example, a trend toward earlier pubertal onset and maturation in both sexes has been shown, and the previously held notion that obese boys might progress to puberty at a slower pace than their nonobese peers is again a matter of debate (**Box 1**).[1,12–17] In contrast, impaired fertility markers and reduced reproductive function have been observed both in obese humans and in animal models of obesity. For example, in the monogenic mouse model of obesity caused by leptin deficiency, mice have central hypogonadism and show reduced fertility.[6,18] In humans, low sperm counts and reduced sperm function have been reported in obese men.[19–21] Adipocytokines and inflammatory cytokines have been discussed as affecting reproductive function and directly interacting with the male reproductive system. For example, nicotinamide phosphoribosyltransferase (NAMPT), a key enzyme of nicotinamide adenine dinucleotide (NAD) metabolism is released from adipocytes but also expressed in the testes. It is thought that NAMPT might be a key player in modulating sperm function in humans.[10,11] At the moment only a few studies and preliminary data exist. In conclusion, obesity affects both pubertal development and fertility and reproduction in men.

SCOPE AND RESEARCH QUESTIONS

It is well established that the start of puberty requires a minimum critical body weight and fat mass. It has been observed that the onset of pubertal changes is earlier in

---

Box 1
Evidence that obesity affects male sexual maturation, sexual functioning, and fertility in humans

Effect of obesity/overweight on male puberty. Obese boys develop earlier onset of:

Testicular growth (volume)

Pubarche

Peak height velocity

Voice break

Effect of obesity/overweight on male gonadal functions. Obese men may have lower:

Testosterone levels/androgen insufficiency

Sperm count

Sperm motility

Coital frequency per week

Levels of testicular nicotinamide adenine dinucleotide

Effect of obesity/overweight on male functioning. Obese men may have:

Sarcopenia

Impaired cognitive functions (not definite)

Increased aromatase activity

Increased estrogen levels

Data from Refs.[1,3,8–11,13,19,22–26,28–35,44]

obese boys, compared with normal-weight children, although it is still unclear whether there is enough evidence to show a direct link between adiposity and puberty.[22–29] In addition, there is still much debate regarding the impact of childhood obesity on testicular development in boys. Importantly, the link between fertility and testicular function and obesity or fat mass has also been suggested but not proved.[30–35] Molecular mechanisms substantiating the link between fat mass and sperm function remain speculative and unproved. Endocrine disruptors may cause increased weight gain and at the same time reduce sperm counts, sperm motility, and hence fertility in men. This article explores the evidence linking adiposity with the timing of puberty in boys, explores the links between obesity and fertility in men, and reciprocally gives some insight into the role of androgens on male obesity.

OBESITY IN CHILDHOOD AND ADOLESCENCE

Childhood overweight and obesity are commonly seen across most developed and developing countries, with a high prevalence of about 15% to 35%. The current view on the cause of accumulation of excess fat mass proposes that weight gain is the result of an exposure to an obesogenic environment, superimposed on a background of genetic susceptibility brought about through evolutionary adaptation.[7,36–42] Children with lifestyle-related obesity tend to be tall throughout childhood, a process thought to be related to nutritionally driven increases in insulinlike growth factor 1 (IGF-I). Nevertheless, these children generally achieve a normal adult final height, a result apparently related to either earlier onset of, and/or advanced progression through, puberty. Although in many industrialized countries, such as in Sweden, France, Germany, and Australia, the prevalence of obesity at early ages is plateauing, the high prevalence of obesity in children and adolescents remains a major concern, given its well-described association with long-term health problems, such as cardiovascular disease, type 2 diabetes, hyperlipidemia, orthopedic problems, and cancer.[39,41,42]

Approximately 40% to 70% of interindividual differences in body weight and composition are thought to be caused by genetic variation. Numerous genes have been identified by genome-wide association studies (GWASs) and candidate gene approaches that seem to be associated with the regulation of body weight.[37] According to the thrifty gene hypothesis, evolutionary selection pressure has selected genes that promote storing of energy in fat depots and genes that promote more thrifty handling of energy, which subsequently allows individuals to survive periods of food deprivation. However, within the modern obesogenic environment, these same genetic susceptibility traits now seem to be detrimental by promoting obesity and its associated metabolic diseases.[37,40–43]

Most genes identified in monogenic cases of obesity, such as the genes encoding for the melanocortin 4 receptor, proopiomelanocorticotropin, or the leptin receptor, seem to be involved in the central regulation of energy intake. Variants of genes involved with energy use, such as those encoding β-adrenergic receptors 2 and 3, hormone-sensitive lipase, and mitochondrial uncoupling proteins 1, 2, and 3, have also been commonly associated with obesity.[37] However, less than 5% of cases of obesity are thought to be caused by monogenic variations. Although GWASs have revealed several candidate genes affecting body weight in both children and adults, the major proportion of genetic influence on obesity remains unexplained.

In parallel it has become obvious that the sociocultural inheritance of body fat mass, weight, and weight control also contributes significantly to the obesity epidemic.[40] A quantitative analysis of the nature and extent of the person-to-person spread of obesity as a possible factor contributing to the obesity epidemic was performed within a densely interconnected social network of 12,067 people repeatedly reassessed as part of the Framingham Heart Study (1971–2003). Longitudinal screening revealed that weight gain in one person was associated with weight gain in that person's friends, siblings, spouse, and neighbors. People's chances of becoming obese increased by 57% if they had a friend who became obese in a given interval, and by 40% among pairs of adult siblings, if 1 sibling became obese. Environmental network phenomena therefore also seem to be relevant to the biological and behavioral traits of obesity, and obesity seems to spread through social ties.[1,30] Thus, both intrinsic (ie, genetic), and extrinsic (socioeconomic and cultural) factors contribute substantially and similarly to the evolution of human obesity.

MALE PUBERTY

Puberty is a developmental process that results in reproductive capability. In boys, normal and true central puberty begins with the activation of the hypothalamic-pituitary-gonadal axis, which is followed by enlargement of the testes, commonly followed by pubic hair development and penile growth. The influences of hypothalamic gonadotropin-releasing hormone (GnRH), the gonadotropins luteinizing hormone (LH) and follicle-stimulating hormone (FSH), and the sex steroid testosterone and its metabolites bring about the manifestations of puberty, which are both external (genital enlargement, hair growth) and internal (testes). Pubic hair may also develop independently of the activation of the hypothalamic-pituitary-gonadal pathways, largely through the effect of weak androgens secreted by the adrenal glands (adrenarche). The physical characteristics of sexual development are a result of a series of events that involve a complex interplay between the central nervous system, endocrine glands, and the adipose tissue.[2,22] The different phases of external pubertal development in boys are conventionally designated as Tanner stages G1 to G5 for testicular enlargement and penile growth and PH1 to PH6 for pubic hair growth, and additionally testicular volume is assessed using orchidometers. Although the tempo and process of sexual development are conserved in human populations and races, the timing of onset of puberty occurs across a wide range of ages in both girls and boys. The molecular mechanisms triggering pubertal onset, and the factors that influence progression and tempo of sexual development, have been elucidated to some extent but remain the focus of intensive research (**Box 2**).[9,14,38]

The increased pulsatile hypothalamic secretion of the decapeptide GnRH is essential for the activation of the pituitary-gonadal axis at puberty. The GnRH secretory

---

Box 2
Hypothetical mechanisms of how obesity might affect onset and tempo of pubertal development and sexual functions

Common genes linking energy metabolism and puberty onset and progress

Nutritional factors (protein, sugars)

Energy supply (calories)

Adipocytokines (signaling)

Insulin/insulinlike growth factor effects

NAMPT and other enzymes providing energy to spermatozoa

Data from Refs.[1,2,10,11,37,40,42,45]

network initially develops and is temporarily active during species-specific periods of fetal/neonatal development up to the first months of life (called minipuberty). Classic puberty represents the secondary reactivation of an existing system. From a neurobiological perspective, the timing of puberty is therefore a function of changes in the neural systems controlling GnRH release, and the large interindividual variability in the onset and progression of puberty indicates that the timing of puberty is not simply a function of chronologic age.[22,31,32,36] Instead, the neurotransmitter and neuromodulatory systems that affect the GnRH secretory network convey information about metabolic fuels; energy stores in the liver, muscles, and adipose tissues; somatic development; and, for many species, information about season and social environment.

MALE FERTILITY

Male fertility is influenced and affected by endocrine, nutritional, environmental, and sociocultural factors, and secular trends. There are recent data and increasing evidence, in particular from the Scandinavian countries, showing that over the last decades sperm counts and sperm motility have decreased in young men.[33–35] However, the number of children fathered by individuals during their lifetimes has not declined visibly during the same period of time. Socioeconomic and cultural circumstances substantially influence the number of children per couple. Hence, no reliable data as to fecundity and fertility in developed nations and their relation to biological and molecular mechanisms exist. It may be that the impact of socioeconomic factors exceeds by far the effects that endocrine disruptors in the environment and/or nutritional factors may have on male fertility in the newer generations.[10,11,30–35]

CHILDHOOD GROWTH, FAT MASS DEVELOPMENT, AND MALE PUBERTY

In the newborn period, height velocity adjusts postnatally and is typically more reflective of genetic endowment than is prenatal growth. It approximates 25 cm/y in the first year, reducing to 12.5 cm/y in the second year. The annual height velocity then decreases on an average to 8 cm (ages 2–4 years) and then 6 cm (ages 4–6 years) during childhood, before a plateau phase of 5.5 cm/y is reached before the onset of puberty. Distinct gender-specific differences in both height and weight accretion already exist in childhood and these are accentuated during puberty. Boys gain height at a prepubertal rate until a mean age of 11 years and then experience a peak height velocity of 9.5 cm/y at approximately 13.5 years of age (corresponding with Tanner genital stages 3 and 4). The overall pubertal increment in stature in boys exceeds that of girls by only 3 to 5 cm, meaning that the mean adult height difference of approximately 13 cm between the sexes is largely caused by a more prolonged period of prepubertal growth in boys.[1] Weight velocity then accelerates rapidly in puberty and is gender specific, with boys gaining a mean of approximately 13.7 g/d (5 kg/y), whereas girls achieve approximately only 11.5 g/d (4.2 kg/y).[1,14]

Newborn boys have about 6.5% more (absolute) fat-free mass (FFM) than newborn girls. This gender difference mirrors the relative paucity of total body fat along with higher birth weights seen in boys. Initially fat mass increases to 25% to 30% of the total body weight by 6 months but then FFM begins to preferentially accumulate. Boys gain approximately 1 kg more absolute FFM than girls before puberty. In puberty, boys normally acquire FFM at a greater rate and for a longer period than girls, and adult values of FFM are attained by approximately 15 to 16 years of age in girls and 2 to 3 years later in boys.[4,13,36]

EFFECTS OF PUBERTY ON OBESITY

The role of puberty and normal variations in pubertal timing for the development of obesity in men remains mostly unclear. One study that did explore this was designed to investigate the impact of pubertal timing and prepubertal body mass index (BMI) (kg/m^2) on young adult BMI and fat mass distribution in more than 500 subjects from the population-based Gothenburg Osteoporosis and Obesity Determinants study. Although age at peak height velocity was an independent negative predictor of young adult BMI and whole-body fat mass, the age at peak height velocity was an independent negative predictor of central, but not peripheral, fat mass. Therefore, early pubertal onset may specifically predict a tendency to more central fat mass distribution, whereas a predominantly subcutaneous obese phenotype is more strongly predicted by a high prepubertal BMI.[1,14,29]

PUTATIVE INFLUENCE OF OBESITY ON TIMING OF PUBERTY

The degree to which these findings translate to earlier puberty being driven by the obesity epidemic is less clear. For example, a Danish study examined the association between prepubertal BMI and pubertal timing, as assessed by age at onset of pubertal growth spurt (OGS) and peak height velocity. Although BMI at the age of 7 years was inversely associated with age at OGS and peak height velocity, there was a downward trend in the age at attaining puberty in both boys and girls, irrespective of BMI. These data therefore suggest that the obesity epidemic may contribute to, but cannot be solely responsible, for the trend.[16,17,24]

However, overall the data on a putative association between body fatness, BMI and obesity, and age of pubertal onset in boys are scarce.[26,27,44] Therefore, indirect evidence has been used to assess these associations, and also to answer the question of whether obese boys enter puberty earlier than lean boys and, if so, whether they progress faster through puberty. For example, a small study of 201 children evaluated for short stature and/or delayed puberty showed an inverse relationship between weight status and pubertal development. This study suggests a slowing effect of malnutrition on pubertal development in boys and, conversely, it could be speculated that overnutrition may therefore accelerate development in boys.[26,27]

More direct evidence regarding the relationship between obesity and accelerated or delayed puberty in boys comes from a comparison of responses to a brief course of testosterone therapy in boys with constitutional delayed puberty, obesity, and possible gonadotropin deficiency, which suggests the importance of testosterone for fat mass development and, conversely, the effect of adipose tissue on androgen levels. Testosterone treatment increased growth rate and mean testis length in the 4 months following testosterone treatment. It was therefore concluded that obese boys constitute a distinct category of boys with pubertal delay in terms of their growth.[44] However, it is unclear whether overweight but otherwise healthy boys with delayed puberty have a variation of constitutional delay of growth and maturation. In one study, at diagnosis of delayed puberty, the overweight boys had a less delayed bone age, greater height standard deviation score (SDS) for chronologic age, and greater height SDS for bone age. Predicted height for the overweight boys exceeded their midparental height, whereas nonoverweight boys were predicted to be less than their midparental height. These observations suggest that, in the context of delayed puberty, being overweight may modulate adult height and/or that the cause of delayed puberty in overweight boys may differ from typical constitutional delay.[1,26,44] However, they do not strongly support an argument that obesity leads to delayed puberty in boys.

To directly examine the impact of childhood BMI on timing of male puberty, adult stature, and obesity, a retrospective school-based cohort follow-up study was performed in 1520 men with serial height and weight measurements from the age of 9 to 18 years. These individuals were followed up in adulthood to a mean age of 63 years. In this study, boys with a higher childhood BMI tended to have an earlier puberty and the childhood BMI correlated strongly and positively with adult adiposity, but inversely with leg length, suggesting again an earlier age of puberty. In contrast, boys with lower BMI had a later puberty, tended to be taller, and were less obese as adults.[1,26]

Voice break is a late but characteristic event in male puberty, and an assessment of age at voice break may be a relevant marker for epidemiologic studies of male pubertal development. The timing of voice break was investigated in 463 Danish choir boys. Over a 10-year period, age at voice break followed a general downward trend. Regarding body weight, the investigators observed a tendency toward early voice break with increasing BMI. Thus boys in the heaviest quartile at 8 years of age had an increased likelihood of early voice break, with this occurring on average approximately 6 years later, compared with boys in the thinnest quartile. However, this trend to earlier voice break could not be exclusively explained by a general increase in BMI during that period. These findings indicate a relationship between prepubertal BMI and the timing of puberty.[1,23]

A subsequent combined cross-sectional and longitudinal study (The Copenhagen Puberty Study) therefore specifically evaluated secular trends in pubertal onset over a 15-year period and their relationship to BMI in boys. Onset of puberty, defined as age at attainment of a testicular volume greater than 3 mL, occurred significantly earlier in 2006 to 2008 than in 1991 to 1993 along with significantly higher LH, but not testosterone, levels. Correspondingly, BMI SDS increased significantly from the years 1991 to 1993 to the years 2006 to 2008 and pubertal onset and LH levels were no longer significantly different between study periods after adjustment for BMI. It was therefore concluded that the estimated mean age at onset of puberty had declined significantly during the 15-year interval and that this decline was associated with the coincident increase in BMI.[16,17,27]

Adrenal androgens may represent a critical link between body fatness and timing of puberty. However, whether or not adrenarche affects the timing of pubertal development is controversial. The association of adrenal androgen secretion with early and late pubertal markers, independent of potential influences of dietary animal protein intake, was investigated in a prospective cohort study of healthy white children, suggesting that a higher animal protein intake may be involved in an earlier pubertal growth spurt and age at peak height velocity, whereas a more intensive adrenarcheal process may precipitate a shorter pubertal growth spurt and a notably earlier onset of breast and genital development in girls and boys, respectively.[13,14,24,33–35]

Therefore, when available data are taken together, our current opinion is that obesity is related to earlier, rather than delayed, pubertal development in boys.

EFFECTS OF OBESITY ON MALE REPRODUCTION

Growing evidence has linked the metabolic syndrome, including central obesity, insulin resistance, dyslipidemia, and hypertension, to the increasing prevalence of male infertility.[19] Obesity and metabolic diseases might contribute to all types of sexual dysfunction, which is known to increase in older age, although the effects of obesity on sexual function might not be evident at younger ages. A recent study has shown that coital frequency is lower in older men with higher BMI and the presence of metabolic disease in older individuals, but that this is not the case in young men.[30] Several studies have shown that testosterone exerted beneficial effects on brain function, including synaptic plasticity and cognitive functions.[31] However, controversial data have been generated as to the roles of testosterone in insulin-resistant obesity and cognitive function. Whether or not increasing fat mass, lowering testosterone levels, and insulin-resistant states affect sexual behavior and hence reproduction is therefore still unclear.[31]

MOLECULAR MECHANISMS OF ADIPOSE TISSUE MODULATION OF MALE PUBERTY AND REPRODUCTION

Genetic variants may also directly account for a link between obesity and pubertal timing. Variations in LIN28B, a human ortholog of the gene-regulating processing of micro-RNAs, were recently reported to be associated with timing of puberty in humans.[1] Genetic variation in LIN28B was associated with earlier voice break and more advanced pubic hair development in boys. In addition, the investigators found a faster tempo of height attainment in girls and boys, and a shorter adult height in those with allelic variation at this site, in keeping with earlier growth cessation caused by advanced epiphyseal closure. These data suggest that genetic influences on pubertal timing may be important and may even be stronger than environmental factors (the impact of which may therefore be more difficult to assess). Many additional studies also indicate that the timing of pubertal onset is under strong genetic control. However, genes controlling pubertal timing in the general population have not yet been clearly identified. A GWAS detected linkage of constitutional delay to a region on chromosome 2p13-2q13, and the pericentromeric region of chromosome 2. This locus may therefore represent a component of the internal clock controlling the timing of onset of puberty.[1,37]

Another important mechanism that contributes to the regulation of puberty by body composition is the interrelationship between gut, fat, and central nervous system hormones and peptides. Lately there has been an increased understanding of how hormones and gut peptides affect energy intake and storage in adipose tissue, and how these interact with the central nervous system to control energy balance. Moreover, some of these peptides have been shown to play important roles in modulating the gonadotropic axis with their absence, or an imbalance in their secretion, being able to disturb pubertal onset or progression. A growing body of evidence from both rodent and human studies suggests that leptin may be the critical link between body fat and earlier puberty. Leptin-deficient mice and humans fail to enter puberty unless leptin is administered,[6] and rodent studies indicate that very low levels of leptin stimulate gonadotropin secretion both at the hypothalamic and the pituitary level.[6] However, current evidence indicates that leptin plays a permissive role rather than acting as the critical metabolic signal initiating puberty. Knowledge concerning the role played by ghrelin, an orexigenic and growth-promoting peptide produced by the digestive tract, on sexual development has also been accumulating[13] and other peptides derived from the digestive tract may also be involved in the regulatory link between energy homeostasis and sexual development.[1]

The involvement of environmental factors, such as endocrine-disrupting chemicals (EDCs), in the timing of onset of puberty has also received much interest lately. Evidence for this comes from recent changes in age at puberty onset and pattern of distribution that are variable among countries, as well as new forms of sexual precocity after immigration to an environment with improved socioeconomic conditions. However, the evidence of association between early or late pubertal timing and exposure to EDCs is weak in humans, possibly because of heterogeneity of effects from mixtures of EDCs, as well as the inability to accurately assess fetal and/or neonatal exposure to these substances. Recent observations also support the concept that EDCs may cause disturbed energy balance and contribute to the obesity epidemic, which adds another layer of complexity to understanding the role that they may play in the timing of puberty. Several aspects link this system and the reproductive axis: this leads to coexisting neuroendocrine and peripheral effects and has a dependency on fetal/neonatal programming. Many factors have recently been discovered that cross-link the 2 systems; for instance, leptin, adiponectin, and agouti-related peptide.[21]

NAMPT represents an essential enzyme of NAD metabolism in somatic cells. This protein regulates cellular NAD+ levels and energy metabolism and is also implicated in the regulation of apoptosis. NAMPT has been linked to both obesity and the development of type 2 diabetes.[10,11,45] NAD+ is possibly required as a cosubstrate for dehydrogenases during spermatogenesis. Moreover, apoptosis signaling is known to be present and can be stimulated in human spermatozoa. It has been suggested that NAMPT may be effective in human spermatozoa as a mediator of sperm viability, motility, fertilization capacity, and apoptosis induction.[10,11,45] First, NAMPT protein was detected in different cell types of human testes, such as spermatogonia, spermatocytes, Sertoli cells, and Leydig cells, as well as in spermatozoa, where the expression levels were significantly higher in immature than in mature ejaculated spermatozoa. Second, NAMPT was secreted into the supernatant of human spermatozoa and its levels were significantly higher in immature spermatozoa compared with mature cells. In contrast, inhibition of NAMPT by FK866, a specific inhibitor of the enzyme, did not influence motility, capacitation, or apoptosis signaling. In summary, NAMPT is present in human spermatozoa in a maturation-dependent manner. However, its impact on spermatozoa maturation and function needs further investigation.[10,11,45]

Another factor that may be important in the link between obesity and pubertal development is the effect of early growth on long-term molecular mechanisms regulating growth and maturation. However, the contribution of rapid weight gain during specific periods in early life on the timing of puberty is still not clear. In a UK longitudinal birth cohort study,[4,28] faster early infancy weight gain was associated with increased body fat mass at 10 years of age and also with earlier age at menarche. In contrast, subsequent weight gain between 9 and 19 months was not associated with later adiposity or age at menarche. The investigators concluded that, in developed settings, rapid weight gain during the first 9 months of life is a risk factor for both increased childhood adiposity and early menarche in girls.[9,14] Several longitudinal studies have also shown that timing of puberty is most closely linked to infancy weight gain, suggesting an early window for programming of growth and development. Earlier puberty was related to smaller size at birth and rapid growth between birth and 2 years. Rapid early weight gain leads to taller childhood stature and higher IGF-I levels, possibly through early induction of growth hormone receptor numbers, and these may have long-term effects on growth and the timing of puberty. However, such children are also at risk of childhood obesity, meaning that associations of early growth with timing of puberty are confounded by adiposity. In the Avon Longitudinal Study of Parents and Children, rapid infancy weight gain was associated with increased risk of obesity at 5 and 8 years, evidence of insulin resistance, exaggerated adrenarche, and reduced levels of sex hormone–binding globulin (SHBG). The increased IGF-I and adrenal androgen levels potentially increased aromatase activity and increased free sex steroid levels consequent to lower SHBG levels, and this could all promote activity of the GnRH pulse generator. In addition, obese children have higher leptin levels, which is a proven permissive factor in initiating LH pulsatility.[31]

Conversely, early pubertal onset might predict predominantly central fat distribution, which is known to be associated with increased risk of cardiovascular disease.[42]

Over the last decade, the evidence linking obesity to impaired reproductive function has grown. As to male reproductive function, fewer data are available, in particular as to the molecular mechanisms that may cause infertility in obese men.[19,45] There is a striking similarity between female androgen excess and male androgen deficiency, both states being associated with reduced fertility.[32] Androgens increase lean and muscle mass and decrease the amount of visceral fat relative to body mass in men. A sedentary lifestyle causes sarcopenia and obesity, leading to abdominal obesity, metabolic disorders, and reduced sex hormone production in men. In addition, reduced sex hormone levels and gonadal dysfunction play an important role in the pathogenesis of obesity and diabetes, and their consequences.[32] Furthermore, exposure to EDCs that have become prevalent in the environment and food chain might be a causative factor for both the development of unhealthy fat mass and gonadal dysfunction.[21]

SUMMARY AND RESEARCH AGENDA

Studies have confirmed a strong relationship between achievement of critical body weight and puberty. In addition, and perhaps most importantly, it is now clear that an excess of body weight during childhood, early in infancy, and even during fetal life seems to have a significant impact on age of pubertal onset and increased testicular volume in boys. This earlier onset of puberty may be directly caused by factors related to body fat mass, such as adipocytokine levels, or alternatively may have other causes, such as genetic variation, social environment, endocrine disruptors, or other environmental factors. In addition, it is interesting to hypothesize that, from an evolutionary point of view, further increases in body weight may not be of any advantage in achieving earlier reproductive competence; they could be deleterious in terms of sexual maturation and reproduction and in addition lead to early cardiovascular and metabolic complications that are associated with obesity.[1,10,11]

ACKNOWLEDGMENTS

The authors received support from the Medical Faculty of the University of Leipzig, Germany, and EFRE, EU, Brussels. They also thank the Saxonian Ministry for Science and Culture, Dresden, Germany, and the Leipzig Children's Hospital Foundation, Leipzig, Germany, for continuously supporting parts of our work.

REFERENCES

1. Wagner IV, Sabin MA, Pfäffle RW, et al. Effects of obesity on human sexual development. Nat Rev Endocrinol 2012;31:246–54.
2. Frisch RE. Pubertal adipose tissue: is it necessary for normal sexual maturation? Evidence from the rat and human female. Fed Proc 1980;39:2395–400.
3. Herman-Giddens ME, Wang L, Koch G. Secondary sexual characteristics in boys: estimates from the national health and nutrition examination survey III, 1988–1994. Arch Pediatr Adolesc Med 2001;155:1022–8.
4. Sandhu J, Ben Shlomo Y, Cole TJ, et al. The impact of childhood body mass index on timing of puberty, adult stature and obesity: a follow-up study based on adolescent anthropometry recorded at Christ's Hospital (1936–1964). Int J Obes 2006;30:14–22.

5. Roelants M, Hauspie R, Hoppenbrouers K. References for growth and pubertal development from birth to 21 years in Flanders, Belgium. Ann Hum Biol 2009; 36:680–94.

6. Kiess W, Reich A, Meyer K, et al. A role for leptin in sexual maturation and puberty? Horm Res 1999;51:55–63.

7. Kiess W, Galler A, Reich A, et al. Clinical aspects of obesity in childhood and adolescence. Obes Rev 2001;2:29–36.

8. Kindblom JM, Lorentzon M, Norjavaara E, et al. Pubertal timing is an independent predictor of central adiposity in young adult males: the Gothenburg Osteoporosis and Obesity Determinants Study. Diabetes 2006;55:3047–52.

9. Wang Y. Is obesity associated with early sexual maturation? A comparison of the association in American boys versus girls. Pediatrics 2004;113:171–2.

10. Thomas S, Kratzsch D, Schaab M, et al. Seminal plasma adipokine levels are correlated with functional characteristics of spermatozoa. Fertil Steril 2013;99:1256–63.

11. Thomas S, Garten A, Schaab M, et al. NAMPT – a maturation marker of human spermatozoa and testes. Exp Clin Endocrinol Diabetes 2013;121:85.

12. Toppari J, Juul A. Trends in puberty timing in humans and environmental modifiers. Mol Cell Endocrinol 2010;324:39–44.

13. Pomerants T, Tillmann V, Jürimäe J, et al. Relationship between ghrelin and anthropometrical, body composition parameters and testosterone levels in boys at different stages of puberty. J Endocrinol Invest 2006;29:962–7.

14. Persson I, Ahlsson F, Ewald U, et al. Influence of perinatal factors on the onset of puberty in boys and girls: implications for interpretation of link with risk of long term diseases. Am J Epidemiol 1999;150:747–55.

15. Karlberg J. Secular trends in pubertal development. Horm Res 2002;57:19–30.

16. Aksglaede L, Juul A, Olsen LW, et al. Age at puberty and the emerging obesity epidemic. PLoS One 2009;4:e8450.

17. Juul A, Teilmann G, Scheike T, et al. Pubertal development in Danish children: comparison of recent European and US data. Int J Androl 2006;29:247–55.

18. Körner A, Kratzsch J, Gausche R, et al. New predictors of the metabolic syndrome in children - role of adipocytokines. Pediatr Res 2007;61:640–5.

19. Morrison CD, Brannigan RE. Metabolic syndrome and infertility in men. Best Pract Res Clin Obstet Gynaecol 2015;29:507–15.

20. Klenov VE, Jungheim ES. Obesity and reproductive function: a review of the evidence. Curr Opin Obstet Gynecol 2014;26:455–60.

21. García-Arevalo M, Alonso-Magdalena P, Rebelo Dos Santos J, et al. Exposure to bisphenol-A during pregnancy partially mimics the effects of a high-fat diet altering glucose homeostasis and gene expression in adult male mice. PLoS One 2014;9:e100214.

22. Marshall WA, Tanner JM. Variations in the pattern of pubertal changes in boys. Arch Dis Child 1970;45:13–23.

23. Greil H, Kahl H. Assessment of developmental age: cross-sectional analysis of secondary sexual characteristics. Anthropol Anz 2005;63:63–75.

24. Sørensen K, Aksglaede L, Petersen JH, et al. Recent changes in pubertal timing in healthy Danish boys: associations with body mass index. J Clin Endocrinol Metab 2010;95:263–70.

25. De Onis M, Dasgupta P, Saha S, et al. The National Center for Health Statistics reference and the growth of Indian adolescent boys. Am J Clin Nutr 2001;74: 248–53.

26. Nathan BM, Sedlmeyer IL, Palmert MR. Impact of body mass index on growth in boys with delayed puberty. J Pediatr Endocrinol Metab 2006;19:971–7.

27. Juul A, Magnusdottir S, Scheike T, et al. Age at voice break in Danish boys: effects of pre-pubertal body mass index and secular trend. Int J Androl 2007;30:537–42.
28. Ahmed ML, Ongg KK, Dunger DB. Childhood obesity and the timing of puberty. Trends Endocrinol Metab 2009;20:237–42.
29. He Q, Karlberg J. BMI gain in childhood and its associations with height gain, timing of puberty, and final height. Pediatr Res 2001;49:815–21.
30. Rurik I, Varga A, Fekete F, et al. Sexual activity of young men is not related to their anthropometric parameters. J Sex Med 2014;11:2264–71.
31. Pintana H, Chattipakorn N, Chattipakorn S. Testosterone deficiency, insulin-resistant obesity and cognitive function. Metab Brain Dis 2015;30(4):853–76.
32. Escobar-Morreale HF, Alvarez-Blasco F, Botella-Carretero JI, et al. The striking similarities in the metabolic associations of female androgen excess and male androgen deficiency. Hum Reprod 2014;29:2083–91.
33. Adamopoulos DA, Pappa A, Billa E, et al. Seasonality in sperm parameters in normal men and dyspermic patients on medical intervention. Andrologia 2009; 41:118–24.
34. Sobreiro BP, Lucon AM, Pasqualotto FF, et al. Semen analysis in fertile patients undergoing vasectomy: reference values and variations according to age, length of sexual abstinence, seasonality, smoking habits and caffeine intake. Sao Paulo Med J 2005;123:161–6.
35. Centola GM, Eberly S. Seasonal variations and age-related changes in human sperm count, 547 motility, motion parameters, morphology, and white blood cell concentration. Fertil Steril 1999;72:803–8.
36. Veldhuis JD, Roemmich JN, Richmond EJ, et al. Endocrine control of body fat composition in infancy, childhood, and puberty. Endocr Rev 2005;26:114–46.
37. Koerner A, Kiess W, Stumvoll M, et al. Polygenic contribution to obesity: genome-wide strategies reveal new targets. Front Horm Res 2008;36:12–36.
38. Boettner A, Kratzsch J, Müller G, et al. Gender differences of adiponectin levels develop during the progression of puberty and are related to serum androgen levels. J Clin Endocrinol Metab 2004;89:4053–61.
39. Sundblom E, Petzold M, Rasmussen F, et al. Childhood overweight and obesity prevalences levelling off in Stockholm but socioeconomic differences persist. Int J Obes 2008;32:1525–30.
40. Cohen-Cole E, Fletcher JM. Is obesity contagious? Social networks vs. environmental factors in the obesity epidemic. J Health Econ 2008;27:1382–7.
41. Grow HM, Cook AJ, Arterburn DE, et al. Child obesity associated with social disadvantage of children's neighbourhoods. Soc Sci Med 2010;71:584–91.
42. Freedman DS, Dietz WH, Srinivasan SR, et al. The relation of overweight to cardiovascular risk factors among children and adolescents: the Bogalusa Heart Study. Pediatrics 1999;103:1175–82.
43. Lipek T, Igel U, Gausche R, et al. Obesogenic environments: environmental approaches to obesity prevention. J Pediatr Endocrinol Metab 2015;28:485–95.
44. Kaplowitz P. Delayed puberty in obese boys: comparison with constitutional delayed puberty and response to testosterone therapy. J Pediatr 1998;133:745–9.
45. Garten A, Schuster S, Penke M, et al. Physiological and pathophysiological roles of NAMPT and NAD metabolism. Nat Rev Endocrinol 2015. [Epub ahead of print].

Psychological Outcomes and Reproductive Issues Among Gender Dysphoric Individuals

Lauren Schmidt, MD[a], Rachel Levine, MD[b],*

KEYWORDS

- Gender dysphoria • Transgender • Gender-affirmation therapy
- Psychiatric comorbidities • Fertility

KEY POINTS

- An increasing number of adolescents identify as transgender, and are seeking treatment consisting of pubertal suppression, cross-sex hormones, and sex reassignment surgery.
- Longitudinal outcome studies of gender dysphoric individuals suggest improved psychological functioning after gender reassignment treatment.
- Interventions for fertility preservation among gender dysphoric individuals are currently limited to cryopreservation of gametes and gonadal tissue banking.

INTRODUCTION

Gender dysphoria is a condition in which a person experiences discrepancy between the anatomic sex assigned at birth and the gender he or she identifies with, resulting in internal distress and a desire to live and be accepted as the preferred gender. Originally regarded exclusively as a mental disorder, gender dysphoria is currently believed to result from interaction among biologic, environmental, psychosocial, and cultural factors. Before the 1950s, sex consisted of a binary system of males and females, and no distinction existed between sex and gender. John William Money, a psychologist at Johns Hopkins University, studied the development of gender identity among infants born with ambiguous genitalia, and advocated for the role of social and environmental factors in the development of gender identity.[1] The term "gender identity" was devised to refer to an individual's internal experience as male or female, and is

The authors report no conflicts of interest.
[a] Department of Psychiatry, Yale University School of Medicine, 500 University Drive, Hershey, PA 17033, USA; [b] Pennsylvania State University College of Medicine, Hershey Medical Center, 500 University Drive, Hershey, PA 17033, USA
* Corresponding author.
E-mail address: Rlevine@hmc.psu.edu

Endocrinol Metab Clin N Am 44 (2015) 773–785
http://dx.doi.org/10.1016/j.ecl.2015.08.001
0889-8529/15/$ – see front matter © 2015 Elsevier Inc. All rights reserved.

endo.theclinics.com

not necessarily binary.[2] The term "transsexual" was created to describe individuals who strive to live in accordance with their preferred gender, facilitated by hormones or surgery.[3]

Transsexualism was first publicized by endocrinologist Harry Benjamin in his 1966 book, *The Transsexual Phenomenon*, in which he presented his patient Christine Jorgensen, the first individual to undergo sex reassignment surgery.[4] In 1979 the Harry Benjamin Gender Dysphoria Association was formed, which established the standards of care to guide the treatment of transsexualism.[1–3] The diagnosis of transsexualism appeared for the first time in the *Diagnostics and Statistical Manual of Mental Disorders* (DSM), 3rd edition, in 1980, under the overarching title of gender identity disorder, which also included gender identity disorder of childhood.[5] Gender identity disorder has recently been renamed gender dysphoria in the DSM-5.[6]

Today, the Harry Benjamin Gender Dysphoria Association is known as the World Professional Association for Transgender Health (WPATH). Almost 50 years after Dr Benjamin introduced transsexualism to society, data on the medical and social needs of gender-nonconforming individuals are limited, especially among the pediatric population. The terms "transgender" and "transsexual" are often used interchangeably. Whereas "transsexual" identifies individuals with a desire to live as a member of the gender opposite than that assigned at birth, "transgender" may also be used to identify individuals whose gender identity does not conform to the conventional male and female roles.[7] Not all individuals who identify as transgender choose to seek endocrine or surgical treatment. An increasing number of children and adolescents now identify as transgender and are pursuing medical services to align their physical characteristics with their preferred gender.[2] As more young individuals receive medical treatment for gender dysphoria, the long-term effects of pubertal suppression and cross-sex hormone therapy on psychological well-being and fertility must be addressed.

EPIDEMIOLOGY

Globally, data suggest that the prevalence of gender dysphoria among natal adult males and natal adult females ranges from 0.002% to 0.0003% and 0.005% to 0.014%, respectively.[6] Although limited data exist regarding the prevalence of transgender youth, multidisciplinary clinics for transgender children and adolescents in North America and Europe report increased demands for services.[8] In general, surveys conducted to assess the prevalence of gender dysphoria are an underestimation of reality, secondary to cultural and societal bias.

ETIOLOGY

Most endocrinology research on gender dysphoria has been conducted in individuals diagnosed with disorders of sex development. Although most patients with gender dysphoria do not have disorders of sex development, populations of patients with disorders of sex development have been used to investigate the role of prenatal and postnatal steroids in gender development.[1] The influence of androgens on behavior was first reported in girls with a history of prenatal exposure to exogenous androgens, leading to masculinization of genitalia and behavior.[2] The incidence of gender dysphoria is increased in females with excessive exogenous androgen production from 46,XX congenital adrenal hyperplasia.[2]

Higher rates of gender dysphoria have also been observed in 46,XY individuals with androgen receptor defects, 46,XY 5α-reductase-2 deficiency, and penile agenesis.[2,9] In humans, androgens are likely the primary steroid hormone contributing to the sexual dimorphism of brain and behavior. Many individuals with 5α-reductase-2 deficiency are born with female-appearing external genitalia and are raised female. Among the largest cohort of patients with 5α-reductase-2 deficiency, 56% to 63% of those surveyed reported female-to-male (FTM) gender change.[9] Similarly, among newborns with 46,XY cloacal exstrophy who underwent castration and were raised as female, most identified as male.[10]

Diffusion-weighted MRI has been used to investigate differences in white matter microstructure between natal males and females. White matter contains androgen receptors and the volume of white matter is known to increase during male adolescence secondary to increase in testosterone.[11] Through the use of diffusion-weighted MRI, Rametti and colleagues[12] determined that the white matter microstructure in FTM individuals, who had not yet initiated cross-sex hormone therapy, more closely resembled that of males than that of their biologic female sex. Additional diffusion-weighted MRI studies have concluded that white matter microstructure in both FTM and male-to-female (MTF) individuals falls halfway between that of genetic females and males.[13]

DIAGNOSIS

Gender dysphoria often emerges in early childhood. Approximately 80% of gender dysphoric youth do not persist in having gender dysphoria as adolescents, but rather become homosexual or bisexual adults.[1,2,14] The onset of worsening gender dysphoria during puberty significantly predicts the persistence of transgenderism throughout adulthood.[14] According to the DSM-5, gender dysphoria is defined as, "A marked incongruence between one's experienced/expressed gender and assigned gender, of at least 6 months' duration, as manifested by at least 6 of 8 criteria in children and 2 of 6 criteria in adolescents and adults" (**Box 1**).[6]

Before initiation of medical therapy, the diagnosis of persistent gender dysphoria must be confirmed by a mental health professional. Individuals with gender dysphoria often present with comorbid behavioral and emotional problems. Transgender youths have a higher risk of depression, anxiety, substance abuse, suicidal ideation, suicidal attempts, and self-injurious behavior than their non–gender dysphoric peers.[15] It is recommended that transgender youths be treated at a multidisciplinary gender dysphoria clinic, consisting of pediatric endocrinologists, urologists, gynecologists, and psychologists. Although an increasing number of multidisciplinary clinics have been established in the United States, management of gender dysphoric youths is still very controversial. The guidelines and standards of care are primarily based on expert opinion as opposed to evidence-based data. The refusal of most insurance companies to cover therapy for transgender individuals has led to a deficit in adequate care and research for gender dysphoria.

TREATMENT

The most widely accepted guidelines for treating gender dysphoria come from the WPATH Standards of Care, the United States Endocrine Society (ES), and the Netherlands Amsterdam Gender Clinic. After a formal diagnosis of gender dysphoria is established, individuals are encouraged to live permanently as their desired gender. This includes adopting a preferred name, hairstyle, clothing, and behavior.

Completely Reversible Interventions

The first phase of hormonal therapy for adolescents is pubertal suppression. According to the WPATH Standards of Care and ES guidelines, pubertal suppression is initiated at Tanner Stage 2 (**Box 2**).[2,3,7,16] Preventing the development of

---

Box 1
Criteria for diagnosing gender dysphoria in individuals

Criteria for Gender Dysphoria in Children

1. A strong desire to be of the other gender or an insistence that he or she is the other gender.

2. In boys (assigned gender), a strong preference for cross-dressing or simulating female attire; or in girls (assigned gender), a strong preference for wearing only typical masculine clothing and a strong resistance to the wearing of typical feminine clothing.

3. A strong preference for cross-gender roles in make-believe play or fantasy play.

4. A strong preference for the toys, games, or activities stereotypically used or engaged in by the other gender.

5. A strong preference for playmates of the other gender.

6. In boys (assigned gender), a strong rejection of typically masculine toys, games, and activities and a strong avoidance of rough-and-tumble play; or in girls (assigned gender), a strong rejection of typically feminine toys, games, and activities.

7. A strong dislike of one's sexual anatomy.

8. A strong desire for the primary and/or secondary sex characteristics that match one's experienced gender.

Criteria for Gender Dysphoria in Adolescents and Adults

1. A marked incongruence between one's experienced/expressed gender and primary/or secondary sex characteristics.

2. A strong desire to be rid of one's primary and/or secondary sex characteristics because of a marked incongruence with one's experienced/expressed gender.

3. A strong desire for the primary and/or secondary sex characteristics of the other gender.

4. A strong desire to be of the other gender (or some alternative gender different from one's assigned gender).

5. A strong desire to be treated as the other gender (or some alternative gender different from one's assigned gender).

6. A strong conviction that one has the typical feelings and reactions of the other gender (or some alternative gender different from one's assigned gender).

Reprinted with permission from the Diagnostic and Statistical Manual of Mental Disorders, Fifth Edition, (Copyright ©2013). American Psychiatric Association. All Rights Reserved.

---

secondary sexual characteristics that are not consistent with a person's preferred gender can lead to decreased body dysphoria and can lessen the need for future surgical reconstruction.[2] Before initiating pubertal suppression, a physical examination documenting testicular volume and penis width or breast size, terminal hair distribution, baseline metabolic laboratory studies, sex steroid levels, and bone age should be completed, in addition to addressing psychological, social, and family issues.[17]

Concerns with the administration of gonadotropin-releasing hormone (GnRH) analogues include detrimental effects on bone mineralization and height. In a study evaluating the Dutch protocol, which recommends GnRH analogue initiation at age 12 and cross-sex hormones at age 16, bone density was decreased during GnRH administration, but was within normal limits following the onset of cross-gender hormones.[18] The authors of the study concluded that the administration of cross-sex hormones counteracts the adverse effects of GnRH analogues.

Box 2
Interventions for pubertal suppression available in the United States for transgender adolescents

A. Interventions for Pubertal Suppression

1. Gonadotropin-releasing hormone analogues: Inhibit the hypothalamic-pituitary-gonadal axis
   a. Leuprolide: Monthly intramuscular injection
   b. Histrelin: Subcutaneous implant, yearly dosing
   c. Nafarelin intranasal spray: Multiple daily doses, has not yet been used for gender dysphoria

2. Less expensive alternative options
   a. Medroxyprogesterone: Inhibition of gonadal steriogenesis; administered either orally (up to 40 mg/day) or intramuscularly (150 mg q 3 months)
   b. Sprironolactone: Inhibits testosterone among MTF; daily oral administration
   c. Finasteride: Inhibits type II 5α-reductase and blocks conversion of testosterone to 5α-dihydrotestosterone among MTF

B. Monitoring Protocol During Pubertal Suppression

1. Every 3 months
   a. Physical examination: Height, weight, sitting height, Tanner stages
   b. Laboratory studies: Luteinizing hormone, follicle-stimulating hormone, estradiol/testosterone

2. Every year
   a. Laboratory studies: Calcium, Phosphate, Alkaline Phosphatase 25-hydroxyvitamin D, renal and liver function tests, lipids, glucose, insulin, glycosylated hemoglobin.
   b. Bone age on radiograph of the left hand

Data from Refs.[2,7,20]

Partially Reversible Interventions

The ES recommends the initiation of cross-sex hormones at the age of 16 years.[7] There are concerns, however, that extending the prepubertal state until 16 years may potentiate adverse consequences for emotional well-being, because many same-age peers will already have begun puberty.[14] Several institutions are currently studying the emotional and physical effects of initiating cross-sex hormone therapy at 14 years.[2] Cross-sex hormones are used to induce desired feminizing or masculinizing secondary sex characteristics, and the effects of these hormones are considered to be partially reversible.

Estrogen is used in MTF individuals to induce puberty and to achieve feminization (**Table 1**A).[7] The goal of treatment is to maintain the serum estradiol at the mean level for premenopausal women (<200 pg/mL), and serum testosterone in the female range (<55 ng/dL).[7] Among adolescents and young adults, oral estradiol treatment is considered safe and is more cost effective than the topical or injectable formulations. Transdermal and injectable forms of estradiol bypass the liver's first-pass effect and do not stimulate hepatic clotting factors, and have been shown to reduce the adverse effects associated with estrogen therapy: deep venous thrombophlebitis, prolactinoma, hypertension, liver disease, and increased risk of breast cancer.[19] Oral ethinyl estradiol and conjugated estrogens should be avoided in older patients who may be at an increased risk of deep venous thrombosis.[7] Many providers refrain from prescribing progesterone because it has been associated with a higher incidence of breast cancer when used in combination with estrogen in postmenopausal women.[20] If a

Table 1
Hormonal interventions for transgender adolescents and adults

A. MTF Cross-Sex Hormone Therapy	
Hormone and Effects	**Administration/Adult Dosage**

17β-Estradiol
  Breast development, redistribution of fat,
    softer skin, alteration in mood
  Reduce male-pattern hair growth,
    erections, and libido
  Induction of female puberty with oral
    estradiol, increase dose every 6 mo (5 μg/
    kg/d, 10 μg/kg/d, 15 μg/kg/d, 20 μg/kg/d,
    2 mg/kg/d)
	Oral: 2.0–8.0 mg/d
	Transdermal patch: 5–30 mg every 2 wk
	Parenteral: 5–30 mg intramuscularly
	  every 2 wk

Progesterone
  Risks and benefits are not well established
  Associated with decreased bone density
    and obesity
	20–60 mg/d

Spironolactone Suppress male-pattern hair growth	100–200 mg/d
Finasteride Reduce balding	1 mg/d

B. FTM Cross-Sex Hormone Therapy	

Testosterone
  Irreversible clitoral enlargement,
    deepening of the voice, male pattern
    hair growth, cessation of menses,
    increase lean muscle mass
  Induction of male puberty with
    intramuscular testosterone, increase
    biweekly dose every 6 mo (25 mg/m^2,
    50 mg/m^2, 75 mg/m^2, 100 mg/m^2)
	Parenteral enanthate or cypionate:
	  100–200 mg intramuscularly every 2 wk
	Topical gel: 1%: 2.5–10 mg/d
	Patch: 2.5–7.5 mg/d
	Patch is changed daily

C. Monitoring Protocol During Cross-Sex Hormonal Therapy

Every 3 mo
  Physical examination: height, weight, Tanner staging, blood pressure
  Hormonal laboratory studies: luteinizing hormone, follicle-stimulating hormone, estradiol/
    testosterone
  Metabolic laboratory studies: calcium, phosphate, alkaline phosphatase, potassium,
    complete blood count, renal and liver function, fasting lipids, glucose, insulin,
    glycosylated hemoglobin
Every year
  Laboratory studies: prolactin
  Bone density on DEXA scan
  Bone age on radiograph of the left hand

(*Data from* Rosenthal SM. Approach to the patient: transgender youth: endocrine considerations. J Clin Endocrinol Metab 2014;10:1919–28; and Hembree WC, Cohen-Kettenis P, Delemarre-van de Waal HA, et al. Endocrine treatment of transsexual persons: an endocrine society clinical practice guideline. J Clin Endocrinol Metab 2009;94(9):3132–54.)

patient begins hormone treatment after the completion of puberty, neither estradiol nor GnRH analogues can affect vocal pitch, laryngeal prominence, or height.[14]

    For FTM adolescents testosterone can be delivered via transdermal or parenteral routes to maintain testosterone levels in the male range (320–1000 ng/dL; see **Table 1**B).[7,14] Transdermal and intramuscular testosterone both result in similar masculinizing effects, but the process is slower with transdermal preparations.[7] Intramuscular testosterone can result in cyclic variation of plasma testosterone level and clinical effects.[7] Transdermal testosterone preparations can be advantageous in maintaining stable testosterone levels. Adverse effects of testosterone therapy include hyperlipidemia, decreased insulin sensitivity, decreased bone density, polycythemia, acne, and infertility (see **Table 1C**).[4,7]

Irreversible Interventions

Sex reassignment surgery is available to individuals who desire a more masculine or feminine appearance. In the United States, sexual reassignment operations are not usually offered to patients younger than 18 years of age. The WPATH and ES both emphasize the importance of living as the preferred gender while undergoing hormone replacement therapy for at least 1 year before considering sexual reassignment surgery. Transgender individuals who have not experienced either physical or psychological satisfaction with cross-sex hormones are strongly discouraged from seeking sexual reassignment surgery.

MTF transgender individuals may elect to undergo vaginoplasty to create female-appearing external genitals. This surgical procedure involves penile inversion, clitoroplasty, and creating of labia from scrotal skin.[21] For MTF individuals, orchidectomy and penectomy are often the first procedures performed.[22] Nerve-sparing techniques have preserved sexual responsiveness postoperatively with moderate to high rates of orgasmic functioning reported by MTF and FTM individuals.[23] Additional surgical procedures available to MTF transgender individuals include breast augmentation, facial feminizing surgery, and fat transplants.

In FTM transgender individuals an elected mastectomy is often the first gender reassignment surgery performed. A mastectomy can be performed as early as 16 years of age, after receiving testosterone therapy for at least 1 continuous year.[20] Additional surgical procedures available to FTM transgender individuals include construction of neoscrotum with testis prosthesis with or without a metoidioplasty, or creation of a microphallus from a hypertrophic clitoris, or phalloplasty.[17] FTM transgender individuals may elect to have a hysterectomy and oophorectomy. Transgender individuals who choose to have their gonads surgically removed can discontinue GnRH analogue treatment.[7]

The number of individuals seeking sexual reassignment surgery in the United States is unknown because most insurance companies classify these procedures as elective and do not cover the costs. From a surgical perspective, the amount of genital skin available for either vaginoplasty or phalloplasty before 18 years of age may be limited, especially post pubertal suppression with GnRH analogues.[16] Many individuals achieve significant improvement of gender dysphoria with hormone therapy alone and choose not to undergo surgery.

PSYCHOLOGICAL OUTCOMES

Pubertal suppression therapy was first introduced nearly 15 years ago, and since has become widely available to adolescents struggling with gender dysphoria.[24] Gender dysphoric adolescents who do not receive counseling or medical therapy are at an increased risk of substance abuse, self-injurious behavior, and suicide.[15] Until recently, no data have been available assessing the quality of life among transgender adolescents. de Vries and colleagues[24] studied psychological well-being among 55 transgender young adults who received pubertal suppression therapy during adolescence at the Center of Expertise on Gender Dysphoria in the Netherlands. Among the participants, gender dysphoria and body image dissatisfaction persisted throughout pubertal suppression and remitted after initiation of cross-sex hormones. In general, transgender females reported more satisfaction with primary sex characteristics compared with transgender males throughout the duration of cross-sex hormone treatment. At 1-year post gender reassignment surgery, all participants reported being either "very or fairly" satisfied with the operative results.[24] The authors concluded that post sex reassignment surgery, psychological functioning and subjective happiness were comparable with that reported by same-age non–gender dysphoric peers.[24] Although this longitudinal study is applicable to gender nonconforming adolescents globally, limited research has been conducted in regards to psychological functioning among young transgender individuals receiving treatment in the United States.

Aside from the study by de Vries and colleagues longitudinal outcome assessments of transgender individuals have so far been limited to adult populations. The quality of life of transgender individuals has been reported to be less favorable than that of the general population.[25,26] Before receiving treatment of gender dysphoria, MTF and FTM individuals suffer from a greater incidence of mental health morbidities.[15,20] FTM transsexuals who receive testosterone self-report a significantly higher quality of life than those who do not receive cross-sex hormones.[25] Similarly, psychological well-being is statistically higher in transgender women who have had sex reassignment surgery, facial feminization surgery, or both, compared with their nonsurgical counterparts either receiving only cross-sex hormones or no treatment.[27] A long-term study at the Karolinska Institute in Sweden followed individuals who had undergone sex reassignment surgery, and found increased mortality among this population from 10 years after surgery onward.[28] However, the mortality rate was only significantly increased for those operated on before 1989, suggesting that improved surgical technique and societal acceptance of gender dysphoria has aided in overall well-being among those seeking treatment.[26]

Stress-induced hypercortisolism is an established risk factor for premature mortality. The evaluation of perceived stress and cortisol awakening plasma levels were studied in transgender patients before and after cross-sex hormone treatment.[29] Following 12 months of cross-sex hormone therapy, elevated levels of morning plasma cortisol detected before treatment had returned to normal range.[28] Among adult transsexuals undergoing treatment of gender dysphoria, family support, cross-sex hormone therapy, and employment were associated with a better quality of life.[30]

Most MTF and FTM individuals elect to continue cross-sex hormone treatment lifelong to prevent the loss of preferred secondary sex characteristics. Even individuals who choose to undergo sex reassignment surgery usually continue low-dose cross-sex hormone therapy. Therefore, it is important to understand the influence cross-sex hormones have on morbidity and mortality. Psychological evaluation has supported the use of hormones and sex reassignment surgery in relieving gender dysphoria. However, some transgender individuals still experience comorbid psychiatric problems, social isolation, and discrimination. Asscherman and colleagues[18] reported that MTF individuals had a 51% increased mortality rate compared with the general male population. This increased mortality rate was attributed to suicide, substance abuse, AIDS, and cardiovascular disease. There was no difference in the mortality rate between FTM individuals and the general female population.[18]

Transgender adolescents undergoing cross-sex hormone treatment are considered to be at an increased risk for metabolic dysfunction. In MTF individuals, androgen suppression and estrogen-replacement therapy contribute to increases in visceral fat, and subsequent increase in triglycerides, hepatic dysfunction, and insulin resistance.[18,31] Increases in blood pressure and arterial stiffness have been observed in MTF undergoing estrogen and antiandrogen treatment.[30] Aside from the increased risk of cardiovascular disease attributable to metabolic dysfunction, MTF individuals receiving estrogen therapy are at an increased risk for venous thrombosis. In the past, long-term ethinyl estradiol use was independently associated with venous thrombosis and a threefold increased risk of cardiovascular disease.[7] Today, ethinyl estradiol is not recommended for cross-sex hormone treatment among transgender patients, and thus the risk of venous thrombosis has decreased.

Hormone-dependent tumors are extremely rare among MTF and FTM individuals receiving cross-sex hormones. There are very few cases of MTF patients who developed breast cancer while receiving estrogen therapy, but breast adenomas have been observed more frequently.[30] Additional research is needed to determine the independent risk of prolonged estrogen exposure on the development of cancer. MTF individuals are strongly urged to have regular breast examinations performed by their physicians. On initiating estrogen and antiandrogen therapy, the prostate decreases in volume. Because of the elevated risk of surgical complications including urinary incontinence, the prostate is not removed during sex reassignment surgery.[30] Few cases of prostate cancer have been reported in MTF patients receiving estrogen replacement. However, it is not clear whether the cancers were estrogen sensitive or were present before hormone replacement initiation.[32] In addition to undergoing regular prostate examinations, MTF individuals should have their serum prolactin levels monitored while taking estrogen. This is because several cases of prolactinomas attributed to high-dose estrogen treatment have been reported.[30] Adult FTM individuals who have not undergone a hysterectomy are at an increased risk of developing endometrial cancer while receiving testosterone therapy, because testosterone can be aromatized to estradiol.[33] It is critical that adolescents and young adults consider reproductive options with their physicians before having a hysterectomy or initiating gender reassignment treatment.

REPRODUCTIVE AND FERTILITY OUTCOMES

Individuals with gender dysphoria who opt to undergo cross-sex hormone and surgical treatments must consider irreversible loss of future reproductive potential. Today, an increasing number of gender dysphoric youths are diagnosed and started on hormone-replacement therapy. Many of these young individuals are neither mature nor old enough to thoroughly consider the effects cross-sex hormones will have on their future fertility. The WPATH and ES strongly recommend that gender dysphoric youth be counseled on options to preserve their ability to have genetically related children as adults. This conversation between the physician and patient should begin during pubertal suppression with GnRH analogues.[7] The use of GnRH analogues not only prevents the development of sexual characteristics that are not consistent with the preferred gender, but also delays fertility. Before initiation of cross-sex hormone treatment, transgender adolescents should be counseled on the suppressive effects of hormonal therapy on gamete production and are encouraged to consider gender interventions for fertility.

In MTF individuals, estrogen therapy decreases spermatogenesis and may eventually lead to azoospermia.[34] MTF individuals have the option of cryopreserving semen before starting hormone therapy. The stored sperm can be used in the future to produce a genetically related offspring through assisted reproductive techniques. Gender dysphoria and sexual orientation are exclusive to one another, and therefore not all options are available for all transgender individuals. Transgender females who have a female partner can use their sperm through intrauterine insemination, in vitro fertilization, or intracytoplasmic sperm injections.[33] Transgender females who are in a relationship with a male will need oocyte donation and a surrogate mother. Unfortunately, the cost of sperm banking is rarely covered by insurance and discourages some individuals from pursuing cryopreservation. In the past many transsexual women chose to forgo fertility preservation to have a faster transition. Some transsexual women believe that sperm preservation prevents them from deidentifying with their male past.[35] As an increasing number of prepubertal males explore gender reassignment treatment, these patients and their families can elect to bank samples of testicular tissue, with the hope that the tissue can be used in the future to derive sperm.[36]

In FTM individuals, testosterone therapy eventually leads to reversible amenorrhea with ovarian follicles remaining in place. Androgen treatment neither depletes nor affects the development of primordial follicles.[36] Before undergoing sexual reassignment surgery, FTM individuals are encouraged to explore options to preserve future fertility. Postpubertal females can elect to undergo oocyte banking. Unfortunately, unlike cryopreservation of sperm, mature oocytes are very sensitive to chromosomal damage from freezing and thawing. Therefore, ovarian tissue banking may be a more realistic future option. Ovarian tissue banking has been used in women and prepubertal females with malignant disease undergoing chemotherapy or radiation treatment.[36] Because FTM individuals retain usable ovarian follicles even after undergoing androgen therapy, ovarian tissue banking can be performed at the time of gonadectomy.[36] Both oocyte and ovarian tissue banking require donor sperm and a recipient uterus. Among women who have undergone chemotherapy or radiation therapy banked ovarian tissues has been autotransplanted into the patients themselves. However, this is not ideal for many FTM individuals who seek to deidentify with the female gender and do not wish to become pregnant. Additionally, sex reassignment surgery in transsexual men includes a hysterectomy.[34] Grafting the tissue into another individual predisposes one to the possibility of immune rejection. In vitro culture of ovarian tissue has been mostly unsuccessful and more research is needed to develop methods to preserve female gametes.

In the United States, hysterectomy and oophorectomy are not necessary for legal sex reassignment.[34] Thus, some transgender men have chosen not to have their ovaries or uterus removed, and have used donor sperm to conceive and gestate genetically related children. In a study aimed to understand the reproductive wishes of transgender men following sex reassignment surgery, most transgender men surveyed still desired to have children either by genetic procreation or adoption.[34] As an increasing number of gender dysphoric individuals present to their health care providers at younger ages, options for preserving fertility will become direr.

The WPATH strongly advocates for parenthood, stating, "Transsexual, transgender, and gender nonconforming people should not be refused reproductive options for any reason."[3] Many transgender individuals have normal loving relationships with their children, and there is no evidence that having a transgender parent negatively impacts a child's development.[33] Although most data available document the overall well-being of transgender individuals after gender reassignment treatment, some medical experts remain critical in regards to the use of assisted reproduction technologies for transgender individuals after gender reassignment.

SUMMARY

Over the last decade, the number of children and adolescents presenting to multidisciplinary gender dysphoria clinics has been increasing. Although most young prepubertal children will not persist in meeting criteria for gender dysphoria in adolescence, those who do often seek treatment of pubertal suppression with GnRH analogues. Both the WPATH and ES support the use of GnRH analogues to suppress the development of unwanted secondary sex characteristics at Tanner stage 2. Those with persistent gender dysphoria can elect to receive cross-sex hormones at 16 years, or sex reassignment surgery as an adult. Although advanced nerve-sparing techniques have aided in the preservation of functionality post sex reassignment surgery, options for preserving future fertility remain limited to either cryopreservation of gametes or gonadal tissue banking. Although most data available have found that psychological health is not only improved, but is comparable with non–gender dysphoric individuals after receiving gender affirmation therapy, some medical experts remain critical in the use of assisted reproduction technologies for transgender individuals. Being equipped to care for transgender patients, especially adolescents, requires not only knowledge of the diagnostic criteria for gender dysphoria, but also a thorough understanding of the transition process and the physical, psychological, reproductive, and societal challenges these individuals encounter.

REFERENCES

1. Meyer-Bahlburg HF. Sex steroids and variants of gender identity. Endocrinol Metab Clin North Am 2013;42:435–52.
2. Rosenthal SM. Approach to the patient: transgender youth: endocrine considerations. J Clin Endocrinol Metab 2014;10:1919–28.
3. Coleman E, Bockting W, Botzer M, et al. Standards of care for the health of transsexual, transgender, and gender-nonconforming people, version 7. Int J Transgenderism 2011;13:165–232.
4. Benjamin H. The transsexual phenomenon. New York: Julian Press Inc Publishers; 1966.
5. American Psychiatric Association (APA). Diagnostic and statistical manual of mental disorder. 3rd edition. Washington, DC: American Psychiatric Association; 1980.
6. American Psychiatric Association (APA). Diagnostic and statistical manual of mental disorders. 5th edition. Arlington (VA): American Psychiatric Association; 2013.
7. Hembree WC, Cohen-Kettenis P, Delemarre-van de Waal HA, et al. Endocrine treatment of transsexual persons: an endocrine society clinical practice guideline. J Clin Endocrinol Metab 2009;94(9):3132–54.
8. de Vries AL, Cohen-Kettenis PT. Clinical management of gender dysphoria in children and adolescents: the Dutch approach. J Homosex 2012;59:301–20.
9. Cohen-Kettenis PT. Gender change in 46,XY persons with 5alpha-reductase-2 deficiency and 17beta-hydroxysteroid dehydrogenase-3 deficiency. Arch Sex Behav 2005;34:399–410.
10. Reiner WG, Gearhart JP. Discordant sexual identity in some genetic males with cloacal exstrophy assigned to female sex at birth. N Engl J Med 2004;350:333–41.
11. Perrin JS, Leonard G, Perron M, et al. Sex differences in the growth of white matter during adolescence. Neuroimage 2009;45:1055–66.
12. Rametti G, Carrillo B, Gomez-Gil E, et al. White matter microstructure in female to male transsexuals before cross-sex hormonal treatment. A diffusion tensor imaging study. J Psychiatr Res 2011;45:199–204.
13. Kranz GS, Hahn A, Kaufmann U, et al. White matter microstructure in transsexuals and controls investigated by diffusion tensor imaging. J Neurosci 2014;34(46): 15466–75.

14. Olson J, Forbes C, Belzer M. Review article: management of the transgender adolescent. Arch Pediatr Adolesc Med 2011;165:171–6.

15. Spack NP, Edwards-Leeper L, Feldman HA, et al. Children and adolescents with gender identity disorder referred to a pediatric medical center. Pediatrics 2012; 129:418–25.

16. Unger CA. Gynecologic care for transgender youth. Curr Opin Obstet Gynecol 2014;26:347–54.

17. Delemarre-van de Waal HA, Cohen-Kettenis PT. Clinical management of gender identity disorder in adolescents: a protocol on psychological and paediatric endocrinology aspects. Eur J Endocrinologya 2006;155:S131–7.

18. Asscherman H, Giltay EJ, Megens JA, et al. A long-term follow-up study of mortality in transsexuals receiving treatment with cross-sex hormones. Eur J Endocrinol 2011;164:635–42.

19. Chlebowski RT, Hendrix SL, Langer RD, et al. Influence of estrogen plus progestin on breast cancer and mammography in healthy postmenopausal women: the Women's Health Initiative Randomized Trial. JAMA 2003;289(24):3242–53.

20. Spack NP. Management of transgenderism. JAMA 2013;309:478–84.

21. Krege S, Bex A, Lummen G, et al. Male-to-female transsexualism: a technique, results and long-term follow-up in 66 patients. BJU Int 2001;88:396–402.

22. Klein C, Gorzalka BB. Sexual functioning in transsexuals following hormone therapy and genital surgery: a review. J Sex Med 2009;6:2922–39.

23. Cohen-Kettenis PT, van Goozen SH. Pubertal delay as an aid in diagnosis and treatment of a transsexual adolescent. Eur Child Adolesc Psychiatry 1998;7(4): 246–8.

24. de Vries AL, McGuire JK, Steensma TD, et al. Young adult psychological outcome after puberty suppression and gender reassignment. Pediatrics 2014;134(4):1–9.

25. Newfield E, Hart S, Dibble S, et al. Female-to-male transgender quality of life. Qual Life Res 2006;15:1447–57.

26. Dhejne C, Lichtenstein P, Boman M, et al. Long-term follow-up of transsexual persons undergoing sex reassignment surgery: cohort study in Sweden. PLoS One 2011;6(2):e16885.

27. Ainsworth TA, Spiegel JH. Quality of life of individuals with and without facial feminization surgery or gender reassignment surgery. Qual Life Res 2010;19(7): 1019–24.

28. Colizzi M, Costa R, Pace V, et al. Hormonal treatment reduces psychobiological distress in gender identity disorder, independently of the attachment style. J Sex Med 2013;10:3049–58.

29. Gomez-Gil E, Zubiaurre-Elorza L, Esteva I, et al. Hormone-treated transsexuals report less social distress, anxiety and depression. Psychoneuroendocrinology 2012;37:662–70.

30. Gooren LJ, Giltay EJ, Bunck MC. Long-term treatment of transsexuals with cross-sex hormones: extensive personal experience. J Clin Endocrinol Metab 2008;93: 19–25.

31. Van Haarst EP, Newling DW, Gooren LJ, et al. Metastatic prostatic carcinoma in a male-to-female transsexual. Br J Urol 1998;81:776.

32. Spinder T, Spijkstra JJ, van den Tweel JG, et al. The effects of long term testosterone administration on pulsatile lutenizing hormone secretion and on ovarian histology in eugonadal female to male transsexual subjects. J Clin Endocrinol Metab 1989;69:151–7.

33. Wierckx K, Stuyver I, Weyers S. Sperm freezing in transsexual women. Arch Sex Behav 2012;41:1069–71.

34. Wierckx K, Caenegem EV, Pennings G, et al. Reproductive wish in transsexual men. Hum Reprod 2012;27(2):483–7.

35. Ginsberg JP, Crlson CA, Lin K, et al. An experimental protocol for fertility preservation in prepubertal boys recently diagnosed with cancer: a report of acceptability and safely. Hum Reprod 2009;25(1):37–41.

36. Van den Broecke R, Van der Elst J, Liu J, et al. The female-to-male transsexual patient: a source for human ovarian cortical tissue for experimental use. Hum Reprod 2001;16:145–7.

Reproductive System Outcome Among Patients with Polycystic Ovarian Syndrome

CrossMark

Enrico Carmina, MD

KEYWORDS

- PCOS • AMH • Ovulatory PCOS • Fertility • Hyperandrogenism • Insulin resistance
- Infertility • Ovarian function

KEY POINTS

- Polycystic ovarian syndrome (PCOS) is a heterogeneous disorder and the anovulatory phenotype, although the most common in patients who are referred to specialized clinics, may not be the most common in general population.
- The association of a derangement of early follicle development and increased insulin level seems to be the main mechanism determining anovulation.
- Because of the role of increased insulin levels in anovulation of women with PCOS, lifestyle represents the first step in any treatment of anovulation in this disorder.
- Changes in ovarian function during later reproductive adult age may be particularly beneficial in women affected by PCOS determining appearance of normal ovulatory cycles and fertility.
- Menopausal age is probably delayed in women with PCOS but long-term follow-up studies are needed to confirm this hypothesis.

REPRODUCTIVE OUTCOME IN POLYCYSTIC OVARY SYNDROME: ANOVULATORY AND OVULATORY PATIENTS

For many years it was believed that polycystic ovary syndrome (PCOS) is characterized by irregular menses and infertility. In the early 1990s the National Institutes of Health definition of PCOS included chronic anovulation as a cardinal symptom of the disorder.[1] However, in the following years several studies indicated that many patients could present a very similar disorder but normal ovulatory cycles.[2–4] Finally, Rotterdam and Androgen Excess definitions of the syndrome acknowledged that ovulatory patients are also part of PCOS.[5,6]

It is now well understood that PCOS may present with different clinical patterns[7–9] and that the anovulatory phenotype, although the most common in patients who are

The author has nothing to disclose.
Reproductive Endocrinology Unit, Department of Mother and Child Health, University of Palermo, Via delle Croci 47, Palermo 90139, Italy
E-mail address: enrico.carmina@ae-society.org

Endocrinol Metab Clin N Am 44 (2015) 787–797
http://dx.doi.org/10.1016/j.ecl.2015.07.006
endo.theclinics.com

referred to specialized clinics,[10,11] may not be the most common in the general population.[12-14] The few epidemiologic studies that have tried to assess the prevalence of PCOS in the general population have found that ovulatory patients with PCOS are as common[12] or more common[13,14] than anovulatory patients with PCOS. Of course, many ovulatory patients are not cured or are not referred to clinics specialized in infertility or in PCOS treatment.

All this information reopens an old question: what is the mechanism of anovulation in PCOS? Why are some patients with PCOS ovulatory, whereas others are anovulatory? A major difficulty in answering this question results from the limited understanding of pathophysiology of PCOS. Although the main elements of the syndrome have been characterized, the causes and the pathophysiologic mechanisms remain largely undetermined. New information coming from genome-wide association studies has confirmed that in most cases PCOS depends on a particular genetic background with some gene polymorphisms (DENND1A, THADA, luteinizing hormone [LH] receptor) being particularly common.[15-17] How this genetic background determines the syndrome is still unclear but initial data suggest that these gene polymorphisms may be based on two main elements of the syndrome: increased ovarian androgen production and derangement of early follicle development.[18-20] No sufficient information exists about the relationship of this genetic background with the ovulatory or anovulatory status, although the large Chinese genome-wide association studies have been performed in patients diagnosed according to Rotterdam criteria and therefore also include ovulatory patients.[15]

MECHANISMS OF ANOVULATION IN POLYCYSTIC OVARY SYNDROME

Most available data suggest that anovulation in PCOS is not the consequence of increased androgen ovarian secretion. Although patients with the classic National Institutes of Health anovulatory phenotype tend to have higher androgen levels than patients with the hyperandrogenic ovulatory phenotype,[21,22] high androgen levels may be found in patients with no PCOS without determining anovulation.[22,23]

It has been suggested that the arrest of antral follicle growth and anovulation are the consequence of the derangement of early follicle development.[24] It has been shown that granulosa cells cultured from follicles derived from anovulatory women with PCOS are hyperresponsive to follicle-stimulating hormone (FSH) in terms of estradiol production.[25,26] When granulosa cells from ovulatory patients with PCOS were evaluated, these cells behaved normally in terms of estradiol response to FSH and responded to LH only when taken from a larger dominant follicle.[27] On the contrary, granulosa cells taken from anovulatory PCOS tended to be hyperresponsive to FSH and in some instances responded to LH also when these cells were taken from small (3–4 mm) follicles.[27] The inappropriate response in small follicles to LH could result in terminal differentiation of the granulosa cells and thence in premature arrest of follicle growth.[24] Because in the same studies there was a large heterogeneity in the behavior of studied follicles of anovulatory women, with granulosa cells of some follicles responding normally to LH,[27] mathematical models have been developed suggesting that in a heterogeneous population of small follicles, if a group of follicles is relatively more mature, anovulatory arrest develops.[24]

However, it is unlikely that the derangement of early follicle development is the only cause of chronic anovulation in PCOS. Genetic studies have been unable to differentiate between ovulatory and anovulatory patients with PCOS.[28] Importantly, most anovulatory women with PCOS become ovulatory when they lose weight, and an increase of body weight may transform an ovulatory woman with PCOS into an anovulatory patient with PCOS.[21,29] It is unclear how this could be possible if the problem just depends on an (inherited) alteration of early follicle development.

Anovulatory patients with PCOS present an endocrine character that may be partially reverted when they lose weight: these patients are more obese and have higher insulin levels than ovulatory patients with PCOS.[8,9,11,22] Ovulation may also occur after administration of most insulin-sensitizing drugs, including metformin and thiazilenediones.

In vitro studies have shown that increased insulin levels, also in a condition of insulin resistance, may affect ovarian steroidogenesis and determine arrest of follicle growth.[30,31] Although obesity reduces fertility by several mechanisms, most obese women have normal ovulatory cycles[32,33] and it suggests that hyperinsulinemia affects follicle growth only in the presence of some previous derangement of follicle development.

Other mechanisms of anovulation may be operative and may be more important in subgroups of patients with PCOS. About one-third of classic hyperandrogenic anovulatory patients with PCOS have normal body weight and 50% of them have normal fat distribution, normal insulin levels, and no insulin resistance.[34] Patients with PCOS with the normoandrogenic phenotype (chronic anovulation, polycystic ovaries, and normal androgen levels) generally present normal body weight, normal insulin, and insulin sensitivity.[8,22,35] Therefore, other mechanisms independent of insulin have to be operative and may determine arrest of follicle growth. No evidence exists on what these mechanisms may be. It has been suggested that increased antimullerian hormone (AMH) values may play a role in the arrest of follicle growth by inhibiting the recruitment of primordial follicles and diminishing the response of recruited follicles to FSH, thus impairing the selection of the dominant follicle.[36] It is possible that, in some patients, a particularly severe alteration of folliculogenesis may result in particularly high levels of AMH sufficient to impair the selection of the dominant follicle. However, in most patients with PCOS, increased AMH does not seem to play a main role in blocking the selection and growth of the dominant follicle and the ovulation.[37] It is consistent with the relatively low AMH values in patients with anovulatory normoandrogenic PCOS.[38] Many questions remain unsolved and only future studies will find new solutions.

In **Fig. 1**, the possible pathophysiologic mechanisms of ovulatory and anovulatory PCOS are summarized. In this model, at least two gene variants produce the main

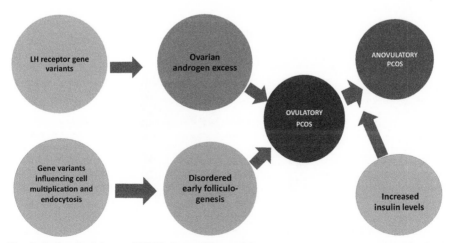

Fig. 1. Pathophysiology of PCOS. A possible model.

characters of PCOS: derangement of early follicle development and ovarian androgen excessive production. The consequence is generally ovulatory PCOS. Increased insulin levels (probably secondary to environmental factors) determine the arrest of follicle growth and transform the ovulatory PCOS to an anovulatory (classic) PCOS.

IMPROVEMENT OF FERTILITY DURING LATE REPRODUCTIVE AGE IN POLYCYSTIC OVARY SYNDROME

For many years it was assumed that anovulatory patients with PCOS remain infertile for all their reproductive age. In fact, it was perceived that the disorder could worsen with age.

However, several studies have shown that many anovulatory patients with PCOS may become ovulatory in their later reproductive years.[39–42] In their initial study, evaluating 205 patients with PCOS, Elting and coworkers[39] found a highly significant linear trend (*P*<.001) for a shorter menstrual cycle length with increasing age with several patients getting normal menstrual cycles after their 40s. This finding has been confirmed by two longitudinal studies of women with PCOS.[40,41] In our large longitudinal study of women with PCOS,[41,42] 193 patients with PCOS have been followed for at least 20 years, from the age of 20 to 25 (mean age, 21.8 ± 1) to an age of 40 to 45. A progressive improvement of menstrual cycles, starting after the age of 35, was found and at their last observational period, in their mid-40s, about 50% of the patients were ovulatory with some patients (about 10%) presenting a complete remission of all clinical and endocrine symptoms (**Fig. 2**).[41,42]

The appearance of ovulatory cycles in women who were anovulatory and had menstrual irregularities from puberty is a surprising phenomenon that may depend on changes of ovarian function that happen during adult age. In fact, moving from the age of 20 to 25 to the age of 40 to 45, normal women present with mild decrease of ovarian androgen secretion (most evident with stimulated androgen secretion), marked decrease of adrenal androgen secretion, and 20% decrease of ovarian size.

In particular, it has been shown that adrenal androgen secretion declines progressively from the age of 25 to 30 until the age of 50 to 60 with smaller changes taking place after the age of 60.[43] Most importantly, ovarian androgen secretion capacity also starts to decline before the age of 30.[44] Because circulating E_2 levels remain

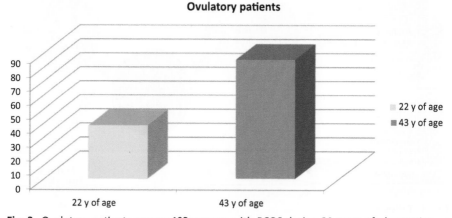

Fig. 2. Ovulatory patients among 193 women with PCOS during 20 years of observation.

normal for years while ovarian androgen secretion (in large part used for estradiol synthesis) progressively declines, it has been hypothesized that compensatory mechanisms, reflected by the gradual rise in serum FSH levels, operate and maintain a normal estrogen ovarian production.[44]

These changes in ovarian androgen production are reflected also by a smaller ovarian volume in women older than 40 compared with younger normal women.[45,46] It has been shown that in normal women ovarian volume shows a negative correlation with age and FSH circulating levels. There is a statistically significant decrease in ovarian volume with each decade of life from age 30 to age 70. In a cross-sectional study, mean ovarian volume was 6.6 ± 0.19 mL in women younger than 30; 6.1 ± 0.06 mL in women 30 to 39; 4.8 ± 0.03 mL in women 40 to 49; and 2.6 ± 0.01 mL in women 50 to 59.[45]

The changes in ovarian function during later reproductive adult age may be particularly important and beneficial for women affected by PCOS. The progressive reduction of ovarian (and adrenal) androgen production may be the main factor determining a disappearance or a substantial improvement of hyperandrogenism several years before menopause.

This hypothesis has been confirmed by several studies. The negative association between dehydroepiandrosterone sulfate (DHEAS) levels and age is preserved in women who are hyperandrogenic[47] and DHEAS reduces by about 50% in women with PCOS moving from young to late reproductive age.[48] In women with PCOS, age has significant negative correlations with total testosterone[49] and circulating testosterone levels significantly decline moving from the years 30s to 40s.[40-42] The ovarian size and the severity of morphologic changes of ovaries in women with PCOS also reduce during late reproductive age.[50,51]

In our 20-year follow-up study,[41,42] moving from 20 to 25 to 40 to 45 years of age, in PCOS the following changes occur: testosterone circulating levels decreased by 30% and in several patients normalized (**Fig. 3**), DHEAS levels decreased by 50% and in most patients normalized (**Fig. 4**), and ovarian volume decreased by about 20% and in most patients normal ovarian size was found.

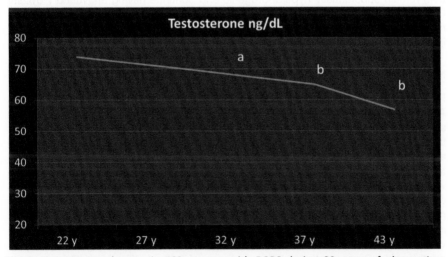

Fig. 3. Testosterone changes in 193 women with PCOS during 20 years of observation. [a] P<.05. [b] P<.01.

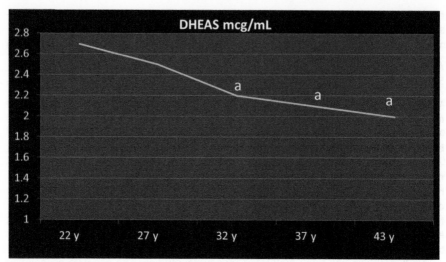

Fig. 4. DHEAS changes in 193 women with PCOS during 20 years of observation. [a] $P<.01$.

These changes influence ovarian function in patients with PCOS and probably explain the occurrence of ovulatory cycles in patients with PCOS during their late reproductive age. Our follow-up is continuing and shows that ovulation occurs in most women with PCOS when they approximate to the menopausal age (Carmina E and colleagues, unpublished data, 2015).

Probably, the improvement occurs earlier in patients with less severe hormonal alteration. In fact, we have demonstrated that the occurrence of ovulatory cycles correlates negatively with AMH values these patients had in their 30s.[52] In most patients the improvement of ovarian function and the progressive decline of androgen production may be sufficient to determine the appearance of ovulatory cycles but some patients (because they were more hyperandrogenic or had a smaller decline of androgen secretion) remain substantially hyperandrogenic and continue having anovulatory cycles. Future studies should be able to determine what are the exact mechanisms that determine the appearance of ovulatory cycles in women with PCOS with aging and if we may influence this naturally occurring phenomenon.

MENOPAUSAL AGE IN WOMEN WITH POLYCYSTIC OVARY SYNDROME

Preliminary data seem to show that menopause may occur later in women with PCOS. Although no longitudinal studies until menopausal age exist, some cross-sectional data suggest that menopause may occur about 2 years later in women with PCOS.[53] In addition, AMH values in women with PCOS tend to be higher in premenopausal age, probably because AMH is higher in these women and the decline to menopausal values takes more time.[54] It suggests that the fertility potential may be more prolonged in women with PCOS and these data, taken together with the appearance of ovulatory cycles during late reproductive age,[41,42] may be consistent with the idea that the spontaneous fertility outcome of women with PCOS may be much better than previously imagined. However, real data are missing and only large longitudinal studies will reveal whether women with PCOS may get normal spontaneous fertility during their late reproductive aging. Cross-sectional data on outcome of in vitro fertilization (IVF) treatment in infertile women of different age groups show that women with PCOS, after their 40s, have the same reduced response in terms of pregnancies and live births as women of similar age with other forms of infertility (tubal infertility).[55]

A RATIONALE APPROACH TO INFERTILITY TREATMENT IN POLYCYSTIC OVARY SYNDROME

Most women with PCOS, particularly those with a mild phenotype or only slightly increased AMH values, cannot wait for a future fertility but wish to have and should have children during their young adult age. Fertility treatment is needed and should be conducted in a way that is as rapid and effective as possible.

All reviews on therapy for infertility in PCOS suggest using diet and lifestyle measures as the first step of the treatment protocol.[56,57] In fact, several studies have shown that about 50% of obese patients with PCOS may obtain ovulatory cycles and regular fertility with a modest weight loss (>5%). Ovulatory cycles are obtained early and may depend more on energy restriction than on weight loss. However, in clinical practice unsatisfactory results are often observed probably because very good organization is needed for keeping low the dropout rate that generally is high.

It may be wise to suggest lifestyle measures (correct diet and physical exercise) to all patients, including normoweight patients, but at the same time to start an ovulation induction treatment. Recent data seem to show that aromatase inhibitors (letrozole) may be the best option for inducing ovulation in PCOS.[58,59] However, in many countries these products are off-label for ovulation induction and clomiphene remains the most common and effective product for inducing ovulation in women with PCOS.[56,57,60]

Clomiphene may induce ovulation in 60% to 80% of women with PCOS but pregnancies and live births occur only in half of ovulating patients.[60] Although some experts prolong treatment with clomiphene up to a year when ovulation is induced but no pregnancy is obtained, it seems more rationale to move to a different treatment when ovulation is induced but no pregnancy is obtained in 6 months.[61]

If no ovulation is induced, higher doses of clomiphene should be used and eventually metformin should be added. Several,[62,63] but not all studies,[60] have shown that metformin, although less effective than clomiphene, may increase the efficacy of clomiphene.

Next step in infertility treatment of women with PCOS, if no pregnancy is obtained with clomiphene, is the use of gonadotropins. Although several protocols have been suggested, better results are obtained with a simple step-up low-dose gonadotropin treatment.[64] In controlled studies, it induces more ovulations with lower rates of ovarian hyperstimulation than other gonadotropin protocols.

If gonadotropin treatment fails, IVF should be suggested. Although other treatments may be used, including ovarian drilling,[65] the results in patients failing to respond to previous treatments are unsatisfactory and IVF should be preferred.[66]

The following rationale approach may be suggested:

- Lifestyle program + clomiphene

Start clomiphene at low doses (50 mg/day × 5 days) increasing doses every 2 months if no ovulation is obtained. If the patient remains anovulatory also with high (150 mg/day × 5 days) clomiphene doses, add metformin (1500 or 1700 mg/day in two or three doses) × 3 months.

If no ovulation is obtained in the following 3 months, move to gonadotropin treatment.

If ovulation but no pregnancy is induced by clomiphene (or clomiphene + metformin) continue the product at the current dose for 3 additional months and then move to gonadotropin treatment.

- Low-dose step-up gonadotropin treatment

If no pregnancy is obtained after three gonadotropin cycles, move to IVF.

- IVF

At the end, most women with PCOS become pregnant and have a child.

REFERENCES

1. Zawadzki JK, Dunaif A. Diagnostic criteria for polycystic ovary syndrome: towards a rationale approach. In: Dunaif A, Givens JR, Haseltine F, et al, editors. Polycystic ovary syndrome. Boston: Blackwell Scientific Publications; 1992. p. 377–84.
2. Carmina E, Lobo RA. Do hyperandrogenic women with normal menses have polycystic ovary syndrome? Fertil Steril 1999;71:319–22.
3. Carmina E, Lobo RA. Polycystic ovaries in women with normal menses. Am J Med 2001;111:602–6.
4. Carmina E. Diagnosing PCOS in women who menstruate regularly. Contemporary OB/GYN 2003;48:53–64.
5. Rotterdam ESHRE/ASRM Sponsored PCOS Consensus Workshop Group. Revised 2003 consensus on diagnostic criteria and long-term health risks related to polycystic ovary syndrome. Fertil Steril 2004;81:19–25.
6. Azziz R, Carmina E, Dewailly D, et al. Position statement: criteria for defining polycystic ovary syndrome as a predominantly hyperandrogenic syndrome: an androgen excess society guideline. J Clin Endocrinol Metab 2006;91:4237–45.
7. Carmina E, Azziz R. Diagnosis, phenotype and prevalence of polycystic ovary syndrome. Fertil Steril 2006;86(Suppl 1):87–9.
8. Welt CK, Gudmundsson JA, Arsson G, et al. Characterizing discrete subsets of polycystic ovary syndrome as defined by the Rotterdam criteria: the impact of weight on phenotype and metabolic features. J Clin Endocrinol Metab 2006;91: 4842–8.
9. Carmina E. The spectrum of androgen excess disorders. Fertil Steril 2006;85: 1582–5.
10. Azziz R, Woods KS, Reyna R, et al. The prevalence and features of the polycystic ovary syndrome in an unselected population. J Clin Endocrinol Metab 2004;89: 2745–9.
11. Carmina E, Rosato F, Jannì A, et al. Relative prevalence of different androgen excess disorders in 950 women referred because of clinical hyperandrogenism. J Clin Endocrinol Metab 2006;91:2–6.
12. March WA, Moore VM, Willson KJ, et al. The prevalence of polycystic ovary syndrome in a community sample assessed under contrasting diagnostic criteria. Hum Reprod 2010;25:544–51.
13. Tehrani FR, Simbar M, Tohidi M, et al. The prevalence of polycystic ovary syndrome in a community sample of Iranian population: Iranian PCOS prevalence study. Reprod Biol Endocrinol 2011;9:39.
14. Yildiz BO, Bozdag O, Yapici Z, et al. Prevalence, phenotype and cardiometabolic risk of polycystic ovary syndrome under different diagnostic criteria. Hum Reprod 2012;27:3067–73.

15. Chen ZJ, Zhao H, He L, et al. Genome-wide association study identifies suscep-tibility loci for polycystic ovary syndrome on chromosome 2p16.3, 2p21 and 9q33.3. Nat Genet 2011;43:55–9.
16. Welt CK, Duran JM. Genetics of polycystic ovary syndrome. Semin Reprod Med 2014;32:177–82.
17. Brower MA, Jones MR, Rotter JI, et al. Further investigation in Europeans of suscep-tibility variants for polycystic ovary syndrome discovered in genome-wide associ-ation studies of Chinese individuals. J Clin Endocrinol Metab 2015;100:E182–6.
18. McAllister JM, Modi B, Miller BA, et al. Overexpression of a DENND1A isoform produces a polycystic ovary syndrome theca phenotype. Proc Natl Acad Sci U S A 2014;111:E1519–27.
19. McAllister JM, Legro RS, Modi BP, et al. Functional genomics of PCOS: from GWAS to molecular mechanisms. Trends Endocrinol Metab 2015;26:118–24.
20. Hsueh AJ, Kawamura K, Cheng Y, et al. Intraovarian control of early folliculogen-esis. Endocr Rev 2015;36:1–24.
21. Carmina E. Mild androgen disorders. Best Pract Res Clin Endocrinol Metab 2006; 20:207–20.
22. Guastella E, Longo RA, Carmina E. Clinical and endocrine characteristics of the main PCOS phenotypes. Fertil Steril 2010;94:2197–201.
23. Franks S. Polycystic ovary syndrome. N Engl J Med 1995;333:853–61.
24. Franks S, Stark J, Hardy K. Follicle dynamics and anovulation in polycystic ovary syndrome. Hum Reprod Update 2008;14:367–78.
25. Erickson GF, Magoffin DA, Garzo VG, et al. Granulosa cells in polycystic ovaries: are they normal or abnormal? Hum Reprod 1992;7:293–9.
26. Mason HD, Willis DS, Beard RW, et al. Estradiol production by granulosa cells of normal and polycystic ovaries: relationship to menstrual cycle history and con-centrations of gonadotropins and sex steroids in follicular fluid. J Clin Endocrinol Metab 1994;79:1355–60.
27. Willis DS, Watson H, Mason HD, et al. Premature response to luteinizing hormone of granulosa cells from anovulatory women with polycystic ovary syndrome: rele-vance to the mechanism of anovulation. J Clin Endocrinol Metab 1998;83: 3984–91.
28. Cui L, Zhao H, Zhang B, et al. Genotype-phenotype correlations of PCOS sus-ceptibility SNPs identified by GWAS in a large cohort of Han Chinese women. Hum Reprod 2013;28:538–44.
29. Huber-Buckholz MM, Carey DG, Norman RJ. Restoration of reproductive poten-tial by lifestyle modification in obese polycystic ovary syndrome: role of insulin sensitivity and luteinizing hormone. J Clin Endocrinol Metab 1999;84:1470–4.
30. Ciaraldi TP, Aroda V, Mudaliar S, et al. Polycystic ovary syndrome is associated with tissue-specific differences in insulin resistance. J Clin Endocrinol Metab 2009;94:157–63.
31. Rice S, Christoforidis N, Gadd C, et al. Impaired insulin-dependent glucose meta-bolism in granulosa-lutein cells from anovulatory women with PCOS. Hum Reprod 2005;20:373–81.
32. Jensen TK, Scheike T, Keiding N, et al. Fecundability in relation to body mass and menstrual cycle patterns. Epidemiology 1999;10:422–8.
33. Pasquali R, Gambineri A. Metabolic effects of obesity on reproduction. Reprod Biomed Online 2006;12:542–51.
34. Carmina E, Bucchieri S, Esposito A, et al. Abdominal fat quantity and distribution in women with polycystic ovary syndrome and extent of its relation to insulin resis-tance. J Clin Endocrinol Metab 2007;92:2500–5.

35. Dewailly D, Catteau-Jonard S, Reyss AC, et al. Oligoanovulation and polycystic ovaries but no overt hyperandrogenism. J Clin Endocrinol Metab 2006;91: 3922–7.
36. Pierre A, Peigné M, Grynberg M, et al. Loss of LH-induced down-regulation of anti-Müllerian hormone receptor expression may contribute to anovulation in women with polycystic ovary syndrome. Hum Reprod 2013;28:762–9.
37. Li J, Li R, Yu H, et al. The relationship between serum anti-Müllerian hormone levels and the follicular arrest for women with polycystic ovary syndrome. Syst Biol Reprod Med 2015;61:103–9.
38. Köninger A, Koch L, Edimiris P, et al. Anti-Mullerian hormone: an indicator for the severity of polycystic ovarian syndrome. Arch Gynecol Obstet 2014;290: 1023–30.
39. Elting MW, Korsen TJ, Rekers-Mombarg LT, et al. Women with polycystic ovary syndrome gain regular menstrual cycles when ageing. Hum Reprod 2000;15:24–8.
40. Brown ZA, Louwers YV, Fong SL, et al. The phenotype of polycystic ovary syndrome ameliorates with aging. Fertil Steril 2011;96:1259–65.
41. Carmina E, Campagna AM, Lobo RA. A 20-year follow-up of young women with polycystic ovary syndrome. Am J Obstet Gynecol 2012;119:263–9.
42. Carmina E, Campagna AM, Lobo RA. Emergence of ovulatory cycles with aging in women with polycystic ovary syndrome (PCOS) alters the trajectory of cardiovascular and metabolic risk factors. Hum Reprod 2013;28:2245–52.
43. Labrie F, Bélanger A, Cusan L, et al. Marked decline in serum concentrations of adrenal C19 sex steroid precursors and conjugated androgen metabolites during aging. J Clin Endocrinol Metab 1997;82:2386–92.
44. Piltonen T, Koivunen R, Ruokonen A, et al. Ovarian age-related responsiveness to human chorionic gonadotropin. J Clin Endocrinol Metab 2003;88:3327–32.
45. Pavlik EJ, DePriest PD, Gallion HH, et al. Ovarian volume related to age. Gynecol Oncol 2000;77:410–2.
46. Oppermann K, Fuchs SC, Spritzer PM. Ovarian volume in pre- and perimenopausal women: a population-based study. Menopause 2003;10:209–13.
47. Morán C, Knochenhauer E, Boots LR, et al. Adrenal androgen excess in hyperandrogenism: relation to age and body mass. Fertil Steril 1999;71:671–4.
48. Goodarzi MO, Carmina E, Azziz R. DHEA, DHEAS and PCOS. J Steroid Biochem Mol Biol 2015;145:213–25.
49. Liang SJ, Hsu CS, Tzeng CR, et al. Clinical and biochemical presentation of polycystic ovary syndrome in women between the ages of 20 and 40. Hum Reprod 2011;26:3443–9.
50. Winters SJ, Talbott E, Guzick DS, et al. Serum testosterone levels decrease in middle age in women with the polycystic ovary syndrome. Fertil Steril 2000; 73:724–9.
51. Koivunen R, Laatikainen T, Tomás C, et al. The prevalence of polycystic ovaries in healthy women. Acta Obstet Gynecol Scand 1999;78:137–41.
52. Carmina E, Campagna AM, Mansueto P, et al. Does the level of serum antimüllerian hormone predict ovulatory function in women with polycystic ovary syndrome with aging? Fertil Steril 2012;98:1043–6.
53. Tehrani FR, Solaymani-Dodaran M, Hedayati M, et al. Is polycystic ovary syndrome an exception for reproductive aging? Hum Reprod 2010;25:1775–81.
54. Piltonen T, Morin-Papunen L, Koivunen R, et al. Serum anti-Mullerian hormone levels remain high until late reproductive age and decrease during metformin therapy in women with polycystic ovary syndrome. Hum Reprod 2005;20:1820–6.

55. Kalra SK, Ratcliffe SJ, Dokras A. Is the fertile window extended in women with polycystic ovary syndrome? Utilizing the Society for Assisted Reproductive Technology registry to assess the impact of reproductive aging on live-birth rate. Fertil Steril 2013;100:208–13.
56. Costello MF, Misso ML, Wong J, et al. The treatment of infertility in polycystic ovary syndrome: a brief update. Aust N Z J Obstet Gynaecol 2012;52:400–3.
57. Jayasena CN, Franks S. The management of patients with polycystic ovary syndrome. Nat Rev Endocrinol 2014;10:624–36.
58. Franik S, Kremer JA, Nelen WL, et al. Aromatase inhibitors for subfertile women with polycystic ovary syndrome. Cochrane Database Syst Rev 2014;(2):CD010287.
59. Legro RS, Brzyski RG, Diamond MP, et al, NICHD Reproductive Medicine Network. Letrozole versus clomiphene for infertility in the polycystic ovary syndrome. N Engl J Med 2014;371:119–29.
60. Legro RS, Barnhart HX, Schlaff WD, et al, Cooperative Multicenter Reproductive Medicine Network. Clomiphene, metformin, or both for infertility in the polycystic ovary syndrome. N Engl J Med 2007;356:551–66.
61. Perales-Puchalt A, Legro RS. Ovulation induction in women with polycystic ovary syndrome. Steroids 2013;78:767–72.
62. Moll E, Korevaar JC, Bossuyt PM, et al. Does adding metformin to clomifene citrate lead to higher pregnancy rates in a subset of women with polycystic ovary syndrome? Hum Reprod 2008;23:1830–4.
63. Misso ML, Teede HJ, Hart R, et al. Status of clomiphene citrate and metformin for infertility in PCOS. Trends Endocrinol Metab 2012;23:533–43.
64. Homburg R, Howles C. Low-dose FSH therapy for anovulatory infertility associated with PCOS: rationale, reflections and refinements. Hum Reprod Update 1999;5:493–9.
65. Mitra S, Nayak PK, Agrawal S. Laparoscopic ovarian drilling: an alternative but not the ultimate in the management of polycystic ovary syndrome. J Nat Sci Biol Med 2015;6:40–8.
66. Costello MF, Ledger WL. Evidence-based management of infertility in women with polycystic ovary syndrome using surgery or assisted reproductive technology. Womens Health (Lond Engl) 2012;8:291–300.

Fertility Preservation in Children and Adolescents

Stephanie J. Estes, MD

KEYWORDS

- Fertility preservation • Infertility • Cryopreservation • Sperm • Egg • Oocyte
- Cancer • Survivorship

KEY POINTS

- Fertility preservation counseling should be discussed and considered in the pediatric and adolescent population.
- Oocyte cryopreservation and embryo cryopreservation are the standard of care for fertility preservation in girls and ovarian tissue cryopreservation is still considered experimental.
- Sperm cryopreservation is the standard of care for fertility preservation in boys, whereas testicular tissue cryopreservation is experimental.
- Oncofertility is the field of medicine in which oncologist and reproductive fertility specialist work together to address the reproductive health of patients with cancer.

INTRODUCTION

Case presentation: A 16-year-old girl presents from an outside institution to see you for management of newly diagnosed Hodgkin lymphoma. Her parents are anxious to begin treatment as soon as possible and the patient's mother is crying off and on throughout the visit. At the end of the appointment, you ask if there are any further questions. The patient tentatively remarks that she has always wanted to have children someday. How do you respond?

Fertility preservation is the process whereby gametes are maintained for the future goal of developing a pregnancy. The ability to maximize fertility potential and options to allow for future fertility is an emerging crucial survivorship issue. Many medical advancements have allowed the pediatric and adolescent population to survive their oncologic conditions[1] and other medical diseases that lead to continuation of life beyond the reproductive years. The American Society of Clinical Oncology

The author has nothing to disclose.
Donor Oocyte Program, Robotic Surgical Services, Division of Reproductive Endocrinology and Infertility, Department of Obstetrics and Gynecology, Pennsylvania State University, College of Medicine, Hershey Medical Center, Mail Code H103, 500 University Drive, Hershey, PA 17033-0850, USA
E-mail address: sestes@hmc.psu.edu

reconfirmed its recommendation to discuss the risk of infertility and fertility preservation options in patients with cancer who are anticipating treatment.[2,3] The American Society for Reproductive Medicine also advocates for informing patients receiving potentially gonadotoxic therapies about fertility preservation and future reproduction options.[4] It is critical to engage our patients in discussions regarding fertility preservation because of the public health impact of this process with regard to the increasing numbers of childhood survivors and increased maternal age at time of pregnancy.[5]

Oncofertility is the multidisciplinary approach of oncologists and reproductive fertility specialists working together to achieve the goals of patients with cancer. This field also incorporates research endeavors, applying new technology to practice, and includes involvement in the psychosocial issues that pervade the process of balancing life-preserving treatment with fertility-preserving options.[6–8] Although there are many reasons for fertility preservation in children and adolescents, cancer is currently the main indication for fertility preservation, and interest in this group of patients has led to development of the oncofertility focus.

INDICATIONS FOR FERTILITY PRESERVATION

The main indications for fertility preservation in children and adolescents encompass medical conditions or treatments that are gonadotoxic or may result in premature ovarian insufficiency or will result in removal of ovarian or testicular tissue (**Box 1**). Cancer and its treatment is a potential significant risk factor for loss of gonadal function and infertility. In 2015, approximately 10,000 children in the United States younger than 15 will be diagnosed with cancer, and cancer is the second leading cause of death in children. Overall, there has been a slight rise in childhood cancer rates over the past few decades. In comparison with 5-year survival rates of approximately 58% in the mid-1970s, more than 80% of children with cancer now survive 5 years or more.[9,10] The following are the types of cancers that occur most often in children[11]:

- Leukemia (30%)
- Brain and central nervous system (CNS) tumors (26%)
- Lymphoma (Hodgkin and non-Hodgkin) (6%)
- Neuroblastoma
- Wilms tumor
- Rhabdomyosarcoma
- Retinoblastoma
- Bone cancer (including osteosarcoma and Ewing sarcoma)

For adolescents ages 15 to 19, the most common types of cancers are Hodgkin lymphoma, thyroid carcinoma, brain and CNS, and testicular germ cell tumors.[12] Cancer accounts for approximately 5% of deaths and is the fourth leading cause of death in the adolescent age group. Survival rates for cancer in teens have not undergone significant change in recent decades, which differs from the advancements seen in many cancers in children. The chance of developing cancer is approximately equal for adolescent boys and girls, but cancer survival rates are slightly higher in girls than in boys. Overall, approximately 85% of girls are still alive 5 years after being diagnosed with cancer, compared with approximately 80% of boys, which may be the result of the type of cancers identified in males and females. The following are the most common cancers in adolescents:

- Lymphomas (Hodgkin lymphoma and non-Hodgkin lymphoma)
- Leukemias (mostly acute lymphocytic leukemia and acute myeloid leukemia)
- CNS tumors

Box 1
Indications for fertility preservation

Cancer diagnoses before chemotherapy or radiation

- Lymphoma
- Leukemia
- Sarcoma
- Malignant bone tumors
- Testicular
- Brain tumors

Turner syndrome

Fragile X

Galactosemia

Other medical diseases before chemotherapy or myeloablative conditioning

- Systemic lupus erythematosus
- Behcet disease
- Rheumatoid arthritis/juvenile idiopathic arthritis
- Multiple sclerosis
- Renal disease
- Hematochromatosis
- Sickle cell disease
- Aplastic anemia
- Heritable bone marrow failure syndromes (Fanconi anemia, Diamond-Blackfan)
- Metabolic conditions (for example, Hurler syndrome)

Before planned removal of ovaries

- Endometriosis
- Ovarian tumors

- Thyroid cancer
- Testicular cancer
- Malignant bone tumors (osteosarcoma and Ewing tumors)
- Soft tissue tumors (sarcomas)
- Melanoma

Other medical conditions that do not involve malignancy may also be an indication for fertility preservation. Organ-specific involvement and chemotherapy exposure in juvenile systemic lupus erythematosus[13,14] and renal diseases, such as nephrotic syndrome,[15,16] are examples. Additionally, female children at risk for premature ovarian insufficiency/failure in cases such as Turner syndrome,[17] galactosemia,[18] and other conditions, such as those with DSD, transgender, those with familial history of early menopause, Kallmann syndrome, and hereditary or acquired hemochromatosis may be candidates for fertility preservation techniques. Surgical resection in the setting of endometriosis[19,20] has been described as another possible indication; however, the exact details of how these patients should be managed are not clearly known.

There is a lack of follow-up for outcomes related to women who cryopreserved oocytes for medical reasons[21] and disease-specific data for nonmalignant conditions is needed.

GAMETE CRYOPRESERVATION

Cryopreservation is the use of very low temperatures to preserve structurally intact living cells and tissues.[22] Cells have an ideal balance with regard to temperature. Freezing and thawing techniques have arisen out of the need to adapt to the requirements necessary for cellular survival. Water crystallization and ice formation begin between -5 and $-15°C$. The cell membrane, up to a point, can prevent intracellular movement of ice crystals; however, in the meantime there is an increasing concentration of solute into the cell relative loss of intracellular water that can lead to cell death. As a result, if cooling is too slow, then there is resultant cellular dehydration. If cooling is too fast, then external ice can cause rupture of plasma membrane and injury to cellular organelles.[23,24] The field of cryobiology has described an inverted "U"-shaped curve that exists for the survival of various cell types as a function of the associated cooling rate. Damage occurs to cells at slow cooling rates due to exposure to high concentrations of nonpermeating salts and at high cooling rates from lack of equilibrium of intracellular/extracellular milieu.[25] The thawing process must also control for these factors.

Human sperm cryopreservation had its underpinnings in 1949, when Polge and colleagues[26] and Sherman and Bunge[27–29] reported the first pregnancies from frozen-thawed sperm in the setting of insemination cycles. Further advancements occurred due to the discovery that storing human sperm in liquid nitrogen (LN2) was a superior technique (storing at temperature of $-196°$ Celsius compared with higher temperatures between -20 and $-75°$ Celsius). Cryoprotectants are necessary for sperm to remain viable and must be able to enter cells with low toxicity. The cryoprotectants increase the total concentration of all solutes in the system, which decreases the amount of ice formed at any given temperature.[22] Sperm need to maintain not only their structural integrity, but also their functional integrity after the thaw. Poor semen quality may have more damage, resulting in decreased ability for fertilization compared with normal samples.[30] Overall, the large surface area and small volume of spermatozoa make them an ideal specimen for cryopreservation, which helped in the early adoption of sperm freezing as a viable fertility preservation method.

The first pregnancy from human oocyte cryopreservation was reported in 1986.[31] Due to oocyte characteristics, such as cell size (**Fig. 1**) and thickened zona pellucida during freezing, the success of fertility preservation with oocytes was initially underwhelming. As with spermatozoa, cryoprotective agents, such as glycerol, 1,2-propanediol, ethylene glycol, and dimethylsulfoxide (DMSO) have been used to help cells survive low temperatures by decreasing the toxic effects of osmotic stress, other abnormal proteins, and concentrated salts.[32] The addition of intracytoplasmic sperm injection (ICSI) in the 1990s and the fast-freeze technique (vitrification) have been important milestones in the field, enabling egg freezing to become viable option for women.[32–34] Vitrification is the solidification of a liquid into a glasslike state, and its purpose is to prevent ice crystal formation.[35] Fast cooling rates are challenging to achieve and cryo-loops are often now used to maximize the surface exposure to liquid nitrogen.

Because of the difficulties with standardizing a successful technique for cryopreservation of the oocyte, along with the physiologic clinical factors of difficult access to the specimen with fewer cells available for study, oocyte cryopreservation was only removed from its experimental status in January 2013.[36,37] Now success rates

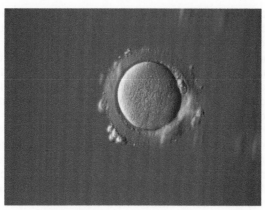

Fig. 1. Mature oocyte, ×200 magnification. (*Courtesy of* Janis Moessner, BS ELD (ABB), IVF Laboratory Director, Penn State Hershey Medical Center, Hershey, PA.)

using cryopreserved oocytes are similar to assisted reproductive techniques with fresh oocytes (fertilization rates of approximately 75% and implantation rates of approximately 40%).[37]

Ethical and Psychosocial Considerations for Fertility Preservation

The concept of future fertility is a highly relevant topic, particularly to those impacted. Group discussions have revealed that adolescent and young adult survivors of childhood cancer were impacted by living with a risk of possible infertility with regard to not only their own well-being, but also intimate relationships.[38] There can be decline in quality of life from an emotional and psychosocial standpoint due to infertility.[39–41] Cancer survivors indicate that they desire to have their own biological children and the significance of this has increased as more individuals survive their cancer.[42,43] Last, health care providers should be aware that future childbearing desires may change and that 1 of 6 patients who have no pretreatment desire to have children changed their opinion about desiring children years after the diagnosis, demonstrating the significance of fertility preservation counseling.[44]

The ethics of fertility preservation involve autonomy of the patient to have options for reproductive choice, and a possible shortened life span is generally not considered a reason to restrict fertility services.[45] The possibility of posthumous desire for reproduction should be discussed, and documentation with the necessary legal provisions is warranted so that lack of proper documentation does not impede future reproductive options.[46,47] Legal counsel and consultation from hospital ethics committees should be encouraged to be used.[48]

The principles of beneficence and nonmaleficence apply with a special focus on minimal risk to children. The concern of justice for having fair treatment for all patients is another ethical quandary for fertility preservation as one considers that only those able to pay for the cost of this option may be able to proceed, giving preference to the wealthy.[49] Health care providers are obligated to address fertility issues in all at-risk patients to review the potential detrimental effects of medical therapy on reproduction and offer fertility preservation consultation.[50,51]

Evaluation of Fertility Potential

The evaluation of female reproductive potential can occur through multiple methods. Anti-Mullerian hormone (AMH), antral follicle counts on transvaginal ultrasound, early follicular serum follicle-stimulating hormone (FSH), and estradiol are routinely used and have been recently reviewed in a Practice Committee Opinion of the American Society for Reproductive Medicine.[52] Chemotherapy and radiation can negatively affect these markers, and a decline in ovarian function may lead to reduced fertility.[53,54] AMH appears to be the most useful indicator, although complete standardization of normal values in pediatrics in relation to fertility is not yet available.[55–61] The ease of use of AMH is enhanced by its lack of significant variability by menstrual cycle dating or exogenous hormones.[62] Unfortunately, there is no absolute value that guarantees future fertility or that denotes complete lack of ability to conceive. Neither menstrual cycles nor FSH levels are reliable predictors of posttreatment conception.[63,64]

For male patients, impaired spermatogenesis can occur as a result of surgery, chemotherapy, and/or radiation.[65] Evaluation is simplified when compared with female patients by being able to evaluate fertility potential by hormone levels such as anti-Mullerian hormone and semen assessment.[66,67]

Fertility Preservation Counseling

It is challenging in the medical field to obtain informed consent, especially in the setting of complex technology such as fertility preservation. Patients and their families may not understand the implications of the information given to them,[68] but an effort must be made to include the most up-to-date and site-specific information possible. Most adolescents (>70%) reported making a decision for enrollment into a research study in combination with a parent,[69] and this process of assent is also important when preservation of fertility options are selected. Children are to be involved in the process of assent "to the extent of their capacity."[70] The essential elements of informed consent include multiple factors[70–72] and include discussing the following:

- Estimate of risk of infertility with proposed treatment
- Overall prognosis for patient
- Risk of delaying treatment (egg or embryo cryopreservation)
- Effect of pregnancy on primary disease or risk of recurrence
- Genetic screening, if indicated
- Use of established versus experimental techniques
- Benefit to minors and ability to give assent
- Any known risks to future offspring

Although all the risks are unknown, it appears that fertility preservation does not worsen prognosis and does not increase the chance of recurrence. Children born to cancer survivors are not at an increased risk of congenital malformations, cancer, or chromosomal syndrome unless the patient's primary cancer was part of a genetic syndrome.[2] Additional counseling regarding procedure-specific issues, such as oocyte and embryo cryopreservation, is recommended (**Box 2**).[46,68,73,74] For experimental methods, full institutional review board consent is required, and this topic is not reviewed here.

There still exists a discrepancy between providers understanding fertility preservation and taking the next step for encouraging a referral to a reproductive endocrinology specialist. The reasons cited for lack of referral included lack of patient interest in fertility preservation, lack of time due to beginning of therapy, and poor prognosis for future fertility.[75] Approximately 61% of providers rarely or never referred patients to a clinician who specializes in fertility.[75]

Barriers to fertility preservation include financial costs of treatment, lack of information and knowledge of options, lack of access or referral to fertility specialists, and limited time until start of therapy for primary diagnosis.[76] Only 13.5% of oncologist

Box 2
Informed consent for oocyte and embryo cryopreservation

Oocyte Cryopreservation

- Ovarian stimulation and retrieval
  - Side effects/risks with medications used and risks of the procedures
  - Need for monitoring, serial laboratory testing, and transvaginal ultrasounds
- Methods that will be used for cryopreservation
- Expected thaw-survival rate for oocytes
  - Risk that no oocyte may survive
  - Requirement for intracytoplasmic sperm injection for future fertilization
  - Expected fertilization rate per surviving thawed oocyte
- Clinic-specific data and outcomes for live birth rate
  - If not enough data for clinic-specific data, then reference peer-reviewed literature
  - Success rates may be lower for women after age 35
  - High likelihood that women who cryopreserve oocytes before age 35 will never use them
- Clear disposition plan for cryopreserved oocytes
- Potential risk of basing important life decisions and expectations on the number of cryopreserved oocytes
- Possibility that the facility may cease operation, need to transfer the oocytes to a different facility, or that the oocytes may be lost as a result of laboratory accident or other event

Embryo Cryopreservation

- Description of procedure
  - Side effects/risks with medications used and risks of the procedures
  - Need for monitoring, serial laboratory testing, and transvaginal ultrasounds
  - Collection of sperm
- Barriers to successful pregnancy
  - Poor response, abnormal oocytes, failure of fertilization
- Clear disposition plan for embryos
- Description of embryo cryopreservation
  - Freezing of embryos
  - Mechanical failure of event leading to loss of embryos
  - Theoretic risk of congenital anomalies and long-term storage
- Expected thaw-survival rate for embryos
  - Risk that no embryo may survive
- Clinic-specific data and outcomes for live birth rate

Adapted from The Practice Committee of the Society for Assisted Reproductive Technology, Practice Committee of the American Society for Reproductive Medicine. Essential elements of informed consent for elective oocyte cryopreservation: a practice committee opinion. Fertil Steril 2007:88(6);1495–6; and The Practice Committee of the Society for Assisted Reproductive Technology, Practice Committee of the American Society for Reproductive Medicine. Elements to be considered in obtaining informed consent for ART. Fertil Steril 2006:86(5);S272–3.

reported "always or often" giving patient educational material about fertility preservation.[77] A systematic approach, including professional education and automated fertility notifications infrastructure, augment the ability to capture the patient population that should receive further counseling/referrals.[78]

Fertility Preservation Treatment Options

There are both standard and experimental options for boys (**Fig. 2**) and girls (**Fig. 3**) for fertility preservation. The options are reviewed in their most appropriate category that follows; however, overlap for some techniques for prepubertal and postpubertal patients will occur. Fertility preservation requires an individualized approach based on the age of the patient, type of medical condition and expected treatment plan, time available, financial considerations, and long-term considerations. Gonadal shielding to reduce radiation to the reproductive organs is a standard practice.[79]

Prepubertal Boys

Testicular tissue freezing
Testicular tissue in prepubertal boys may be obtained via surgical procedure under anesthesia and cryopreserved for future use.[80] This technique is considered experimental and is the only option for fertility preservation in prepubertal boys. Protocols are being investigated to enable intratesticular grafting of tissue or infusion of testicular cell suspension into the seminiferous tubules.[81,82] Cryopreserved testicular tissue has been shown to maintain spermatogonia.[80]

Spermatogonial stem cell transplantation, xenotransplantation, and in vitro maturation of sperm
Testicular tissue from prepubertal boys has been cryopreserved, thawed, and then xenografted into mice showing the survival of spermatogonia.[83] Retrieval of spermatogonial stem cells with a plan for subsequent reimplantation or in vitro maturation for development into mature spermatozoa has been investigated in animal models.[84–86] In vitro spermatogenesis would avoid the chance of cotransplanting tumor cells.[81,87]

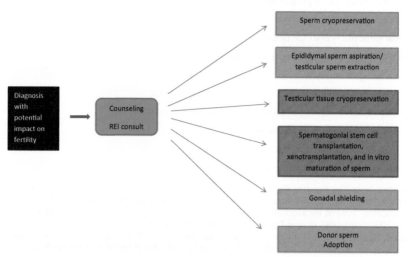

Fig. 2. Fertility preservation discussion for boys. REI, reproductive endocrinology and infertility. Orange box indicates standard of care; red box indicates experimental.

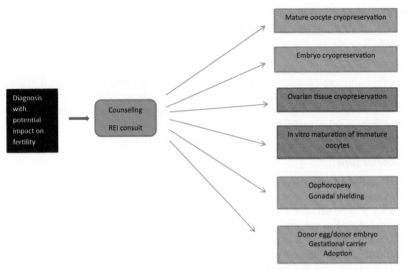

Fig. 3. Fertility preservation discussion for girls. REI, reproductive endocrinology and infertility. Orange box indicates standard of care; red box indicates experimental.

Postpubertal Boys

Sperm cryopreservation

Sperm cryopreservation is a standard fertility preservation option in in postpubertal boys and continues to be effective (**Fig. 4**).[88–94] There is a potential higher risk of DNA damage in sperm after chemotherapy, so collection of the specimen should occur before initiation of therapy.[2] Continued efforts to discuss and offer sperm cryopreservation to postpubertal children and adolescents is necessary.[95] Penile vibratory

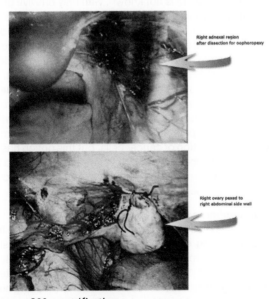

Fig. 4. Spermatozoa, ×200 magnification.

stimulation or electroejaculation can be used if masturbation is unsuccessful.[96,97] Live birth has been achieved with sperm that had been cryopreserved for as long as 28 years.[98]

Testicular sperm extraction

Testicular sperm extraction can remove sperm under general anesthesia if masturbation and electroejaculation do not result in adequate specimen for cryopreservation.[99,100] Surgical sperm extraction can also occur by percutaneous epididymal sperm aspiration, testicular sperm aspiration, and microepididymal sperm aspiration.[101]

Prepubertal Girls

Ovarian tissue cryopreservation

Ovarian tissue cryopreservation is the process by which ovarian tissue is obtained, usually by a laparoscopic procedure for freezing of either cortical strips or the whole ovary.[102] This is the only option for fertility preservation in prepubertal girls and can be used in postpubertal girls who cannot undergo delay in start of oncologic therapy. The ovarian cortex contains primordial follicles that can be used to obtain immature oocytes or transplanted at a later date. The benefit of this option is immediate collection without delay in chemotherapy and in addition to fertility, there can be return of hormonal function to allow endogenous secretion of hormones. This process is considered experimental. Whole ovary transplantation has had limited success.

Ovarian cortical tissue can be transplanted to a heterotopic location such as the subcutaneous tissue in the forearm or abdomen. There are reports of return of endocrine function and cases of embryos created[103,104]; however, only one case of a delivery of twins has been documented with the unfortunate concomitant finding of macroscopic evidence of tumor (granulosa cell) noted at the time of cesarean delivery.[105] Heterotopic transplantation has the advantages of being a simple procedure and results in easy access for follicular monitoring and oocyte collection. Disadvantages are that an in vitro fertilization (IVF) procedure is necessary, and the effect of the local environment on the oocyte is not known, with only one live birth published.[106]

Ovarian cortical tissue can undergo orthotopic transplantation. The ovarian tissue is placed at the site of the ovary or in the region of the broad ligament/ovarian fossa.[104] Autografts do not have unlimited survival, but placement in the pelvis can allow for natural conception. Approximately 50 live births have been reported worldwide; however, only one patient had been premenarchal at the time of ovarian tissue collection.[104,106–108] Immature oocytes can be obtained from ovarian tissue; however, total in vitro maturation of oocytes from cryopreserved tissue has not yet been successful.

Reimplantation of ovarian tissue may allow return of cancer cells with possible risk of recurrence.[109–112] Xenotransplantation of ovarian tissue into animals could eliminate the possibility of reintroduction of cancer cells, but this option has not been investigated beyond the stage of follicular/oocyte development.[113,114] The future may hold promise for an "artificial ovary" made of alginate matrigel matrix onto which preantral follicles and ovarian cells can be grafted.[106]

Ovarian transposition/oophoropexy

Ovarian transposition is used to surgically move the ovaries out of the field of radiation. In children, the most common cancer indications are rhabdomyosarcomas of the bladder, vagina, or uterus or sarcomas of pelvic soft tissue/bone. Pelvic or abdominal radiation doses of greater than 15 Gy in prepubertal girls and greater than 10 Gy in postpubertal girls has a significant risk of resultant amenorrhea and subsequent infertility.[53,115] Often, the ovaries are moved to a lateral location in the paracolic gutter by a laparoscopic technique (**Fig. 5**); unilateral or bilateral oophoropexy can be performed depending on the location of disease and anticipated site of radiotherapy. Complications can include ovarian torsion, bowel obstruction, and abdominal pain. Success rates have been reported to be as high as 80%, but long-term results have not been well studied in children.[116,117] Consideration of simultaneous ovarian transposition and ovarian tissue cryopreservation has been proposed.

Postpubertal Girls

Mature oocyte cryopreservation

Oocyte cryopreservation involves stimulating the ovaries with gonadotropins with monitoring by transvaginal ultrasound (**Fig. 6**) and serum hormone levels until the appropriate time for oocyte retrieval. Historically, these cycles were started on a certain day of the menstrual cycle, which increased the time needed to complete the oocyte cryopreservation process. Currently, random-start protocols are used that do not compromise oocyte yield and decrease the interval to which treatment may begin.[118–123] Randomized trials in good prognosis populations have demonstrated that implantation and pregnancy rates are similar between frozen vitrified oocytes and fresh oocytes.[37,124,125] Mature oocyte cryopreservation is now a standard practice and is no longer experimental.[37] Additionally, in clinical situations that would benefit from decreased estrogen exposure, using an aromatase inhibitor, such as letrozole, during the stimulation cycle can result in significantly lower peak estradiol levels without affecting the cycle outcomes.[126,127] Long-term oocyte cryopreservation (3.5 years) does not appear to impact live birth outcomes or increase chromosomal abnormalities.[128]

In vitro maturation of immature oocytes

Although the first successful pregnancy from in vitro maturation (IVM) was reported in 1989,[129] and multiple births have resulted from this technique in various clinical scenarios, maturation rates and pregnancy rates have traditionally been lower than conventional IVF. Although outcomes may be improving,[130] IVM is still considered experimental. For fertility preservation, IVM can be used to maximize the number of oocytes at the time of oocyte retrieval, as an independent method to obtain oocytes in patients who cannot undergo a stimulated cycle or who need immediate treatment, or as an adjunct to ovarian tissue cryopreservation.[131] The first live birth in a

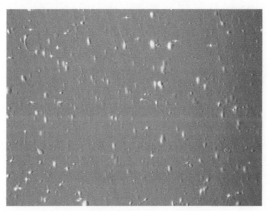

Fig. 5. Right oophoropexy for fertility preservation. (*Courtesy of* Janis Moessner, BS ELD (ABB), IVF Laboratory Director, Penn State Hershey Medical Center, Hershey, PA.)

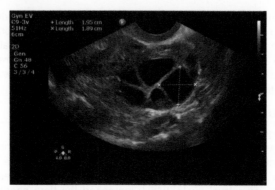

Fig. 6. Transvaginal ultrasound demonstrating the measurement of an ovarian follicle of a stimulated ovary undergoing monitoring for planned oocyte retrieval.

fertility-preserving effort for a patient with ovarian cancer from cryopreserved embryo obtained from in vitro–matured, ex vivo–harvested oocytes has been documented.[132] The outlook for use of IVM of oocytes is promising and deserves further investigation.[133]

Embryo cryopreservation

Embryo cryopreservation has been the standard technique for fertility preservation.[71] This process is similar to oocyte cryopreservation for ovarian stimulation and oocyte retrieval. Partner or donor sperm is necessary to create embryos (**Figs. 7** and **8**), making this a less applicable option for children and adolescents. According to the Centers for Disease Control and Prevention/Society for Assistive Reproductive Technology data for 2012, 47.3% of transfers using frozen nondonor embryos resulted in pregnancy and 37.5% resulted in live birth. These data are representative of the infertility population, as fertility preservation cycles are not listed separately. There were 18,585 egg and embryo banking cycles (which includes fertility preservation) in 2012, which

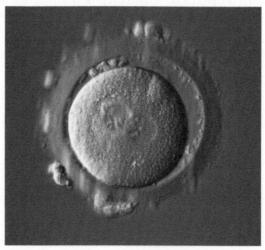

Fig. 7. 2pn (pronuclei) embryo, ×200 magnification. (*Courtesy of* Janis Moessner, BS ELD (ABB), IVF Laboratory Director, Penn State Hershey Medical Center, Hershey, PA.)

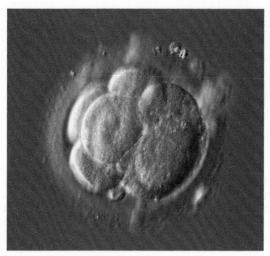

Fig. 8. Eight-cell embryo, ×200 magnification.

accounts for 10.5% of all assisted reproductive technology cycles in the United States in 2012.[134]

Trachelectomy

Radical trachelectomy is a procedure during which the cervix is removed in the setting of low-stage (1A1, 1A2, or 1B1) cervical cancers. It can be performed laparoscopically, vaginally, or abdominally.[135–137] A cerclage is usually placed at the time of surgery and cesarean is indicated for delivery. Of those attempting to become pregnant, approximately 60% were able to conceive; however, there is an increased risk of preterm delivery and second trimester loss.[138] Routine postpartum hysterectomy is not usually recommended and risk of recurrence is less than 4%.

Medical gonadal suppression

Gonadal suppression by gonadotropin-releasing hormone analogues (GnRHa) is one of the most controversial topics in fertility preservation. Protective effect was seen in early animal studies and in nonrandomized human trials. Other studies, such as the German Hodgkin Study Group randomized trial and multiple attempts at review of this topic, do not show an effect or have mixed results.[139–147] Some investigators suggest that because breast, ovary, and endometrium express GnRH receptors, that it cannot be concluded that GnRHa do not reduce the efficacy of chemotherapy by effect on GnRH receptors or by inducing glutathione S-transferases.

A recent meta-analysis of 9 randomized studies was performed by Del Mastro and colleagues.[148] This summary found a statistically significant reduction in the risk of premature ovarian failure (POF) with the use of GnRHa; however, each study defined POF differently, with many using menstruation as the only surrogate for ovarian function and follow-up varied between 6 and 36 months. Although the hope for medical management options for fertility preservation continues, the American Society of Clinical Oncology and European Society for Medical Oncology do not consider use of GnRHa a standard application for all patients.[2,149] Even though there does not seem to be a significant benefit with regard to fertility, GnRHa can decrease menstrual bleeding during cancer treatments, which may be advantageous.

Uterine transplantation

Uterine transplantation has been performed and may be helpful in the setting of pelvic radiation. This technique is experimental. One live birth has been described in a case of congenital absence of the uterus.[150]

Posttreatment options

Posttreatment options include donor sperm, donor egg (oocyte), donor embryo, gestational carrier, or adoption. Child-free living is also a choice that could be made.

SUMMARY

In review, fertility preservation techniques continue to advance the opportunities for children and adolescents to have reproductive potential for the future. Oocyte cryopreservation is no longer experimental and offers postpubertal girls an additional option for fertility preservation. All patients receiving therapy that may affect fertility should receive education and counseling regarding fertility preservation and risk of infertility. Continued clinical trials are necessary, especially in the pediatric and adolescent populations.

REFERENCES

1. Pui CH, Gajjar AJ, Kane JR, et al. Challenging issues in pediatric oncology. Nat Rev Clin Oncol 2011;8(9):540–9.
2. Loren AW, Mangu PB, Beck LN, et al. Fertility preservation for patients with cancer: American Society of Clinical Oncology clinical practice guideline update. J Clin Oncol 2013;31(19):2500–10.
3. Lee SJ, Schover LR, Partridge AH, et al. American Society of Clinical Oncology recommendations on fertility preservation in cancer patients. J Clin Oncol 2006; 24(18):2917–31.
4. Ethics Committee of American Society for Reproductive Medicine. Fertility preservation and reproduction in patients facing gonadotoxic therapies: a committee opinion. Fertil Steril 2013;100(5):1224–31.
5. Murk W, Seli E. Fertility preservation as a public health issue: an epidemiological perspective. Curr Opin Obstet Gynecol 2011;23(3):143–50.
6. Woodruff TK. The Oncofertility Consortium–addressing fertility in young people with cancer. Nat Rev Clin Oncol 2010;7(8):466–75.
7. Woodruff TK. The emergence of a new interdiscipline: oncofertility. Cancer Treat Res 2007;138:3–11.
8. Waimey KE, Duncan FE, Su HI, et al. Future directions in oncofertility and fertility preservation: a report from the 2011 Oncofertility Consortium Conference. J Adolesc Young Adult Oncol 2013;2(1):25–30.
9. Ries LAG, Smith MA, Gurney JG, et al, editors. Cancer incidence and survival among children and adolescents: United States SEER program 1975-1995. Bethesda (MD): National Cancer Institute, SEER Program; 1999. Vol NIH Pub. No. 99-4649.
10. Howlader N, NA, Krapcho M, et al, editors. SEER cancer statistics review, 1975-2011. Bethesda (MD): National Cancer Institute. Available at: http://seer.cancer.gov/csr/1975_2011/. Based on November 2013 SEER data submission, posted to the SEER web site. April 2014.
11. What are the most common types of childhood cancers? American Cancer Society; 2015. Available at: http://www.cancer.org/cancer/cancerinchildren/detailedguide/cancer-in-children-types-of-childhood-cancers. Accessed March 9, 2015.

12. A snapshot of adolescent and young adult cancers. National Cancer Institute; 2014. Available at: http://www.cancer.gov/researchandfunding/snapshots/adolescent-young-adult. Accessed March 9, 2015.

13. Silva CA, Brunner HI. Gonadal functioning and preservation of reproductive fitness with juvenile systemic lupus erythematosus. Lupus 2007;16(8):593–9.

14. Mersereau J, Dooley MA. Gonadal failure with cyclophosphamide therapy for lupus nephritis: advances in fertility preservation. Rheum Dis Clin North Am 2010;36(1):99–108, viii.

15. Miller SD, Ginsberg JP, Caplan A, et al. Sperm banking in adolescent males with nephrotic syndrome: defining the limits of access to fertility preservation. Arch Dis Child 2012;97(9):765–6.

16. Gajjar R, Miller SD, Meyers KE, et al. Fertility preservation in patients receiving cyclophosphamide therapy for renal disease. Pediatr Nephrol 2014;30(7): 1099–106.

17. Oktay K, Bedoschi G. Oocyte cryopreservation for fertility preservation in post-pubertal female children at risk for premature ovarian failure due to accelerated follicle loss in Turner syndrome or cancer treatments. J Pediatr Adolesc Gynecol 2014;27(6):342–6.

18. van Erven B, Gubbels CS, van Golde RJ, et al. Fertility preservation in female classic galactosemia patients. Orphanet J Rare Dis 2013;8:107.

19. Rodolakis A, Akrivos N, Haidopoulos D, et al. Abdominal radical trachelectomy for treatment of deep infiltrating endometriosis of the cervix. J Obstet Gynaecol Res 2012;38(4):729–32.

20. Bedoschi G, Turan V, Oktay K. Fertility preservation options in women with endometriosis. Minerva Ginecol 2013;65(2):99–103.

21. Dahhan T, Dancet EA, Miedema DV, et al. Reproductive choices and outcomes after freezing oocytes for medical reasons: a follow-up study. Hum Reprod 2014;29(9):1925–30.

22. Pegg DE. Principles of cryopreservation. Methods Mol Biol 2015;1257:3–19.

23. Mazur P. Freezing of living cells: mechanisms and implications. Am J Physiol 1984;247(3 Pt 1):C125–42.

24. Fujikawa S, Miura K. Ultrastructural preservation of plasma membranes by non-lethal slow freezing to liquid nitrogen temperature. Cell Struct Funct 1987;12(1): 63–72.

25. Mazur P, Leibo SP, Chu EH. A two-factor hypothesis of freezing injury. Evidence from Chinese hamster tissue-culture cells. Exp Cell Res 1972;71(2):345–55.

26. Polge C, Smith AU, Parkes AS. Revival of spermatozoa after vitrification and dehydration at low temperatures. Nature 1949;164(4172):666.

27. Sherman JK, Bunge RG. Observations on preservation of human spermatozoa at low temperatures. Proc Soc Exp Biol Med 1953;82(4):686–8.

28. Bunge RG, Sherman JK. Fertilizing capacity of frozen human spermatozoa. Nature 1953;172(4382):767–8.

29. Sherman JK, Bunge RG. Effect of glycerol and freezing on some staining reactions of human spermatozoa. Proc Soc Exp Biol Med 1953;84(1):179–80.

30. Borges E, Rossi LM, Locambo de Freitas CV, et al. Fertilization and pregnancy outcome after intracytoplasmic injection with fresh or cryopreserved ejaculated spermatozoa. Fertil Steril 2007;87(2):316–20.

31. Chen C. Pregnancy after human oocyte cryopreservation. Lancet 1986;1(8486): 884–6.

32. Gosden RG. General principles of cryopreservation. Methods Mol Biol 2014; 1154:261–8.

33. Gosden RG, Gosden LL. Eggs come in from the cold. Trends Endocrinol Metab 2012;23(10):498–500.

34. Cil AP, Bang H, Oktay K. Age-specific probability of live birth with oocyte cryopreservation: an individual patient data meta-analysis. Fertil Steril 2013;100(2): 492–9.e493.

35. Fahy GM, Wowk B. Principles of cryopreservation by vitrification. Methods Mol Biol 2015;1257:21–82.

36. ACOG: Committee Opinion No. 584: oocyte cryopreservation. Obstet Gynecol 2014;123(1):221–2.

37. Practice Committees of American Society for Reproductive Medicine, Society for Assisted Reproductive Technology. Mature oocyte cryopreservation: a guideline. Fertil Steril 2013;99(1):37–43.

38. Nilsson J, Jervaeus A, Lampic C, et al. 'Will I be able to have a baby?' Results from online focus group discussions with childhood cancer survivors in Sweden. Hum Reprod 2014;29(12):2704–11.

39. Tschudin S, Bitzer J. Psychological aspects of fertility preservation in men and women affected by cancer and other life-threatening diseases. Hum Reprod Update 2009;15(5):587–97.

40. Canada AL, Schover LR. The psychosocial impact of interrupted childbearing in long-term female cancer survivors. Psychooncology 2012;21(2):134–43.

41. Crawshaw MA, Sloper P. 'Swimming against the tide'–the influence of fertility matters on the transition to adulthood or survivorship following adolescent cancer. Eur J Cancer Care (Engl) 2010;19(5):610–20.

42. Schover LR, Rybicki LA, Martin BA, et al. Having children after cancer. A pilot survey of survivors' attitudes and experiences. Cancer 1999;86(4):697–709.

43. Schover LR. Psychosocial aspects of infertility and decisions about reproduction in young cancer survivors: a review. Med Pediatr Oncol 1999;33(1):53–9.

44. Armuand GM, Wettergren L, Rodriguez-Wallberg KA, et al. Desire for children, difficulties achieving a pregnancy, and infertility distress 3 to 7 years after cancer diagnosis. Support Care Cancer 2014;22(10):2805–12.

45. Robertson JA. Cancer and fertility: ethical and legal challenges. J Natl Cancer Inst Monogr 2005;(34):104–6.

46. Fertility preservation and consent. Lancet Oncol 2014;15(4):361.

47. Ethics Committee of the American Society for Reproductive Medicine. Posthumous collection and use of reproductive tissue: a committee opinion. Fertil Steril 2013;99(7):1842–5.

48. Ayensu-Coker L, Essig E, Breech LL, et al. Ethical quandaries in gamete-embryo cryopreservation related to oncofertility. J Law Med Ethics 2013;41(3): 711–9.

49. Bower B, Quinn GP. Fertility preservation in cancer patients: ethical considerations. Adv Exp Med Biol 2012;732:187–96.

50. Nass SJ, Beaupin LK, Demark-Wahnefried W, et al. Identifying and addressing the needs of adolescents and young adults with cancer: summary of an Institute of Medicine workshop. Oncologist 2015;20:186–95.

51. Linkeviciute A, Boniolo G, Chiavari L, et al. Fertility preservation in cancer patients: the global framework. Cancer Treat Rev 2014;40(8):1019–27.

52. Practice Committee of the American Society for Reproductive Medicine. Testing and interpreting measures of ovarian reserve: a committee opinion. Fertil Steril 2015;103(3):e9–17.

53. Levine JM, Kelvin JF, Quinn GP, et al. Infertility in reproductive-age female cancer survivors. Cancer 2015;121(10):1532–9.

54. Gracia CR, Sammel MD, Freeman E, et al. Impact of cancer therapies on ovarian reserve. Fertil Steril 2012;97(1):134–40.e131.
55. Bath LE, Wallace WH, Shaw MP, et al. Depletion of ovarian reserve in young women after treatment for cancer in childhood: detection by anti-Müllerian hormone, inhibin B and ovarian ultrasound. Hum Reprod 2003;18(11): 2368–74.
56. Dewailly D, Andersen CY, Balen A, et al. The physiology and clinical utility of anti-Mullerian hormone in women. Hum Reprod Update 2014;20(3):370–85.
57. Lie Fong S, Baart EB, Martini E, et al. Anti-Müllerian hormone: a marker for oocyte quantity, oocyte quality and embryo quality? Reprod Biomed Online 2008;16(5):664–70.
58. Brougham MF, Crofton PM, Johnson EJ, et al. Anti-Müllerian hormone is a marker of gonadotoxicity in pre- and postpubertal girls treated for cancer: a prospective study. J Clin Endocrinol Metab 2012;97(6):2059–67.
59. Committee opinion no. 607: Gynecologic concerns in children and adolescents with cancer. Obstet Gynecol 2014;124(2 Pt 1):403–8.
60. Hagen CP, Aksglaede L, Sørensen K, et al. Serum levels of anti-Müllerian hormone as a marker of ovarian function in 926 healthy females from birth to adulthood and in 172 Turner syndrome patients. J Clin Endocrinol Metab 2010; 95(11):5003–10.
61. Hagen CP, Aksglaede L, Sørensen K, et al. Individual serum levels of anti-Müllerian hormone in healthy girls persist through childhood and adolescence: a longitudinal cohort study. Hum Reprod 2012;27(3):861–6.
62. Metzger ML, Meacham LR, Patterson B, et al. Female reproductive health after childhood, adolescent, and young adult cancers: guidelines for the assessment and management of female reproductive complications. J Clin Oncol 2013; 31(9):1239–47.
63. Knight S, Lorenzo A, Maloney AM, et al. An approach to fertility preservation in prepubertal and postpubertal females: a critical review of current literature. Pediatr Blood Cancer 2015;62(6):935–9.
64. Morgan S, Anderson RA, Gourley C, et al. How do chemotherapeutic agents damage the ovary? Hum Reprod Update 2012;18(5):525–35.
65. Magelssen H, Brydøy M, Fosså SD. The effects of cancer and cancer treatments on male reproductive function. Nat Clin Pract Urol 2006;3(6):312–22.
66. Centola GM. Semen assessment. Urol Clin North Am 2014;41(1):163–7.
67. Practice Committee of the American Society for Reproductive Medicine. Diagnostic evaluation of the infertile male: a committee opinion. Fertil Steril 2015; 103(3):e18–25.
68. Grady C. Enduring and emerging challenges of informed consent. N Engl J Med 2015;372(9):855–62.
69. Grady C, Wiener L, Abdoler E, et al. Assent in research: the voices of adolescents. J Adolesc Health 2014;54(5):515–20.
70. Informed consent, parental permission, and assent in pediatric practice. Committee on Bioethics, American Academy of Pediatrics. Pediatrics 1995;95(2): 314–7.
71. Jeruss JS, Woodruff TK. Preservation of fertility in patients with cancer. N Engl J Med 2009;360(9):902–11.
72. Bartholome WG. Informed consent, parental permission, and assent in pediatric practice. Pediatrics 1995;96(5 Pt 1):981–2.
73. Practice Committee of Society for Assisted Reproductive Technology, Practice Committee of American Society for Reproductive Medicine. Essential elements

of informed consent for elective oocyte cryopreservation: a practice committee opinion. Fertil Steril 2008;90(5 Suppl):S134–5.

74. Practice Committee of the American Society for Reproductive Medicine, Practice Committee of the Society for Assisted Reproductive Technology. Elements to be considered in obtaining informed consent for ART. Fertil Steril 2006;86(5 Suppl 1):S272–3.

75. Forman EJ, Anders CK, Behera MA. A nationwide survey of oncologists regarding treatment-related infertility and fertility preservation in female cancer patients. Fertil Steril 2010;94(5):1652–6.

76. Trudgen K, Ayensu-Coker L. Fertility preservation and reproductive health in the pediatric, adolescent, and young adult female cancer patient. Curr Opin Obstet Gynecol 2014;26(5):372–80.

77. Quinn GP, Vadaparampil ST, Malo T, et al. Oncologists' use of patient educational materials about cancer and fertility preservation. Psychooncology 2012; 21(11):1244–9.

78. Reinecke JD, Kelvin JF, Arvey SR, et al. Implementing a systematic approach to meeting patients' cancer and fertility needs: a review of the Fertile Hope Centers of Excellence program. J Oncol Pract 2012;8(5):303–8.

79. Rodriguez-Wallberg KA, Oktay K. Options on fertility preservation in female cancer patients. Cancer Treat Rev 2012;38(5):354–61.

80. Keros V, Hultenby K, Borgström B, et al. Methods of cryopreservation of testicular tissue with viable spermatogonia in pre-pubertal boys undergoing gonadotoxic cancer treatment. Hum Reprod 2007;22(5):1384–95.

81. Tournaye H, Dohle GR, Barratt CL. Fertility preservation in men with cancer. Lancet 2014;384(9950):1295–301.

82. Goossens E, Van Saen D, Tournaye H. Spermatogonial stem cell preservation and transplantation: from research to clinic. Hum Reprod 2013;28(4): 897–907.

83. Wyns C, Van Langendonckt A, Wese FX, et al. Long-term spermatogonial survival in cryopreserved and xenografted immature human testicular tissue. Hum Reprod 2008;23(11):2402–14.

84. Hart R. Preservation of fertility in adults and children diagnosed with cancer. BMJ 2008;337:a2045.

85. Valli H, Phillips BT, Shetty G, et al. Germline stem cells: toward the regeneration of spermatogenesis. Fertil Steril 2014;101(1):3–13.

86. Sadri-Ardekani H, Atala A. Testicular tissue cryopreservation and spermatogonial stem cell transplantation to restore fertility: from bench to bedside. Stem Cell Res Ther 2014;5(3):68.

87. Goossens E, Tournaye H. Male fertility preservation, where are we in 2014? Ann Endocrinol (Paris) 2014;75(2):115–7.

88. Hourvitz A, Goldschlag DE, Davis OK, et al. Intracytoplasmic sperm injection (ICSI) using cryopreserved sperm from men with malignant neoplasm yields high pregnancy rates. Fertil Steril 2008;90(3):557–63.

89. Romerius P, Ståhl O, Moëll C, et al. Sperm DNA integrity in men treated for childhood cancer. Clin Cancer Res 2010;16(15):3843–50.

90. Salonia A, Gallina A, Matloob R, et al. Is sperm banking of interest to patients with nongerm cell urological cancer before potentially fertility damaging treatments? J Urol 2009;182(3):1101–7.

91. Chang HC, Chen SC, Chen J, et al. Initial 10-year experience of sperm cryopreservation services for cancer patients. J Formos Med Assoc 2006;105(12): 1022–6.

92. Edge B, Holmes D, Makin G. Sperm banking in adolescent cancer patients. Arch Dis Child 2006;91(2):149–52.
93. Bahadur G, Ling KL, Hart R, et al. Semen production in adolescent cancer patients. Hum Reprod 2002;17(10):2654–6.
94. Ginsberg JP, Ogle SK, Tuchman LK, et al. Sperm banking for adolescent and young adult cancer patients: sperm quality, patient, and parent perspectives. Pediatr Blood Cancer 2008;50(3):594–8.
95. Daudin M, Rives N, Walschaerts M, et al. Sperm cryopreservation in adolescents and young adults with cancer: results of the French national sperm banking network (CECOS). Fertil Steril 2015;103(2):478–86.e471.
96. Adank MC, van Dorp W, Smit M, et al. Electroejaculation as a method of fertility preservation in boys diagnosed with cancer: a single-center experience and review of the literature. Fertil Steril 2014;102(1):199–205.e191.
97. Gat I, Toren A, Hourvitz A, et al. Sperm preservation by electroejaculation in adolescent cancer patients. Pediatr Blood Cancer 2014;61(2):286–90.
98. Katz DJ, Kolon TF, Feldman DR, et al. Fertility preservation strategies for male patients with cancer. Nat Rev Urol 2013;10(8):463–72.
99. Berookhim BM, Mulhall JP. Outcomes of operative sperm retrieval strategies for fertility preservation among males scheduled to undergo cancer treatment. Fertil Steril 2014;101(3):805–11.
100. Furuhashi K, Ishikawa T, Hashimoto H, et al. Onco-testicular sperm extraction: testicular sperm extraction in azoospermic and very severely oligozoospermic cancer patients. Andrologia 2013;45(2):107–10.
101. Practice Committee of American Society for Reproductive Medicine. Fertility preservation in patients undergoing gonadotoxic therapy or gonadectomy: a committee opinion. Fertil Steril 2013;100(5):1214–23.
102. Practice Committee of American Society for Reproductive Medicine. Ovarian tissue cryopreservation: a committee opinion. Fertil Steril 2014;101(5):1237–43.
103. Stern CJ, Toledo MG, Hale LG, et al. The first Australian experience of heterotopic grafting of cryopreserved ovarian tissue: evidence of establishment of normal ovarian function. Aust N Z J Obstet Gynaecol 2011;51(3):268–75.
104. Donnez J, Jadoul P, Squifflet J, et al. Ovarian tissue cryopreservation and transplantation in cancer patients. Best Pract Res Clin Obstet Gynaecol 2010;24(1):87–100.
105. Stern CJ, Gook D, Hale LG, et al. Delivery of twins following heterotopic grafting of frozen-thawed ovarian tissue. Hum Reprod 2014;29(8):1828.
106. Donnez J, Dolmans MM. Transplantation of ovarian tissue. Best Pract Res Clin Obstet Gynaecol 2014;28(8):1188–97.
107. Dittrich R, Hackl J, Lotz L, et al. Pregnancies and live births after 20 transplantations of cryopreserved ovarian tissue in a single center. Fertil Steril 2015;103(2):462–8.
108. Imbert R, Moffa F, Tsepelidis S, et al. Safety and usefulness of cryopreservation of ovarian tissue to preserve fertility: a 12-year retrospective analysis. Hum Reprod 2014;29(9):1931–40.
109. Dolmans MM, Marinescu C, Saussoy P, et al. Reimplantation of cryopreserved ovarian tissue from patients with acute lymphoblastic leukemia is potentially unsafe. Blood 2010;116(16):2908–14.
110. Resetkova N, Hayashi M, Kolp LA, et al. Fertility preservation for prepubertal girls: update and current challenges. Curr Obstet Gynecol Rep 2013;2(4):218–25.
111. Meirow D, Biederman H, Anderson RA, et al. Toxicity of chemotherapy and radiation on female reproduction. Clin Obstet Gynecol 2010;53(4):727–39.

112. Rosendahl M, Andersen MT, Ralfkiær E, et al. Evidence of residual disease in cryopreserved ovarian cortex from female patients with leukemia. Fertil Steril 2010;94(6):2186–90.
113. Kim SS, Kang HG, Kim NH, et al. Assessment of the integrity of human oocytes retrieved from cryopreserved ovarian tissue after xenotransplantation. Hum Reprod 2005;20(9):2502–8.
114. Lotz L, Liebenthron J, Nichols-Burns SM, et al. Spontaneous antral follicle formation and metaphase II oocyte from a non-stimulated prepubertal ovarian tissue xenotransplant. Reprod Biol Endocrinol 2014;12:41.
115. Levine J, Canada A, Stern CJ. Fertility preservation in adolescents and young adults with cancer. J Clin Oncol 2010;28(32):4831–41.
116. Irtan S, Orbach D, Helfre S, et al. Ovarian transposition in prepubescent and adolescent girls with cancer. Lancet Oncol 2013;14(13):e601–8.
117. Ayensu-Coker L, Bauman D, Lindheim SR, et al. Fertility preservation in pediatric, adolescent and young adult female cancer patients. Pediatr Endocrinol Rev 2012;10(1):174–87.
118. Sönmezer M, Türkçüoğlu I, Coşkun U, et al. Random-start controlled ovarian hyperstimulation for emergency fertility preservation in letrozole cycles. Fertil Steril 2011;95(6):2125.e9–11.
119. von Wolff M, Thaler CJ, Frambach T, et al. Ovarian stimulation to cryopreserve fertilized oocytes in cancer patients can be started in the luteal phase. Fertil Steril 2009;92(4):1360–5.
120. Keskin U, Ercan CM, Yilmaz A, et al. Random-start controlled ovarian hyperstimulation with letrozole for fertility preservation in cancer patients: case series and review of literature. J Pak Med Assoc 2014;64(7):830–2.
121. Martínez F, Clua E, Devesa M, et al. Comparison of starting ovarian stimulation on day 2 versus day 15 of the menstrual cycle in the same oocyte donor and pregnancy rates among the corresponding recipients of vitrified oocytes. Fertil Steril 2014;102(5):1307–11.
122. Cakmak H, Katz A, Cedars MI, et al. Effective method for emergency fertility preservation: random-start controlled ovarian stimulation. Fertil Steril 2013; 100(6):1673–80.
123. Nayak SR, Wakim AN. Random-start gonadotropin-releasing hormone (GnRH) antagonist-treated cycles with GnRH agonist trigger for fertility preservation. Fertil Steril 2011;96(1):e51–4.
124. Cobo A, Meseguer M, Remohí J, et al. Use of cryo-banked oocytes in an ovum donation programme: a prospective, randomized, controlled, clinical trial. Hum Reprod 2010;25(9):2239–46.
125. Rienzi L, Romano S, Albricci L, et al. Embryo development of fresh 'versus' vitrified metaphase II oocytes after ICSI: a prospective randomized sibling-oocyte study. Hum Reprod 2010;25(1):66–73.
126. Oktay K. Further evidence on the safety and success of ovarian stimulation with letrozole and tamoxifen in breast cancer patients undergoing in vitro fertilization to cryopreserve their embryos for fertility preservation. J Clin Oncol 2005;23(16): 3858–9.
127. Oktay K, Hourvitz A, Sahin G, et al. Letrozole reduces estrogen and gonadotropin exposure in women with breast cancer undergoing ovarian stimulation before chemotherapy. J Clin Endocrinol Metab 2006;91(10):3885–90.
128. Goldman KN, Kramer Y, Hodes-Wertz B, et al. Long-term cryopreservation of human oocytes does not increase embryonic aneuploidy. Fertil Steril 2015; 103(3):662–8.

129. Cha KY, Koo JJ, Ko JJ, et al. Pregnancy after in vitro fertilization of human follicular oocytes collected from nonstimulated cycles, their culture in vitro and their transfer in a donor oocyte program. Fertil Steril 1991;55(1):109–13.
130. Chang EM, Song HS, Lee DR, et al. In vitro maturation of human oocytes: its role in infertility treatment and new possibilities. Clin Exp Reprod Med 2014;41(2): 41–6.
131. Chian RC, Uzelac PS, Nargund G. In vitro maturation of human immature oocytes for fertility preservation. Fertil Steril 2013;99(5):1173–81.
132. Prasath EB, Chan ML, Wong WH, et al. First pregnancy and live birth resulting from cryopreserved embryos obtained from in vitro matured oocytes after oophorectomy in an ovarian cancer patient. Hum Reprod 2014;29(2):276–8.
133. Combelles CM, Chateau G. The use of immature oocytes in the fertility preservation of cancer patients: current promises and challenges. Int J Dev Biol 2012; 56(10–12):919–29.
134. Centers for Disease Control and Prevention, American Society for Reproductive Medicine, Society for Assisted Reproductive Technology. 2012 assisted reproductive technology national summary report. Atlanta (GA): US Dept of Health and Human Services; 2014.
135. Li J, Li Z, Wang H, et al. Radical abdominal trachelectomy for cervical malignancies: surgical, oncological and fertility outcomes in 62 patients. Gynecol Oncol 2011;121(3):565–70.
136. Ramirez PT, Pareja R, Rendón GJ, et al. Management of low-risk early-stage cervical cancer: should conization, simple trachelectomy, or simple hysterectomy replace radical surgery as the new standard of care? Gynecol Oncol 2014; 132(1):254–9.
137. Rendón GJ, Ramirez PT, Frumovitz M, et al. Laparoscopic radical trachelectomy. JSLS 2012;16(3):503–7.
138. Pareja R, Rendón GJ, Sanz-Lomana CM, et al. Surgical, oncological, and obstetrical outcomes after abdominal radical trachelectomy—a systematic literature review. Gynecol Oncol 2013;131(1):77–82.
139. Behringer K, Wildt L, Mueller H, et al. No protection of the ovarian follicle pool with the use of GnRH-analogues or oral contraceptives in young women treated with escalated BEACOPP for advanced-stage Hodgkin lymphoma. Final results of a phase II trial from the German Hodgkin Study Group. Ann Oncol 2010; 21(10):2052–60.
140. Oktay K, Sönmezer M. Gonadotropin-releasing hormone analogs in fertility preservation—lack of biological basis? Nat Clin Pract Endocrinol Metab 2008;4(9): 488–9.
141. Bedoschi G, Turan V, Oktay K. Utility of GnRH-agonists for fertility preservation in women with operable breast cancer: is it protective? Curr Breast Cancer Rep 2013;5(4):302–8.
142. Oktay K, Sönmezer M, Oktem O, et al. Absence of conclusive evidence for the safety and efficacy of gonadotropin-releasing hormone analogue treatment in protecting against chemotherapy-induced gonadal injury. Oncologist 2007; 12(9):1055–66.
143. Demeestere I, Brice P, Peccatori FA, et al. Gonadotropin-releasing hormone agonist for the prevention of chemotherapy-induced ovarian failure in patients with lymphoma: 1-year follow-up of a prospective randomized trial. J Clin Oncol 2013;31(7):903–9.
144. Kim SS, Lee JR, Jee BC, et al. Use of hormonal protection for chemotherapy-induced gonadotoxicity. Clin Obstet Gynecol 2010;53(4):740–52.

145. Bedaiwy MA, Abou-Setta AM, Desai N, et al. Gonadotropin-releasing hormone analog cotreatment for preservation of ovarian function during gonadotoxic chemotherapy: a systematic review and meta-analysis. Fertil Steril 2011;95(3). 906–914.e901-904.
146. Chen H, Li J, Cui T, et al. Adjuvant gonadotropin-releasing hormone analogues for the prevention of chemotherapy induced premature ovarian failure in premenopausal women. Cochrane Database Syst Rev 2011;(11):CD008018.
147. Yang B, Shi W, Yang J, et al. Concurrent treatment with gonadotropin-releasing hormone agonists for chemotherapy-induced ovarian damage in premenopausal women with breast cancer: a meta-analysis of randomized controlled trials. Breast 2013;22(2):150–7.
148. Del Mastro L, Ceppi M, Poggio F, et al. Gonadotropin-releasing hormone analogues for the prevention of chemotherapy-induced premature ovarian failure in cancer women: systematic review and meta-analysis of randomized trials. Cancer Treat Rev 2014;40(5):675–83.
149. Peccatori FA, Azim HA, Orecchia R, et al. Cancer, pregnancy and fertility: ESMO Clinical Practice Guidelines for diagnosis, treatment and follow-up. Ann Oncol 2013;24(Suppl 6):vi160–70.
150. Brännström M, Johannesson L, Bokström H, et al. Livebirth after uterus transplantation. Lancet 2015;385(9968):607–16.

Fertility Issues for Patients with Hypogonadotropic Causes of Delayed Puberty

 CrossMark

Jia Zhu, MD[a], Yee-Ming Chan, MD, PhD[a,b],*

KEYWORDS

- Delayed puberty • Idiopathic hypogonadotropic hypogonadism
- Functional hypogonadotropic hypogonadism • Hypothalamic amenorrhea • Fertility
- Height • Bone mineral density

KEY POINTS

- Although self-limited delayed puberty (also called constitutional delay) is generally thought benign, studies suggest that adult height and bone mineral density (BMD) may be compromised, and fertility has not been formally studied.
- Hypothalamic amenorrhea (HA) is thought to resolve with removal of the inciting stressor, but studies show that this is not always the case. Fertility can be achieved in most women with pharmacologic therapies.
- Most men and women with idiopathic hypogonadotropic hypogonadism (IHH) can achieve fertility with pharmacologic therapy, and in some cases spontaneously, but some individuals fail to respond to treatment.

INTRODUCTION

Delayed puberty is commonly defined as the lack of breast development in girls or testicular growth in boys by an age that is 2 or more SDs above the population mean,[1] with cutoffs of 13 years for girls and 14 years for boys traditionally used in clinical practice. In most cases of delayed puberty, no underlying cause is identified and the pubertal delay resolves spontaneously prior to age 18 years, a condition referred to as *self-limited delayed puberty* in this review; other terms include *constitutional delay of puberty*[2,3] and *constitutional delay of growth and puberty*, which technically describes cases that occur in the context of delayed prepubertal growth.[4,5]

Disclosure Summary: Y.-M.C. received support from a Doris Duke Charitable Foundation Clinical Scientist Development Award (2013110).

[a] Division of Endocrinology, Department of Medicine, Boston Children's Hospital, 300 Longwood Avenue, Boston, MA 02115, USA; [b] Department of Pediatrics, Harvard Medical School, 25 Shattuck Street, Boston, MA 02115, USA
* Corresponding author. Boston Children's Hospital, 333 Longwood Avenue, 6th Floor, Boston, MA 02115.
E-mail address: Yee-Ming.Chan@childrens.harvard.edu

Pubertal delay can also be due to functional hypogonadotropic hypogonadism, in which an underlying stressor, such as psychological stress, weight loss, or exercise, impairs function of the reproductive endocrine axis.[6,7] Although this phenomenon has been observed in both sexes, it is more common and has been more extensively studied in girls and women, in whom it is commonly referred to as HA.[1] Individuals can present with delayed puberty, primary amenorrhea, or secondary amenorrhea. In some cases, no clear stressor is identified and puberty has occurred normally, but later reproductive endocrine function is compromised; in these cases, a presumptive diagnosis of HA is often made and is sometimes referred to as idiopathic HA.[8,9]

In rare cases, failure to enter puberty by a typical age can be due to IHH. Individuals with IHH fail to enter puberty or to progress normally through puberty by adult age (commonly defined as 18 years) and in most cases require lifelong sex steroid replacement therapy.[10] Other names for IHH include congenital hypogonadotropic hypogonadism, congenital gonadotropin-releasing hormone (GnRH) deficiency, and isolated GnRH deficiency.[12]

Other causes of delayed or absent puberty include hypogonadotropic hypogonadism due to an anatomic defect or injury in the region of the hypothalamus/pituitary gland (not discussed in this article) and primary gonadal insufficiency, which can be readily recognized from a pattern of hypergonadotropic hypogonadism.[1] Gonadal insufficiency can be due to Turner syndrome, Klinefelter syndrome, chemotherapy, radiation, or galactosemia, which are discussed in articles elsewhere in this issue.[1]

Although self-limited delayed puberty, HA, and IHH are generally considered distinct conditions, it can sometimes be difficult to distinguish the disorders clinically. Individuals with self-limited delayed puberty and IHH have similar initial presentations and are distinguished only retrospectively, because patients with self-limited delay eventually have complete pubertal development. HA due to subtle inciting stressors that are not readily identified may be difficult to distinguish from self-limited delayed puberty or IHH, particularly because some women with IHH can undergo spontaneous breast development and even menarche.[13]

In addition to overlap in clinical presentation, there may be physiologic overlap between the hypogonadotropic causes of delayed puberty. For example, some patients with IHH undergo reversal and achieve normal reproductive endocrine function in adulthood, a clinical phenotype that resembles self-limited delayed puberty except for the age at pubertal onset.[14–17] Furthermore, a recent study reported a genetic link between IHH and self-limited delayed puberty, suggesting a shared pathophysiology for at least some cases,[18] and a genetic link has previously been suggested between HA and IHH.[19]

In general, self-limited delayed puberty is thought to be a benign developmental variant, HA is thought to be a reversible condition if the inciting stressor is removed, and IHH is thought to be a permanent disorder in most cases. This review examines whether the existing data support these widely held concepts.

IS SELF-LIMITED DELAYED PUBERTY BENIGN?

Self-limited delayed puberty is widely thought to have no long-term consequences. This concept has been challenged, however, by findings, reviewed in this article, that suggest that height and BMD may be compromised. These data raise the possibility that reproductive endocrine function in adulthood may be subtly compromised as well. Although no overt reproductive endocrine dysfunction has been reported, no study has formally evaluated adult reproductive endocrine function or fertility in individuals with a history of self-limited delayed puberty.

Adult Height

Early observational studies in children with self-limited delayed puberty suggested that they eventually reach their genetic target height (as calculated by the midparental height).[2,4,5,20,21] Other studies, however, have reported that these individuals attain a final height significantly lower than their genetic target height,[22–30] ranging from 0.6 to 1.5 SDs (approximately 4–11 cm) below target.[27,28]

Several studies have examined the effects of sex steroid treatment on final height. In both individuals with self-limited delayed puberty who reach their genetic target height[2,5,21,31–33] and those who fall short of their genetic target,[29,30] no difference in final height was observed between those who were treated with sex steroids and those who were not. Thus, the failure to attain target height cannot be attributed solely to the delayed appearance of sex steroids.

Bone Mineral Density and Fracture

Two independent studies by Finkelstein and colleagues and Kindblom and colleagues observed that young adult men with a history of frank pubertal delay or a later timing of puberty, respectively, had lower areal BMD (aBMD), measured by dual-energy x-ray absorptiometry (DXA), than men with normal pubertal timing.[34–37] Although 2 other studies also observed a lower aBMD in men with delayed puberty compared with controls, the studies found no difference in volumetric BMD (vBMD), calculated from DXA.[2,3]

One potential explanation for the variability in findings is that aBMD is influenced by bone dimensions and skeletal growth, which can be compromised by self-limited delayed puberty.[2] Finkelstein and colleagues' finding, however, of a lower BMD in men with a history of delayed puberty persisted even after correcting for bone size.[36] Furthermore, Kindblom and colleagues reported lower radial and tibial vBMD, as directly measured by peripheral quantitative CT (pQCT), in men with pubertal timing in the late tertile compared with that in the average tertile, although vBMD for men with frankly delayed puberty was not specifically reported.[37] Resolution of this question may require direct measurement of vBMD by methods such as pQCT in a population with frankly delayed puberty.

Early studies in women provided observational evidence that the risk of osteoporosis may be influenced by the age of menarche in both premenopausal[38–41] and postmenopausal women.[38,39,42–44] Similar to these earlier studies, a recent prospective study of healthy premenopausal women found that menarche later than the median age was associated with lower total distal radial vBMD.[45] vBMD in woman with frankly delayed puberty, however, was not reported, and it is unclear if these findings were attributable to a benefit of earlier pubertal timing or to a harm of later pubertal timing.

Although BMD is used as a measure of bone health and risk of osteoporosis, the primary clinical concern is risk of fracture. Two studies, one in young adult men and another in young adult women, found that an increased age at pubertal onset was associated with an increased fracture risk, although the risk associated with frankly delayed puberty was not reported.[37,46] In later adulthood, the European Prospective Osteoporosis Study reported an association of late menarche (≥ 15 y) with increased risk of vertebral[47] and Colles fracture,[48] and the Mediterranean Osteoporosis Study reported similar results for hip fracture.[49]

Sex steroid therapy has been suggested as a treatment to mitigate the possible compromise of BMD in individuals with self-limited delayed puberty. Two small studies reported that androgen administration did not affect BMD in young adult men with a history of delayed puberty.[2,3] The effects of sex steroid therapy on BMD or fracture risk in women or in men in later adulthood have not been reported.

Self-limited delayed puberty

- Some, but not all, studies have shown that individuals with self-limited delayed puberty fail to achieve their genetic target height. Final height does not seem to be affected (positively or negatively) by sex steroid therapy.

- Similarly, some, but not all, studies have shown that individuals with self-limited delayed puberty have lower BMD than controls; this does not seem influenced by sex steroid therapy and may correlate with increased risk of fracture.

- Thus, self-limited delayed puberty may not be as benign as generally thought. Although no overt reproductive endocrine dysfunction has been reported in adults with a history of self-limited delayed puberty, this has not been formally studied.

FUNCTIONAL HYPOGONADOTROPIC HYPOGONADISM

Inadequate nutrition, excessive exercise, chronic illness, or psychological stress can all suppress hypothalamic GnRH secretion through mechanisms that are not fully clear, resulting in functional hypogonadotropic hypogonadism.[6,7] Although this phenomenon has been reported (eg, by Winston and Wijeratne[50]) in men, it is more common in girls and women, also for unclear reasons, and the term *HA* refers to functional hypogonadotropic hypogonadism in girls and women. Because of this female predominance, studies on reproductive endocrine function and fertility outcomes of functional hypogonadotropic hypogonadism to date have been limited to women.

HA is conventionally thought to resolve with removal of the inciting stressor. Many women with HA, however, have lingering reproductive endocrine defects even after removal of the inciting factor. Thus, ongoing clinical follow-up is important to try to establish a definitive diagnosis and address potential reproductive endocrine issues.

Several observational studies of HA have described outcomes for the disorder; however, the women are often appropriately treated with hormonal therapy, so it is difficult to study the true natural history of HA. Also, because not all women in these studies sought fertility, resumption of menses and/or ovulation induction have often been used as outcome measures.

Resumption of Menses

Observational studies

In studies of adolescents and young women with varying causes of HA, the reported rates of recovering menses range from 29% to 100% over a 10-year follow-up period[8,9,51–53]; 2 of 3 studies that specifically examined multiple underlying causes of HA found that the rate of recovering menses differed by underlying cause,[8,9] with cases associated with a specific inciting factor having a higher rate of recovering menses than those with a presumptive diagnosis of idiopathic HA[9]; the third study used different etiologic categories and may not be directly comparable.[53] Other studies have examined fertility outcomes for specific causes of HA.

In HA associated with weight loss, Nakamura and colleagues reported a spontaneous recovery rate of 30% after 3 years of follow-up[51] and Hirvonen reported a rate of 72% after 6 years.[8] Not all patients in these 2 studies had complete recovery of body weight, although Nakamura and colleagues did not find any significant association between recovery of body weight and recovering menses.[51] Specifically, even in cases of complete recovery of body weight, Nakamura and colleagues reported that 71% of women remained amenorrheic.[51] In contrast, Perkins and colleagues found that 6 of 6 subjects with HA associated with stress and/or weight loss, all of whom reported resolution of the inciting factor, recovered menses over a 10-year follow-up period.[9] These findings in women with HA secondary to weight loss provide evidence that not all women recover reproductive endocrine function with resolution of the stressor, suggesting a separate cause for their reproductive endocrine dysfunction.

Studies of HA associated with anorexia nervosa have primarily been observational studies during and after multidisciplinary care for eating disorders. Golden and colleagues found that adolescents with anorexia nervosa (mean age 17 years) who underwent combination treatment consisting of medical, nutritional, and psychiatric intervention had a recovery rate of menses of 68% at 1 year and 95% at 2 years.[52] van Elburg and colleagues, however, reported 1-year recovery rates of only 39% in their total study population and 57% in subjects who recovered their weight.[54] Hirvonen similarly reported a rate of recovering menses of 56% after 6 years (with 77% recovery of anorexia nervosa)[8] and Perkins and colleagues reported a rate of 60% after 10 years (with 100% recovery of anorexia nervosa).[9]

Some studies have examined outcomes of idiopathic HA. One caveat for these studies is that because HA is defined as having an inciting factor, these cases of presumptive HA either may be due to a subtle stressor that was not identified on clinical evaluation or may be cases of IHH. Hirvonen reported a 60% recovery rate of menses over a 6-year period for idiopathic amenorrhea,[8] whereas Perkins and colleagues found that only 1 of 6 women with idiopathic amenorrhea spontaneously recovered menses over a 10-year follow-up period.[9]

Interventional studies
Cognitive behavioral therapy (CBT) and hypnotherapy have been explored as potential treatments of idiopathic HA. This population has been shown to have more perfectionism, need for social approval, and altered eating attitudes than women with normal menstrual cycles, and thus these psychological treatments may address an occult underlying stressor.[55,56] In a 20-week randomized control trial in 16 women with HA and no clear cause, 6 of 8 women who received CBT resumed ovulation compared with 1 of 8 women in the observation group.[57] In an uncontrolled study of hypnotherapy in 12 women, 75% of subjects resumed menses within a 12-week follow-up period.[58]

Clomiphene citrate is a selective estrogen receptor modulator that blocks estrogen negative feedback on the hypothalamus and/or pituitary gland and thus can increase gonadotropin secretion in some individuals.[59] A study of clomiphene citrate in women with HA due to anorexia nervosa, however, reported that only 27% of the total study population and 50% of those who recovered weight resumed menses.[60] This poor response in women with HA has been attributed to low underlying hypothalamic drive, consistent with the HA label.[59] A recent uncontrolled study of clomiphene citrate in 8 women with HA due to various causes, however, showed that priming with estrogen and progestin resulted in recovery of menses in all 8 women after 2 cycles of therapy.[59]

Preliminary studies have explored leptin, opioid antagonists, and kisspeptin as experimental treatments to restore reproductive endocrine activity in women with HA. A pilot study of leptin therapy found that 3 of 8 women achieved an ovulatory menstrual cycle,[61] and a follow-up randomized, double-blind, placebo-controlled trial reported that 7 of 10 women who received leptin therapy resumed menstruation compared with 2 of 9 women on placebo over a 36-week period.[62] In an early neuroendocrine study investigating the impact of the opioid antagonist naloxone in women with HA, an increase in luteinizing hormone (LH) pulse frequency was seen in 12 of 15 subjects (80%).[63] In 3 subsequent trials of the oral opioid antagonist naltrexone in women with HA, 3 of 3 (100%),[64] 12 of 24 (50%),[65] and 18 of 24 (75%)[66] ovulated. Pilot studies of kisspeptin in HA (each with 5 subjects) have suggested that kisspeptin can elicit increases in gonadotropin secretion,[67–69] but ovulation or resumption of menses was not achieved.[68,69]

Pregnancy

The rates of conception among women with HA have been predominantly limited to studies of pharmacologic treatments. Hirvonen observed a total conception rate of 79% (28 of 34) over 6 years,[8] and Perkins and colleagues reported a rate of more than 95% over 10 years (21 of 22).[9] Approximately 71%[8] and 82%[9] of women with HA in these 2 studies, respectively, received treatment with clomiphene citrate, tamoxifen, gonadotropins, pulsatile GnRH, or a combination of these therapies; however, conception rates associated with specific therapies or causes of HA were not reported.[8,9] For pulsatile GnRH therapy and gonadotropin therapy, Martin and colleagues reported conception rates of 95% and 72%, respectively, over 6 cycles of treatment of women with HA.[69] The conception rate in an uncontrolled trial of naltrexone therapy over 13 weeks in women with HA was reported to be 29%.[66]

Prognostic Factors for Recovery

In addition to the etiology of HA, several biochemical markers have been studied as potential predictors of reproductive endocrine outcomes in women with HA (**Table 1**). In an 8-year study in 93 women with HA (approximately 65% of cases secondary to weight loss), Falsetti and colleagues reported that a higher basal body mass index (BMI) and lower basal cortisol values were associated with a shorter time to recovering menses.[52] In a study of 61 patients with anorexia nervosa, van Elburg and colleagues reported that higher baseline values of the ovarian endocrine markers follicle-stimulating hormone (FSH), inhibin B, and antimüllerian hormone (AMH) were associated with a shorter time to recovering ovarian function.[53] These various factors likely reflected the cause of the amenorrhea, the severity of this underlying cause, and/or the degree of reproductive endocrine suppression. Perkins and colleagues found that other potential markers of severity, including initial presentation (primary amenorrhea, oligomenorrhoea, or normal menarche) and baseline LH patterns (apulsatile, low amplitude, low frequency, low-frequency/low amplitude, and normal), were not associated with recovering menses in 28 women with HA due to various causes.[9]

Functional hypogonadotropic hypogonadism and hypothalamic amenorrhea

- Studies have shown that not all women with HA recover menses and achieve fertility with resolution of their inciting stressor.

- More than 70% of women with HA achieve fertility with conventional gonadotropin or pulsatile GnRH therapy. Investigational studies have proposed CBT and hypnotherapy as psychological treatment approaches and leptin, opioid antagonists, and kisspeptin as promising experimental therapies.

- Studies have suggested that the recovery of reproductive endocrine function in women with HA is associated with the following prognostic factors: cause of amenorrhea, BMI, cortisol, FSH, inhibin B, and AMH.

Table 1
Prognostic factors for fertility in hypothalamic amenorrhea

Study Reference, Year	Etiology of Hypothalamic Amenorrhea	Intervention	n	Observation
Hirvonen,[8] 1977	Mixed	None	356	HA due to AN had 56% rate of resuming menses; HA due to psychogenic factors or weight loss had 72% rate.
Perkins et al,[9] 2001	Mixed	None	28	Idiopathic HA was less likely to recover menses than HA with an identifiable cause; $P<.05$. Initial presentation with primary amenorrhea, irregular menses, or secondary amenorrhea had no association with recovery. Baseline LH pattern (apulsatile, low frequency, low amplitude, or normal) had no association with recovery.
Falsetti et al,[53] 2002	Mixed (no AN)	None	93	Cause of HA had no association with recovery. Each 1 kg/m² increase in baseline BMI was associated with a 34% increased chance of recovery: RR 1.34; $P = .027$. Each 27.6 nmol/L (1.0 μg/dL) reduction in baseline cortisol was associated with a 24% increased chance of recovery: RR 0.76; $P = .008$.
Van Elburg et al,[54] 2007	AN	Specialized program for AN	61	Each 1 SD increase in baseline FSH was associated with a 91% increased rate of recovering menses: HR 1.91; CI, 1.20–3.03. Each 1 SD increase in baseline inhibin B was associated with a 106% increased rate of recovering menses: HR 2.06; CI, 1.21–3.52 Each 1 SD increase in baseline AMH was associated with a 74% increased rate of recovering menses: HR 1.74; CI, 1.13–2.69.

Abbreviations: AN, anorexia nervosa; HR, hazard ratio; RR, relative risk.

IDIOPATHIC HYPOGONADOTROPIC HYPOGONADISM

In most cases of IHH, achieving fertility requires treatment with gonadotropins or pulsatile GnRH, although fertility can occur spontaneously in cases of IHH with reversal. Gonadotropin regimens include human chorionic gonadotropin (hCG), an alternative ligand for the LH receptor, given alone or in combination with an FSH formulation, such as human menopausal gonadotropin (hMG) or recombinant FSH. In theory, replacing GnRH and/or gonadotropins should bypass the GnRH deficiency of IHH, but not all individuals respond to treatment. One potential explanation for this is that additional pituitary and/or gonadal defects can be demonstrated in a sizable proportion of men and women with IHH.[71,72]

Women

The first available treatment for ovulation induction in women with IHH used human gonadotropins (hMG/hCG combination therapy), with reported pregnancy rates ranging from 9% to 30% per treatment cycle and in 22% to 87% of treated women.[73] Similar rates have been reported for recombinant gonadotropin therapy.[73]

Higher rates of ovulation and conception and lower rates of multiple pregnancies have been reported with pulsatile GnRH therapy compared with gonadotropin therapy.[73] Ovulation rates with GnRH are reported to be more than 90%, with a cumulative pregnancy rate of 96% after 6 cycles of therapy.[70,74]

Men

In a study of 28 men with IHH who received 18 months of gonadotropin treatment (combination of hCG and FSH), spermatogenesis was achieved in 25 patients (89%).[75] In another study with a similar gonadotropin therapy regimen, however, only 50% (9 of 18) men with IHH achieved sperm production.[76] Two studies of pulsatile GnRH therapy reported spermatogenesis rates of 70% (24 of 31 men) and 86% (6 of 7 men).[11,77]

Two studies have specifically focused on conception outcomes in men with IHH. In 1 of these studies of pulsatile GnRH therapy, successful conception was achieved in 4 of 5 cycles in 3 subjects.[77] In the same study, of the IHH men treated with gonadotropin therapy (combination hCG and hMG), 90% (18 of 20 men) achieved spermatogenesis, which resulted in conception in 6 of 10 cycles in 3 subjects.[77] Although these results suggest that GnRH therapy might be superior in inducing conception, the small number of subjects desiring conception and the absence of fertility evaluations for female partners limit the conclusions that can be drawn. Furthermore, in a second study in Australia, a 30-year follow-up of 72 men with IHH who desired fertility and had partners with no adverse fertility factors, only 53% (38 men) fathered children with pulsatile GnRH therapy.[78]

Prognostic Factors for Fertility

Three studies have sought to identify factors associated with the successful induction of spermatogenesis and fertility in men, whereas no studies, to the authors' knowledge, have examined prognostic factors for fertility in women. Initial testicular size was associated with increased testicular growth during treatment in all 3 studies,[11,76,78] with a larger testicular volume (>4 mL) associated with higher sperm counts in 1 study[76] and a shorter time to spermatogenesis in another (**Table 2**).[11] In 1 of these studies, low inhibin B (<60 pg/mL) and a history of cryptorchidism were associated with a lower rate of spermatogenesis, whereas anosmia and prior testosterone therapy were not found to be independent predictors.[11] In contrast, another study reported that prior androgen exposure was associated with a 62% decrease in the rate of induction of spermatogenesis and was associated with slower rates of conception (**Table 2**).[78]

Because testosterone therapy is a commonly used treatment in boys with self-limited delayed puberty, the finding that prior androgen exposure may compromise future fertility in patients with IHH raises a potential concern for self-limited delayed puberty and may present a case for more physiologic approaches to treatment. There is no existing evidence, however, on the effects of androgen therapy on future fertility in self-limited delayed puberty.

Idiopathic hypogonadotropic hypogonadism

- More than 90% of women and 50% of men with IHH achieve fertility with pulsatile GnRH therapy. Fertility rates with gonadotropin therapy seem slightly lower and more variable for women but comparable for men.

- Although replacing GnRH and/or gonadotropins should bypass the GnRH deficiency of IHH, studies have shown that not all individuals respond to treatment, which could be due to the presence of additional defects in the reproductive endocrine axis.

- Studies have suggested that larger testicular volume is a favorable prognostic factor for spermatogenesis in men with IHH, whereas low inhibin B and a history of cryptorchidism are negative factors. The effect of prior androgen therapy on fertility outcomes remains unclear.

Table 2
Prognostic factors for fertility in idiopathic hypogonadotropic hypogonadism

Study Reference, Year	Treatment	n	Observation
Pitteloud et al,[11] 2002	Pulsatile GnRH	76 Men	History of partial pubertal development was associated with higher chance of testicular growth: β 4.3; $P = .002$. Cryptorchidism was associated with lower chance of testicular growth: β -1.9; $P = .05$. Baseline inhibin B <60 pg/mL was associated with a lower chance of testicular growth: β: -3.7; $P = .009$. Anosmia not significantly associated with chance of testicular growth: β -1.2; $P = .4$. Prior testosterone therapy was not significantly associated with chance of testicular growth: β -1.9; $P = .09$.
Liu et al,[78] 2009	hCG $\pm$ FSH	75 Men	Prior androgen therapy was associated with a 62% decrease in the chance of spermatogenesis: HR 0.379; 95% CI, 0.203–0.707. A combined TV $\geq$20 mL was associated with a 7.4 increase in odds of achieving spermatogenesis: OR 7.4; 95% CI, 1.9–27.9. A combined TV $\geq$20 mL was associated with a 2.37 increase in odds of achieving conception: OR 2.37; 95% CI, 1.04–5.40
Miyagawa et al,[76] 2005	hCG and hMG	36 Men	A greater initial TV was associated with a higher sperm count: correlation coefficient $r = 0.388$; $P = .003$.

Abbreviations: HR, hazard ratio; TV, testicular volume.

SUMMARY

Self-limited delayed puberty is generally thought to carry no long-term consequences, but studies of adult height and BMD challenge the widely held concept that this entity is a benign developmental variant. Future studies are needed to determine if reproductive endocrine function in these individuals may also be compromised. In hypothalamic amenorrhea, reproductive endocrine function is thought to recover with resolution of the stressor. Studies show, however, that this is not always the case, regardless of the underlying cause. IHH is considered, in most cases, a permanent disorder with infertility caused by defects in the action or secretion of GnRH. Although fertility in IHH individuals can be achieved with hormonal therapy in most cases, some patients do not respond to treatment whereas others achieve fertility spontaneously. Future studies are needed to further identify the various extrinsic and intrinsic factors, in particular modifiable factors, that can have an impact on fertility outcomes in individuals with self-limited delayed puberty, HA, and IHH.

REFERENCES

1. Palmert MR, Dunkel L. Clinical practice. Delayed puberty. N Engl J Med 2012; 366(5):443–53.
2. Bertelloni S, Baroncelli GI, Ferdeghini M, et al. Normal volumetric bone mineral density and bone turnover in young men with histories of constitutional delay of puberty. J Clin Endocrinol Metab 1998;83(12):4280–3.
3. Yap F, Hogler W, Briody J, et al. The skeletal phenotype of men with previous constitutional delay of puberty. J Clin Endocrinol Metab 2004;89(9):4306–11.
4. von Kalckreuth G, Haverkamp F, Kessler M, et al. Constitutional delay of growth and puberty: do they really reach their target height? Horm Res 1991;35(6): 222–5.
5. Arrigo T, Cisternino M, Luca De F, et al. Final height outcome in both untreated and testosterone-treated boys with constitutional delay of growth and puberty. J Pediatr Endocrinol Metab 1996;9(5):511–7.
6. Gordon CM. Clinical practice. Functional hypothalamic amenorrhea. N Engl J Med 2010;363(4):365–71.
7. Woolf PD, Hamill RW, McDonald JV, et al. Transient hypogonadotropic hypogonadism caused by critical illness. J Clin Endocrinol Metab 1985;60(3):444–50.
8. Hirvonen E. Etiology, clinical features and prognosis in secondary amenorrhea. Int J Fertil 1977;22(2):69–76.
9. Perkins RB, Hall JE, Martin KA. Aetiology, previous menstrual function and patterns of neuro-endocrine disturbance as prognostic indicators in hypothalamic amenorrhoea. Hum Reprod 2001;16(10):2198–205.
10. Hoffman AR, Crowley WF Jr. Induction of puberty in men by long-term pulsatile administration of low-dose gonadotropin-releasing hormone. N Engl J Med 1982;307(20):1237–41.
11. Pitteloud N, Hayes FJ, Dwyer A, et al. Predictors of outcome of long-term GnRH therapy in men with idiopathic hypogonadotropic hypogonadism. J Clin Endocrinol Metab 2002;87(9):4128–36.
12. Sykiotis GP, Pitteloud N, Seminara SB, et al. Deciphering genetic disease in the genomic era: the model of GnRH deficiency. Sci Transl Med 2010;2(32):32rv2.
13. Shaw ND, Seminara SB, Welt CK, et al. Expanding the phenotype and genotype of female GnRH deficiency. J Clin Endocrinol Metab 2011;96(3):E566–76.
14. Finkelstein JS, Spratt DI, O'Dea LS, et al. Pulsatile gonadotropin secretion after discontinuation of long term gonadotropin-releasing hormone (GnRH)

administration in a subset of GnRH-deficient men. J Clin Endocrinol Metab 1989; 69(2):377–85.

15. Quinton R, Cheow HK, Tymms DJ, et al. Kallmann's syndrome: is it always for life? Clin Endocrinol (Oxf) 1999;50(4):481–5.

16. Raivio T, Falardeau J, Dwyer A, et al. Reversal of idiopathic hypogonadotropic hypogonadism. N Engl J Med 2007;357(9):863–73.

17. Sidhoum VF, Chan YM, Lippincott MF, et al. Reversal and relapse of hypogonadotropic hypogonadism: resilience and fragility of the reproductive neuroendocrine system. J Clin Endocrinol Metab 2014;99(3):861–70.

18. Zhu J, Choa RE, Guo MH, et al. A shared genetic basis for self-limited delayed puberty and idiopathic hypogonadotropic hypogonadism. J Clin Endocrinol Metab 2015;100(4):E646–54.

19. Caronia LM, Martin C, Welt CK, et al. A genetic basis for functional hypothalamic amenorrhea. N Engl J Med 2011;364(3):215–25.

20. Volta C, Ghizzoni L, Buono T, et al. Final height in a group of untreated children with constitutional growth delay. Helv Paediatr Acta 1988;43(3):171–6.

21. Rensonnet C, Kanen F, Coremans C, et al. Pubertal growth as a determinant of adult height in boys with constitutional delay of growth and puberty. Horm Res 1999;51(5):223–9.

22. Bramswig JH, Fasse M, Holthoff ML, et al. Adult height in boys and girls with untreated short stature and constitutional delay of growth and puberty: accuracy of five different methods of height prediction. J Pediatr 1990;117(6):886–91.

23. LaFranchi S, Hanna CE, Mandel SH. Constitutional delay of growth: expected versus final adult height. Pediatrics 1991;87(1):82–7.

24. Crowne EC, Shalet SM, Wallace WH, et al. Final height in boys with untreated constitutional delay in growth and puberty. Arch Dis Child 1990;65(10):1109–12.

25. Crowne EC, Shalet SM, Wallace WH, et al. Final height in girls with untreated constitutional delay in growth and puberty. Eur J Pediatr 1991;150(10):708–12.

26. Albanese A, Stanhope R. Does constitutional delayed puberty cause segmental disproportion and short stature? Eur J Pediatr 1993;152(4):293–6.

27. Albanese A, Stanhope R. Predictive factors in the determination of final height in boys with constitutional delay of growth and puberty. J Pediatr 1995;126(4):545–50.

28. Sperlich M, Butenandt O, Schwarz HP. Final height and predicted height in boys with untreated constitutional growth delay. Eur J Pediatr 1995;154(8):627–32.

29. Kelly BP, Paterson WF, Donaldson MD. Final height outcome and value of height prediction in boys with constitutional delay in growth and adolescence treated with intramuscular testosterone 125 mg per month for 3 months. Clin Endocrinol (Oxf) 2003;58(3):267–72.

30. Poyrazoglu S, Gunoz H, Darendeliler F, et al. Constitutional delay of growth and puberty: from presentation to final height. J Pediatr Endocrinol Metab 2005; 18(2):171–9.

31. Zucchini S, Wasniewska M, Cisternino M, et al. Adult height in children with short stature and idiopathic delayed puberty after different management. Eur J Pediatr 2008;167(6):677–81.

32. Wehkalampi K, Vangonen K, Laine T, et al. Progressive reduction of relative height in childhood predicts adult stature below target height in boys with constitutional delay of growth and puberty. Horm Res 2007;68(2):99–104.

33. Wehkalampi K, Pakkila K, Laine T, et al. Adult height in girls with delayed pubertal growth. Horm Res Paediatr 2011;76(2):130–5.

34. Finkelstein JS, Neer RM, Biller BM, et al. Osteopenia in men with a history of delayed puberty. N Engl J Med 1992;326(9):600–4.

35. Finkelstein JS, Klibanski A, Neer RM. A longitudinal evaluation of bone mineral density in adult men with histories of delayed puberty. J Clin Endocrinol Metab 1996;81(3):1152–5.

36. Finkelstein JS, Klibanski A, Neer RM. Evaluation of lumber spine bone mineral density (BMD) using dual energy x-ray absorptiometry (DXA) in 21 young men with histories of constitutionally-delayed puberty. J Clin Endocrinol Metab 1999; 84(9):3400–1.

37. Kindblom JM, Lorentzon M, Norjavaara E, et al. Pubertal timing predicts previous fractures and BMD in young adult men: the GOOD study. J Bone Miner Res 2006; 21(5):790–5.

38. Ribot C, Pouilles JM, Bonneu M, et al. Assessment of the risk of post-menopausal osteoporosis using clinical factors. Clin Endocrinol (Oxf) 1992;36(3):225–8.

39. Tuppurainen M, Kroger H, Saarikoski S, et al. The effect of gynecological risk factors on lumbar and femoral bone mineral density in peri- and postmenopausal women. Maturitas 1995;21(2):137–45.

40. Rosenthal DI, Mayo-Smith W, Hayes CW, et al. Age and bone mass in premenopausal women. J Bone Miner Res 1989;4(4):533–8.

41. Ito M, Yamada M, Hayashi K, et al. Relation of early menarche to high bone mineral density. Calcif Tissue Int 1995;57(1):11–4.

42. Fox KM, Magaziner J, Sherwin R, et al. Reproductive correlates of bone mass in elderly women. Study of Osteoporotic Fractures Research Group. J Bone Miner Res 1993;8(8):901–8.

43. Orwoll ES, Bauer DC, Vogt TM, et al. Axial bone mass in older women. Study of Osteoporotic Fractures Research Group. Ann Intern Med 1996;124(2):187–96.

44. Varenna M, Binelli L, Zucchi F, et al. Prevalence of osteoporosis by educational level in a cohort of postmenopausal women. Osteoporos Int 1999;9(3):236–41.

45. Chevalley T, Bonjour JP, Ferrari S, et al. Deleterious effect of late menarche on distal tibia microstructure in healthy 20-year-old and premenopausal middle-aged women. J Bone Miner Res 2009;24(1):144–52.

46. Chevalley T, Bonjour JP, van Rietbergen B, et al. Fractures in healthy females followed from childhood to early adulthood are associated with later menarcheal age and with impaired bone microstructure at peak bone mass. J Clin Endocrinol Metab 2012;97(11):4174–81.

47. Roy DK, O'Neill TW, Finn JD, et al. Determinants of incident vertebral fracture in men and women: results from the European Prospective Osteoporosis Study (EPOS). Osteoporos Int 2003;14(1):19–26.

48. Silman AJ. Risk factors for Colles' fracture in men and women: results from the European Prospective Osteoporosis Study. Osteoporos Int 2003;14(3):213–8.

49. Johnell O, Gullberg B, Kanis JA, et al. Risk factors for hip fracture in European women: the MEDOS Study. Mediterranean Osteoporosis Study. J Bone Miner Res 1995;10(11):1802–15.

50. Winston AP, Wijeratne S. Hypogonadism, hypoleptinaemia and osteoporosis in males with eating disorders. Clin Endocrinol (Oxf) 2009;71(6):897–8.

51. Nakamura Y, Yoshimura Y, Oda T, et al. Clinical and endocrine studies on patients with amenorrhoea associated with weight loss. Clin Endocrinol (Oxf) 1985;23(6): 643–51.

52. Golden NH, Jacobson MS, Schebendach J, et al. Resumption of menses in anorexia nervosa. Arch Pediatr Adolesc Med 1997;151(1):16–21.

53. Falsetti L, Gambera A, Barbetti L, et al. Long-term follow-up of functional hypothalamic amenorrhea and prognostic factors. J Clin Endocrinol Metab 2002; 87(2):500–5.

54. van Elburg AA, Eijkemans MJ, Kas MJ, et al. Predictors of recovery of ovarian function during weight gain in anorexia nervosa. Fertil Steril 2007; 87(4):902–8.
55. Giles DE, Berga SL. Cognitive and psychiatric correlates of functional hypothalamic amenorrhea: a controlled comparison. Fertil Steril 1993;60(3):486–92.
56. Marcus MD, Loucks TL, Berga SL. Psychological correlates of functional hypothalamic amenorrhea. Fertil Steril 2001;76(2):310–6.
57. Berga SL, Marcus MD, Loucks TL, et al. Recovery of ovarian activity in women with functional hypothalamic amenorrhea who were treated with cognitive behavior therapy. Fertil Steril 2003;80(4):976–81.
58. Tschugguel W, Berga SL. Treatment of functional hypothalamic amenorrhea with hypnotherapy. Fertil Steril 2003;80(4):982–5.
59. Borges LE, Morgante G, Musacchio MC, et al. New protocol of clomiphene citrate treatment in women with hypothalamic amenorrhea. Gynecol Endocrinol 2007; 23(6):343–6.
60. Wakeling A, Marshall JC, Beardwood CJ, et al. The effects of clomiphene citrate on the hypothalamic-pituitary-gonadal axis in anorexia nervosa. Psychol Med 1976;6(3):371–80.
61. Welt CK, Chan JL, Bullen J, et al. Recombinant human leptin in women with hypothalamic amenorrhea. N Engl J Med 2004;351(10):987–97.
62. Chou SH, Chamberland JP, Liu X, et al. Leptin is an effective treatment for hypothalamic amenorrhea. Proc Natl Acad Sci U S A 2011;108(16):6585–90.
63. Perkins RB, Hall JE, Martin KA. Neuroendocrine abnormalities in hypothalamic amenorrhea: spectrum, stability, and response to neurotransmitter modulation. J Clin Endocrinol Metab 1999;84(6):1905–11.
64. Wildt L, Leyendecker G. Induction of ovulation by the chronic administration of naltrexone in hypothalamic amenorrhea. J Clin Endocrinol Metab 1987;64(6): 1334–5.
65. Leyendecker G, Waibel-Treber S, Wildt L. Pulsatile administration of gonadotrophin releasing hormone and oral administration of naltrexone in hypothalamic amenorrhoea. Hum Reprod 1993;8(Suppl 2):184–8.
66. Wildt L, Leyendecker G, Sir-Petermann T, et al. Treatment with naltrexone in hypothalamic ovarian failure: induction of ovulation and pregnancy. Hum Reprod 1993; 8(3):350–8.
67. Jayasena CN, Abbara A, Veldhuis JD, et al. Increasing LH pulsatility in women with hypothalamic amenorrhoea using intravenous infusion of Kisspeptin-54. J Clin Endocrinol Metab 2014;99(6):E953–61.
68. Jayasena CN, Nijher GM, Chaudhri OB, et al. Subcutaneous injection of kisspeptin-54 acutely stimulates gonadotropin secretion in women with hypothalamic amenorrhea, but chronic administration causes tachyphylaxis. J Clin Endocrinol Metab 2009;94(11):4315–23.
69. Jayasena CN, Nijher GM, Abbara A, et al. Twice-weekly administration of kisspeptin-54 for 8 weeks stimulates release of reproductive hormones in women with hypothalamic amenorrhea. Clin Pharmacol Ther 2010;88(6): 840–7.
70. Martin KA, Hall JE, Adams JM, et al. Comparison of exogenous gonadotropins and pulsatile gonadotropin-releasing hormone for induction of ovulation in hypogonadotropic amenorrhea. J Clin Endocrinol Metab 1993;77(1):125–9.
71. Sykiotis GP, Hoang XH, Avbelj M, et al. Congenital idiopathic hypogonadotropic hypogonadism: evidence of defects in the hypothalamus, pituitary, and testes. J Clin Endocrinol Metab 2010;95(6):3019–27.

72. Abel BS, Shaw ND, Brown JM, et al. Responsiveness to a physiological regimen of GnRH therapy and relation to genotype in women with isolated hypogonadotropic hypogonadism. J Clin Endocrinol Metab 2013;98(2):E206–16.

73. Messinis IE. Ovulation induction: a mini review. Hum Reprod 2005;20(10): 2688–97.

74. Homburg R, Eshel A, Armar NA, et al. One hundred pregnancies after treatment with pulsatile luteinising hormone releasing hormone to induce ovulation. BMJ 1989;298(6676):809–12.

75. Efficacy and safety of highly purified urinary follicle-stimulating hormone with human chorionic gonadotropin for treating men with isolated hypogonadotropic hypogonadism. European Metrodin HP Study Group. Fertil Steril 1998;70(2): 256–62.

76. Miyagawa Y, Tsujimura A, Matsumiya K, et al. Outcome of gonadotropin therapy for male hypogonadotropic hypogonadism at university affiliated male infertility centers: a 30-year retrospective study. J Urol 2005;173(6):2072–5.

77. Buchter D, Behre HM, Kliesch S, et al. Pulsatile GnRH or human chorionic gonadotropin/human menopausal gonadotropin as effective treatment for men with hypogonadotropic hypogonadism: a review of 42 cases. Eur J Endocrinol 1998; 139(3):298–303.

78. Liu PY, Baker HW, Jayadev V, et al. Induction of spermatogenesis and fertility during gonadotropin treatment of gonadotropin-deficient infertile men: predictors of fertility outcome. J Clin Endocrinol Metab 2009;94(3):801–8.

Adolescent Varicoceles and Infertility

Jessica T. Casey, MS, MD*, Rosalia Misseri, MD

KEYWORDS

• Varicocele • Infertility • Adolescent • Semen analysis • Varicocelectomy

KEY POINTS

- Varicoceles are associated with testicular atrophy and abnormal spermatogenesis, and varicocele-related testicular damage is thought to be progressive in nature.
- The main indications for varicocele repair include male infertility, adolescents with ipsilateral reduced testicular size or abnormal semen parameters, pain, and low testosterone.
- It is unknown whether adolescent varicoceles are associated with adult infertility and benefit from early repair, because 80% of adult men with varicoceles are fertile.
- Adolescents likely demonstrate asynchronous testicular growth and multiple ultrasound evaluations should be used to demonstrate stable, worsening or improving asymmetry before proceeding with varicocelectomy.
- A meta-analysis demonstrated that sperm density, motility, and morphology were decreased in adolescents with varicoceles; varicocele repair led to improvement in sperm density and motility.

INTRODUCTION

A varicocele is a tortuous dilation of the testicular veins of the spermatic cord (plexus pampiniform) palpable within the scrotum owing to high venous back pressure. The majority of varicoceles occur on the left side given the insertion of the left gonadal vein into the left renal vein and its associated higher venous pressure than the inferior vena cava.

Although varicoceles are rare in prepubertal children (3% in <10 years old), the incidence approaches 15% in those 10 to 19 years old, similar to the incidence in adults.[1,2] Varicoceles are the most common cause of male factor infertility, found in up to 40% of men with infertility.[3] Although the treatment of a varicocele in a man desiring paternity is warranted, the treatment of varicoceles in adolescent males is controversial.

The authors have nothing to disclose.
Department of Pediatric Urology, Riley Hospital for Children, 705 Riley Hospital Drive, Suite 4230, Indianapolis, IN 46202, USA
* Corresponding author.
E-mail address: jetcasey@iupui.edu

Endocrinol Metab Clin N Am 44 (2015) 835–842
http://dx.doi.org/10.1016/j.ecl.2015.07.007
0889-8529/15/$ – see front matter © 2015 Elsevier Inc. All rights reserved.

Varicoceles are associated with testicular atrophy and abnormal spermatogenesis, and varicocele-related testicular damage is thought to be progressive in nature.[4] Infertile adult men with varicoceles have been found to have decreased sperm density, decreased spermatic motility, and abnormal sperm morphology. Additionally, varicoceles are associated with low testosterone and high follicle-stimulating hormone levels in adult men.[5] In the adolescent population, varicoceles are worrisome given the concern for progressive effects on testicular growth, ongoing spermatogenesis, and future fertility.

Varicoceles can be associated with a feeling of "heaviness" after a prolonged period of standing. However, most varicoceles are asymptomatic, and fewer than 5% of adolescents present with symptoms of scrotal or testicular pain.[1] Adult varicoceles are often detected on an evaluation for infertility. In adolescents, they are most often detected during a well-child visit or by self-examination, possibly related to asymmetry in testicular size or the mass itself.

Physical examination to identify varicocele should be performed in both the supine and standing positions. Palpable varicoceles feel like a "bag of worms" in the upper scrotum. When supine, the size of the varicocele should reduce. For a thorough examination or when a varicocele is not obvious, the clinician should have the patient stand and perform a Valsalva maneuver.

Varicoceles are graded on a scale described by Dubin and Amelar.[6] Grade I/III varicoceles are palpable only during or after a Valsalva maneuver. Grade II/III varicoceles are palpable on routine physical examination without the need for a Valsalva maneuver. Grade III/III varicoceles are visible to the eye and palpable on routine physical examination. Subclinical varicoceles are not detected on physical examination and found by radiologic examination, most commonly scrotal ultrasonography. Subclinical varicoceles have been shown to have no impact on fertility, and repair of subclinical varicoceles has not been shown to improve fertility rates.[7] However, subclinical varicoceles in the pediatric population have been shown to progress over time and may require long-term follow-up.[8]

If a unilateral, right-sided varicocele that does not decompress while supine is palpated, one should suspect a retroperitoneal mass and undergo cross-sectional imaging.

In the adolescent population, relative testicular size should be assessed by physical examination using an orchidometer and verified by ultrasound. Ultrasound has been shown to be superior for assessment of volume differentials, a necessary component for evaluation of the adolescent varicocele.[9]

PATHOPHYSIOLOGY OF VARICOCELES

The theories behind varicocele-associated abnormal spermatogenesis and impaired fertility include elevated temperature effects on spermatogenesis and increased levels of oxidants/gonadotoxins.[10] The prevailing theory is that poor venous drainage associated with varicoceles leads to disruption of the countercurrent heat exchange along the spermatic cord, leading to elevated scrotal temperatures, which leads to impaired spermatogenesis.[10] Higher scrotal temperatures have been associated with decreased production of testosterone by Leydig cells, altered Sertoli cell function and morphology, injury to the germinal cell membrane, as well as decreased protein synthesis and decreased amino acid transport.[11-15]

Other theories include oxygen deprivation leading to impaired spermatogenesis, increased levels of gonadotropins owing to impaired drainage from poor venous drainage, and increased levels of oxidants within the semen.[10] Seminal reactive oxygen species levels have been shown to be higher in the semen of patients with higher grade varicoceles (grades II and III compared with grade I)[16] and in patients with infertility compared with fertile men.[17] Additionally varicocele repair has been shown to reduce seminal reactive oxygen species levels.[17]

INDICATIONS FOR TREATMENT OF VARICOCELES

There are 4 main possible indications for the treatment of varicoceles: (1) scrotal pain related to the varicocele, (2) low testosterone levels in adult men, (3) adult male factor infertility, and (4) adolescents with ipsilateral reduced testicular size and/or abnormal semen analyses.

Varicocele-Associated Pain

Men and adolescents who present with painful clinical varicoceles should first attempt conservative treatment consisting of scrotal support, oral nonsteroidal antiinflammatory medications, and limitation of strenuous activity. In those who do not respond to conservative treatment and have clinically palpable varicoceles with the associated characteristic pain (chronic dull ache, dragging pain, or throbbing pain that worsens with prolonged standing or physical activity), varicocele repair is an option. However, pain may not resolve despite resolution of the palpable varicocele.[18]

Varicocele-Associated Hypogonadism

Additionally, varicocele repair has been shown to lead to significant testosterone level improvements in adult men who are hypogonadal.[19–21]

Varicocele and Adult Male Infertility

The Male Infertility Best Practice Policy Committee of the American Urologic Association recommends that varicocele repair be considered for the male partner of a couple trying to conceive if the following 4 conditions are met: (1) the couple has documented infertility based on regular intercourse for more than 12 months, (2) the female partner has normal fertility or a correctable cause of infertility, (3) the varicocele is clinically palpable on physical examination, and (4) the male partner has 1 or more abnormal semen parameters or sperm function tests.[22] Additionally, men who have a palpable varicocele and abnormal semen analyses who are not currently attempting conception but desire future fertility are candidates for varicocele repair. Men with palpable varicoceles but normal semen analyses who desire future fertility should be offered semen analysis every 1 to 2 years to detect early signs of abnormal spermatogenesis from progressive testicular dysfunction.[22]

Varicocele repair in adult men has been show to improve not only sperm motility, density, and morphology, but also specific functional sperm defects (sperm penetration assay, oxidant determination, and DNA fragmentation).[5,23–26] In addition, varicocele repair has been show to improve serum follicle-stimulating hormone and testosterone levels.[5,27]

Although there remains some controversy as to whether varicocele repair truly improves semen parameters and paternity rates in adult men, meta-analyses limited to studies of men with clinical varicoceles with abnormal semen parameters (and excluding men with subclinical varicoceles or normal semen analyses) demonstrate a benefit to varicocele repair.[28,29] In the age of assisted reproductive techniques, varicocele repair can allow couples to "downgrade" the level of complexity of assisted reproductive techniques needed and allow for the potential for spontaneous pregnancy for those with nonobstructive azospermia.[30]

Adolescent Varicoceles

Given the association between adult male varicoceles and infertility, and the known progressive nature of varicoceles on spermatogenesis, adolescents with varicoceles are a cause for concern. However, it is unknown whether varicoceles that present in adolescence will lead to adult infertility and benefit from early repair, because 80% of adult men with varicoceles do not have associated infertility. Many studies have attempted to identify criteria by which to determine which adolescents would benefit from varicocele repair. Criteria have included varicocele grade, testicular size discrepancy, total testicular volume, and semen parameters.

Initial studies demonstrated a correlation between testicular asymmetry and higher varicocele grade. More recent studies have shown no correlation between testicular asymmetry and varicocele grade[31] or semen parameters and varicocele grade.[32]

Historically, testicular asymmetry has been the main indication for varicocele repair in the adolescent population, because there have been no objective measures of impaired spermatogenesis, for example, semen analysis and paternity. Kass and Belman[33] demonstrated increases in testicular volume after varicocele repair. However, debate remains regarding the precise volume difference to be used, the duration of follow-up before intervention, and the significance of spontaneous catch-up growth. Various studies use different testicular size discrepancy measurements to indicate clinically relevant asymmetry as an indication for varicocele repair. These measurements include 10%, 15%, or 20% relative volume differences or a 2- to 3-mL absolute volume difference between the affected and unaffected testicle.[31,34–36] In a recent survey of pediatric urologists' clinical practice, 85% reported greater than 20% testicular size discrepancy to be their criteria for a "significant" difference; 2.5% reported they used the definition of 2 mL absolute volume difference.[37]

Once significant asymmetry is found (using whichever definition is preferred), the next question is how long to follow these patients before intervening with varicocele repair. Investigators have shown that a large percentage of patients with initial asymmetry become more symmetric with time.[38] Conversely, some found that a large percentage of patients with initial symmetry become more asymmetric with time.[39,40]

Kolon and colleagues[38] followed 71 boys with varicoceles and a history of 3 or more ultrasounds and no intervening varicocele repair. They found that 71% of those with an initial asymmetry of greater than 15% demonstrated spontaneous testicular growth and no longer met the criteria for surgical intervention (<15% asymmetry) over a 3-year period. Therefore, the authors recommend at least 2, preferably 3, testicular volume measurements 1 year apart to establish stability of testicular asymmetry. Poon and colleagues[40] followed 181 patients expectantly and found that 35% of those with initial asymmetry of less than 20% asymmetry developed greater than 20% asymmetry. Of those with initial asymmetry of less than 20%, 53% remained in that range over a 12-month period. Korets and colleagues[39] followed 89 patients with initially less than 15% asymmetry and demonstrated that 42% had progression of their asymmetry over an 18-month period. Adolescents likely demonstrate asynchronous testicular growth and multiple ultrasound evaluations should be used to demonstrate stable, worsening or improving asymmetry before proceeding with varicocele repair. In a recent survey of pediatric urologists, after seeing a patient with "significant" (personal definition) testicular size discrepancy, 33% would proceed with varicocele repair and the remainder would schedule a follow-up ultrasound at 6 or 12 months.[37]

Because using testicular asymmetry as a surrogate marker for abnormal spermatogenesis may not be ideal, recent research has attempted to correlate adolescent semen parameters with testicular asymmetry. In a study of 57 Tanner stage V adolescent males aged 14 to 20 with clinically apparent varicoceles (grades I-III), those with greater than 20% asymmetry had significantly lower sperm concentration, total motile sperm count, and percent motile sperm.[41] In a more recent study, Christman and colleagues[42] found that total testicular volume at the end of adolescence correlated more with total motile sperm count than either prior total testicular volumes or testicular volume differentials. Additionally, the overall suboptimal semen parameters (66% with low total motile sperm counts) in this population of adolescents with varicocele on active surveillance made these authors call into question the use of serial monitoring of testicular volume differential to identify surgical candidates. They now rely more heavily on semen analysis parameters to determine the need for varicocele repair. Other studies by this group have demonstrated that the semen analysis parameters of youths (median age, 18.5 years) with uncorrected varicoceles more closely resemble those of treated bilateral cryptorchidism than unilateral cryptorchidism, possibly reflecting poorer future fertility outcomes than previously thought.[43]

A recent meta-analysis evaluated the effect of varicoceles and varicocele repair on semen analysis of youths (defined as 15–24 years old).[44] After an analysis of 10 studies including 357 varicocele and 427 control patients, they demonstrated that sperm density, motility, and morphology were decreased significantly in patients with varicoceles. Additionally, an analysis of another 10 studies including 379 treated and 270 untreated patients demonstrated significant improvement in sperm density and motility after varicocele repair. Therefore, without the advantage of a large, randomized trial, there is good evidence that varicoceles affect spermatogenesis in adolescents and some improvement can be seen with varicocele repair.

Despite the use of semen analyses in research to stratify the effect of varicoceles on adolescent spermatogenesis, it does not seem to have crossed the line into clinical use. In a survey of 74 pediatric urologists, 57% reported having never sent a patient for a semen analysis.[37] In another survey of 131 pediatric urologists, only 39% report having used altered semen parameters as an indication for varicocele repair.[45]

The ultimate predictor of the benefit of varicocele repair in adolescents is eventual paternity. Salzhauer and colleagues[46] surveyed 50 patients who underwent varicocele repair and were now more than 21 years old. Of the 18 patients who had attempted paternity, all 18 were successful, demonstrating a lack of harm from varicocele repair. However, this study does not demonstrate evidence for infertility in the unrepaired adolescent varicocele. Bogaert and colleagues[47] demonstrated no improvement in paternity after varicocelectomy versus observation in a cohort of adolescents screened for varicoceles. In this group, only 8% of those undergoing varicocelectomy had testicular asymmetry. These studies shed some light onto the effect of adolescent varicoceles on eventual paternity, but are incomplete studies with mixed populations.

Given the controversy surrounding adolescent varicocele management, it is not surprising that surveys of pediatric urologists have revealed a lack of consensus on diagnostic approaches, treatment decisions and operative approaches.[37,45]

APPROACH TO VARICOCELE REPAIR

Surgical treatments for varicocele repair include open retroperitoneal (Palomo), laparoscopic retroperitoneal (artery-sparing or non–artery-sparing), inguinal approach (Ivanissevich), and the subinguinal approach. The addition of the surgical microscope and intraoperative Doppler ultrasonography has led to a decrease in postoperative complications (testicular artery injury, hydrocele formation, and varicocele recurrence). Additionally, interventional radiology varicocele repair procedures include percutaneous embolization and sclerotherapy. In a recent survey of pediatric urologists, 38% performed laparoscopic retroperitoneal varicocelectomies, 28% subinguinal microsurgical, 14% inguinal, 13% open retroperitoneal, 5% embolization, and 3% sclerotherapy.[45]

SUMMARY

Adult varicoceles are common in men with infertility and varicocele repair in this population has demonstrated improved semen parameters and paternity outcomes. However, without solid objective endpoints (reproducible semen analyses, paternity), the indications for adolescent varicocele repair remain controversial.

REFERENCES

1. Diamond DA, Gargollo PC, Caldamone AA. Current management principles for adolescent varicocele. Fertil Steril 2011;96(6):1294–8.
2. Zampieri N, Cervellione RM. Varicocele in adolescents: a 6-year longitudinal and followup observational study. J Urol 2008;180(4 Suppl):1653–6.
3. Nagler HM, Marinis FG. Varicocele. In: Lipshultz LI, Howards S, editors. Infertility in the male. St Louis (MO): Mosby Year Book; 1997. p. P336–59.
4. Greenberg SH, Lipshultz LI, Wein AJ. Experience with 425 subfertile male patients. J Urol 1978;119(4):507–10.
5. Cayan S, Kadioglu A, Orhan I, et al. The effect of microsurgical varicocelectomy on serum follicle stimulating hormone, testosterone and free testosterone levels in men with varicoceles. BJU Int 1999;84(9):1046–9.
6. Dubin L, Amelar RD. Varicocele size and results of varicocelectomy in selected subfertile men with varicocele. Fertil Steril 1979;21(8):606–9.
7. Jarow JP, Ogle SR, Eskew LA. Seminal improvement following repair of ultrasound detected subclinical varicoceles. J Urol 1996;155(4):1287–90.
8. Cervellione RM, Corroppolo M, Bianchi A. Subclinical varicocele in the pediatric age group. J Urol 2008;179(2):717–9.
9. Diamond DA, Paltiel HJ, DiCanzio J, et al. Comparative assessment of pediatric testicular volume: orchidometer verses ultrasound. J Urol 2000;164(3 Pt 2): 1111–4.
10. Khera M, Lipshultz LI. Evolving approach to the varicocele. Urol Clin North Am 2008;35(2):183–9.
11. Fujisawa M, Yoshida S, Matsumoto O, et al. Deoxyribonucleic acid polymerase activity in the testes of infertile men with varicocele. Fertil Steril 1988;50(5): 795–800.
12. Fujisawa M, Yoshida S, Kojima K, et al. Biochemical changes in testicular varicocele. Arch Androl 1989;22(2):149–59.
13. Gorelick JI, Goldstein M. Loss of fertility in men with varicocele. Fertil Steril 1993; 59(3):613–6.
14. Mieusset R, Bujan L. Testicular heating and its possible contributions to male infertility: a review. Int J Androl 1995;18(4):169–84.
15. Simsek D, Turkeri L, Cevik I, et al. Role of apoptosis in testicular tissue damage caused by varicocele. Arch Esp Urol 1998;51(9):947–50.
16. Allamaneni SS, Naughton CK, Sharma RK, et al. Increased seminal reactive oxygen species levels in patients with varicoceles correlate with varicocele grade but not with testis size. Fertil Steril 2004;82(6):1684–6.
17. Khera M, Najari B, Alkul J, et al. The effect of varicocele repair on semen reactive oxygen species activity in infertile men [abstract]. Fertil Steril 2007;88(Suppl 1): S387–8.

18. Abrol N, Panda A, Kekre NS. Painful varicoceles: role of varicocelectomy. Indian J Urol 2014;40(4):359–73.
19. Abdel-Meguid TA, Farsi HM, Al-Sayyad A, et al. Effects of varicocele on serum testosterone and changes of testosterone after varicocelectomy: a prospective controlled study. Urology 2014;84(5):1081–7.
20. Hsiao W, Rosoff JS, Pale JR, et al. Varicocelectomy is associated with increases in serum testosterone independent of clinical grade. Urology 2013;81(6):1213–7.
21. Tanrikut C, Goldstein M, Rosoff JS, et al. Varicocele as a risk factor for androgen deficiency and effect of repair. BJU Int 2011;108(9):1480–4.
22. Male Infertility Best Practice Policy Committee of the American Urological Association, Practice Committee of the American Society for Reproductive Medicine. Report on varicocele and infertility [abstract]. Fertil Steril 2004;82(Suppl):S142–5.
23. Baker M, McGill J, Sharma R, et al. Pregnancy after varicocelectomy: impact of postoperative motility and DFI. Urology 2013;81(4):760–6.
24. Mostafa T, Anis TH, El-Nashar A, et al. Varicocelectomy reduces reactive oxygen species levels and increases antioxidant activity of seminal plasma from infertile men with varicocele. Int J Androl 2001;24(5):261–5.
25. Ohl D, McCarthy JD, Schuster TG. The effect of varicocele on optimized sperm penetration assay [abstract]. Fertil Steril 2007;76:S48.
26. Schatte EC, Hirshberg SJ, Fallick MD, et al. Varicocelectomy improves sperm strict morphology and motility. J Urol 1998;160(4):1338–40.
27. Su LM, Goldstein M, Schlegel PN. The effect of varicocelectomy on serum testosterone levels in interfile men with varicocele. J Urol 1995;154(5):1752–5.
28. Agarwal A, Deepinder F, Cocuzza M, et al. Efficacy of varicocelectomy in improving semen parameters: new meta-analytical approach. Urology 2007;70(3):532–8.
29. Marmar JP, Agarwal A, Prabakaran S, et al. Reassessing the value of varicocelectomy as a treatment for male subfertility with a new meta-analysis. Fertil Steril 2007;88(3):639–48.
30. McIntyre M, Hsieh TC, Lipshultz L. Varicocele repair in the era of modern assisted reproductive techniques. Curr Opin Urol 2012;22(6):517–20.
31. Alukal JP, Zurakowski D, Atala A, et al. Testicular hypotrophy does not correlate with grade of adolescent varicocele. J Urol 2005;174(6):2367–70.
32. Mori MM, Bertolla RP, Fraietta R, et al. Does varicocele grade determine extent of alteration to spermatogenesis in adolescents? Fertil Steril 2008;90(5):1769–73.
33. Kass EJ, Bellman AB. Reversal of testicular growth failure by varicocele ligation. J Urol 1987;137(3):475–6.
34. Costabile RA, Skoog S, Radoqhich M. Testicular volume assessment in the adolescent with a varicocele. J Urol 1992;147(5):1348–50.
35. Kass EJ, Freitas JE, Bour JB. Adolescent varicocele: objective indications for treatment. J Urol 1989;142(2 Pt 2):579–82.
36. Thomas JC, Elder JS. Testicular growth arrest and adolescent varicocele: dose varicocele size make a difference? J Urol 2002;168(4 Pt 2):1689–91.
37. Coutinho K, McLeod D, Stensland K, et al. Variations in the management of asymptomatic adolescent grade 2 or 3 left varicoceles: a survey of practitioners. J Pediatr Urol 2014;10(3):430–4.
38. Kolon TF, Clement MR, Cartwright L, et al. Transient asynchronous testicular growth in adolescent males with a varicocele. J Urol 2008;180(3):1111–4.
39. Korets R, Woldu S, Nees SN, et al. Testicular symmetry and adolescent varicocele – does it need followup? J Urol 2011;186(4 Suppl):1614–9.
40. Poon SA, Gjertson CK, Mercado MA, et al. Testicular asymmetry and adolescent varicoceles managed expectantly. J Urol 2010;183(2):731–4.

41. Diamond DA, Zurakowski D, Bauer SB, et al. Relationship of varicocele grade and testicular hypotrophy to semen parameters in adolescents. J Urol 2007; 178(4 Pt 2):1584–8.

42. Christman MS, Zderic SA, Canning DA, et al. Active surveillance of the adolescent with varicocele: predicting semen outcomes from ultrasound. J Urol 2014; 191(5):1401–6.

43. Christman MS, Zderic SA, Kolon TF. Comparison of semen analyses in youths with a history of cryptorchidism or varicocele. J Urol 2013;190(4 Suppl):1561–6.

44. Nork JJ, Berder JH, Crain DS, et al. Youth varicocele and varicocele treatment: a meta-analysis of semen outcome. Fertil Steril 2014;102(2):381–7.

45. Pastuszak AW, Kuman V, Shah A, et al. Diagnostic and management approaches to pediatric and adolescent varicocele: survey of pediatric urologists. Urology 2014;84(2):450–6.

46. Salzhauer EW, Sokol A, Glassberg K. Paternity after adolescent varicocele repair. Pediatrics 2004;114(6):1631–3.

47. Bogaert G, Oyre C, De Win G. Pubertal screening and treatment for varicocele do not improve chance of paternity as adult. J Urol 2013;189(6):2298–304.

Testis Development and Fertility Potential in Boys with Klinefelter Syndrome

Shanlee M. Davis, MD[a],*, Alan D. Rogol, MD, PhD[b],
Judith L. Ross, MD[c,d]

KEYWORDS

- Testis development • Reproductive options • Klinefelter syndrome
- Testicular function • Spermatogenesis • X-chromosome
- Sex chromosome aneuploidy

KEY POINTS

- Klinefelter syndrome (KS) is common but underdiagnosed; noninvasive prenatal testing may increase the diagnosis rate by 4- to 5-fold, thereby increasing the demand for evidence-based research in the near future.
- Testis development and function are abnormal from infancy and worsen with age; however, the underlying molecular mechanisms for this have not been elucidated.
- Because of a lack of clinical trials, androgen supplementation practices vary between clinicians. Most often, testosterone injections or gel is initiated in midpuberty, when luteinizing hormone increases above the normal range.
- Small numbers of germ cells are present in around half of prepubertal, pubertal, and adults male subjects with KS.
- With testicular sperm extraction, sperm can be obtained for fertilization in around half of the men with KS.

INTRODUCTION

Klinefelter syndrome (KS), defined by one or more extra X chromosomes in male individuals, is the leading genetic cause of primary hypogonadism and infertility.[1,2] The clinical phenotype has expanded beyond the original description of infertility, small

The authors have nothing to disclose. Consultant to: SOV Therapeutics, Trimel Pharmaceuticals, NovoNordisk, Versartis, AbbVie (A.D. Rogol).
[a] Department of Pediatrics, Children's Hospital Colorado, University of Colorado, 13123 East 16th Avenue, B264, Aurora, CO 80045, USA; [b] Department of Pediatrics, University of Virginia, 685 Explorers Road, Charlottesville, VA 22911, USA; [c] Department of Pediatric Endocrinology, A.I. DuPont Hospital for Children, 1600 Rockland Road, Wilmington, DE 19803, USA; [d] Department of Pediatrics, Thomas Jefferson University, 833 Chestnut Street, Philadelphia, PA 19107, USA
* Corresponding author.
E-mail address: Shanlee.Davis@childrenscolorado.org

Endocrinol Metab Clin N Am 44 (2015) 843–865
http://dx.doi.org/10.1016/j.ecl.2015.07.008
0889-8529/15/$ – see front matter © 2015 Elsevier Inc. All rights reserved.

endo.theclinics.com

testes, and gynecomastia.[3] Animal models, epidemiologic studies, and clinical research of male subjects of all ages with KS have allowed the better characterization of the variable phenotype of this condition. Scientific advances have led to fertility potential in about half of men with KS. Despite this, the molecular mechanisms underlying the nearly universal finding of primary gonadal failure remain elusive. If noninvasive prenatal testing becomes part of routine prenatal care as many suggest, the diagnosis of KS will increase by 4- to 5-fold, thereby raising the demand for high-quality, evidence-based research to improve outcomes in boys and men with KS.[4]

EPIDEMIOLOGY

Population-based studies on newborns as well as adjusted prenatal screening rates yield an incidence of KS in ~1 of 650 male newborns.[5–7] Approximately 3075 infants with KS are born in the United States every year.[8] Based on historic data, it is reasonable to assume more than 2000 of those infants will never be diagnosed. These statistics stem from a study in the United Kingdom in the 1990s that reported 10% of boys with KS are diagnosed prenatally, 7% in childhood or adolescence, and another 17% in adulthood, with the remaining 66% of individuals with KS never receiving a diagnosis.[9] As expected, the reasons for diagnosis depend on age, with developmental and behavioral concerns more common in younger children, pubertal delay in adolescence, and infertility in adulthood.[10] Diagnosis rates likely vary based on time period and geography and therefore may be different in the United States in 2015 than it was in Europe 20 years ago. It is also very probable that prenatal diagnoses will increase in the near future because of the increased utilization of noninvasive prenatal testing that can screen for fetal aneuploidy with a simple maternal blood sample.[4] The actual incidence of KS may be increasing as well because of rising maternal age correlating with the risk for nondisjunction errors during meiosis, resulting in fetal aneuploidy.[5,11,12] In fact, the most recent epidemiologic study found the prevalence of KS to be 1 in 448 male births, along with an overall higher rate of lifetime diagnosis of 50%.[13]

CLINICAL FEATURES

Hypergonadotropic hypogonadism and infertility are nearly universal in adult men with KS.[14] These features together with tall stature, eunuchoid body habitus, and gynecomastia define the cardinal findings described in the earliest literature on KS.[3] For most affected men and boys, manifestations are subtle and nonspecific, therefore falling below the threshold of clinical suspicion, particularly in childhood and early adolescence. Studies consistently report a higher prevalence of type 2 diabetes mellitus, dyslipidemia, fatty liver disease, hypercoagulability, and osteoporosis in adults, with evidence the metabolic dysfunction begins in childhood or adolescence.[10,15–19] Neurodevelopmental, behavioral, and psychosocial deficits are reported throughout the lifespan.[18–21] Toddlers with KS are at risk for motor and language developmental delays, while learning disabilities, internalizing and externalizing behaviors, and social difficulties may arise in school age and beyond.[21–25] Adolescents and adults can struggle with adaptive functioning skills including poor self-care.[26] Cognitive ability is usually in the normal range but lower than sibling controls, and verbal scores are about 10 points lower than performance domains.[27–30] Individuals ascertained by prenatal diagnosis may have fewer neurodevelopmental and psychosocial difficulties than those diagnosed postnatally, highlighting the importance of accounting for selection bias in research studies.[31] Although 80% to 90% of male subjects with KS have a nonmosaic 47,XXY karyotype, a smaller percentage will have mosaicism that is often associated with a milder phenotype, or alternatively, have more than one extra sex chromosome

(48,XXYY, 48,XXXY, 49,XXXXY, 49,XXXYY), generally conferring a more severe phenotype.[32–35]

PATHOPHYSIOLOGY

The phenotypic heterogeneity in male subjects with KS is likely influenced by genetic, epigenetic, and environmental factors. Furthermore, given the universal testicular dysfunction in KS, it is difficult to determine what clinical features are due to hypogonadism and therefore modifiable by androgen supplementation, and what clinical features are manifestations of the aneuploidy itself. In adult men with KS, the presence of physical features, such as higher body fat percentage, type 2 diabetes, decreased left temporal lobe gray matter, and autoimmune disease, correlate with degree of hypogonadism or lack of androgen supplementation; however, these associations do not indicate causality.[18,36–39] Randomized controlled trials investigating androgen replacement in adults with KS have not been done, although several randomized controlled trials in children with KS are underway or recently completed.[40–42] In the KS mouse model, replacement of testosterone improves psychosocial dysfunction but not osteopenia or metabolic dysfunction.[43,44] More research is needed to understand the pathophysiology of the multiple phenotypic features associated with KS.

With the genetic basis for KS, based on an extra X chromosome, most of the focus is the more than 1000 genes on the X chromosome that influence gonadal development, growth, and brain development. It is logical to assume the KS phenotype is secondary to a gene-dosage effect of extra genetic material on the X chromosome that escapes X-inactivation or polymorphisms of specific genes on the X chromosomes, such as the trinucleotide repeat length of the androgen receptor gene.[36,45–47] However, the complexity increases as gene expression on autosomes seems to be influenced by the presence of an extra X chromosome. In a microarray gene expression analysis in the lymphocytes of 10 male subjects, half with 47,XXY, 480 autosomal genes were upregulated in male subjects with KS and more than 200 were downregulated.[48] Similar findings were found in testis transcriptome analysis with significant deregulation of gene expression in Sertoli and Leydig cells as well as germ cells.[49] Tissue-specific differences in autosomal DNA methylation and gene expression were identified in the postmortem brain of a male subject with 47,XXY, including the gene SPAG1 (sperm associated antigen 1) on the long arm of chromosome 8 that codes for a protein thought to be essential for signal transduction pathways in spermatogenesis.[50,51] Differential gene expression of 35 genes correlated with clinical findings of insulin resistance, dyslipidemia, and coagulability.[52] Therefore, aneuploidy itself may result in epigenetic modulation of autosomal genes in a tissue-specific manner, contributing to the complexity in KS pathophysiology. As the knowledge of genetics and epigenetics advances, a better understanding will be gained of the underlying molecular mechanisms yielding gonadal failure as well as the other clinical features commonly found in men with this syndrome.

TESTICULAR DEVELOPMENT, FUNCTION, AND PATHOLOGY

Case series and observational studies at various ages shed light on the natural history of testicular changes throughout the lifespan in individuals with KS. Although it is clear the supernumerary X chromosome is the underlying cause of testicular failure, the molecular mechanisms by which this occurs have not been fully elucidated. Although eventual germ cell failure is evident, it remains unknown whether the germ cells have a primary defect or germ cell maturation is disrupted due to an abnormal gonadal milieu. Future investigation aimed at elucidating the underlying mechanisms will ultimately help develop measures to preserve testicular function.

The authors have synthesized the currently available literature on testicular development in male subjects with KS, including testis size, histologic findings, and serologic gonadal function biomarkers in **Table 1**. Much of the knowledge is based on evidence of marginal quality with small sample sizes, participant selection bias, and poor hormone assay quality. Many reports have been retrospective case series with significant interstudy and even intrastudy methodologic variability, limiting both the comparability and the generalizability of the findings.

Fetal

The increased incidence of underdeveloped genitalia and cryptorchidism increase the concern for fetal androgen insufficiency, particularly during the second or third trimester.[14,53,54] Examinations of testes in second-trimester fetuses with KS have had variable findings with approximately half reporting reduced germ cell numbers and half with normal histology.[55–61] Testosterone concentrations in amniotic fluid have been examined in 6 studies, with 4 of the 6 reporting no differences in total testosterone concentrations between male fetuses with 47,XXY (total n = 33) and 46,XY.[60,62–66] In the largest of these studies, 2 of the 20 subjects with 47,XXY had testosterone levels in the female range; therefore, there may be a minority of male subjects with KS who have a defect in testosterone production in utero.[62] Testosterone levels in cord blood have been reported to be low (n = 3) compared with controls (n = 3); however, this is far too small a sample size from which to draw conclusions.[67] None of these studies measured testosterone concentrations by liquid chromatography mass spectrometry, a method that has increased sensitivity and accuracy compared with older methods, particularly with testosterone concentrations less than 100 ng/dL ($\sim$3.5 mmol/L).[68] There have not been any studies examining other biomarkers of testicular function, such as products of Sertoli cells or insulin-like peptide 3 (INSL3), a hormone produced by Leydig cells and critical for testicular descent.[69] At this time, there is insufficient evidence to determine if hypogonadism is present in the fetus with KS.

Infancy

Penile growth in the first months of life has been considered a biomarker for androgen exposure during the neonatal surge or mini-puberty of infancy.[70] Slow penile growth in the first year of life in boys with KS provides clinical evidence to support relative androgen deficiency in infancy.[70–72] Hypotonia, although certainly not specific for androgen deficiency, is frequently observed in infants with KS.[73] Testes are often small in infancy.[46,73,74] Testicular biopsies have shown a lower number of spermatogonia in all case reports that included quantitative analysis; however, the histologic appearance of Sertoli and Leydig cells was typically normal.[75–79] Five studies report testosterone levels during the mini-puberty period of infancy, all concluding activation of the pituitary-gonadal axis does occur in infants with KS.[73–75,80,81] Three of these (total n = 68) report lower median testosterone levels in KS, whereas the other 2 (total n = 16) found normal or even high-normal testosterone levels. The single study that assessed testosterone concentrations with liquid chromatography/tandem mass spectrometry reported 87% of 38 infants with KS 16 to 120 days of life were less than the median for controls and $\sim$20% decreased below the normal range.[80] Given the variability of the timing and peak of postnatal testosterone levels in normal infant boys and the cross-sectional design of most of these studies in boys with KS, it is very difficult to determine if subtle deficits in the hypothalamic-pituitary-gonadal

Table 1
Summary and synthesis of primary literature on testicular development in Klinefelter syndrome

Testicular Volume	Histology	Leydig Cell Biomarkers	Sertoli Cell Biomarkers
Fetal			
No studies	*Quality:* Poor, ~6 case reports only *Summary:* Approximately half of the case reports conclude reduced germ cell number[55–61] *Conclusion:* Reduced germ cell numbers may be present in some boys with KS before birth	*Quality:* Marginal, 6 studies, total 33 subjects *Summary:* Mean total testosterone (TT) was normal; however, TT was in the female range for 4/33 (12%) *Conclusion:* Amniotic TT is normal for majority, but a deficit in T production may be present in a subset (10%–20%)	No studies
Infancy			
Quality: Marginal, testicular volume mentioned, but usually not compared with controls *Summary:* Older studies generally report normal testes size at birth with lack of enlargement.[79] Two studies found lower testicular volumes than expected in infants (SDS -1.1)[46,75] *Conclusion:* Testicular volume may be normal at birth with less growth over the first year	*Quality:* Poor, <10 case reports/series in infants <12 mo *Summary:* Most with normal appearance but quantitatively fewer germ cells. Germ cells inversely correlate with age *Conclusion:* Although support cells appear normal, germ cell depletion is already present in infancy and is possibly progressive	*Quality:* Adequate, 5 total studies with 83 subjects *Summary:* TT lower than expected in 3 of 5 studies (n = 67),[73,80,81] normal in one (n = 6),[79] and high-normal in another (n = 10).[75] LH normal in all. INSL3 normal in one *Conclusion:* Most likely subnormal serum TT during mini-puberty in most infants with KS	*Quality:* Marginal, 3 studies with N ~ 90 *Summary:* FSH, AMH, and INHB usually within the normal ranges.[81,84] INHB low in ~20% in one study, few boys with high AMH[80] *Conclusion:* Potentially Sertoli cell dysfunction in a subset (<20%)

(continued on next page)

Table 1
(continued)

Testicular Volume	Histology	Leydig Cell Biomarkers	Sertoli Cell Biomarkers
Childhood			
Quality: Adequate, reported in many studies *Summary:* Multiple studies report small testes in most boys; often <1 mL,[10,71,92,150] mean, −1.2 SDS[46,85] *Conclusion:* Testes are smaller prepubertally	*Quality:* Marginal, case reports or series, N ~ 20, +selection bias *Summary:* Fewer germ cells in all,[76,87,90] number inversely correlates with age[86], no germ cells were found in a case series including cryptorchidism.[76] Seminiferous tubules smaller,[87] Leydig and Sertoli cells normal, but interstitial fibrosis and hyalinization occurs in boys nearing puberty[90] *Conclusion:* Depletion of germ cells occurs throughout childhood; degenerative changes in support cells may be beginning	*Quality:* Marginal, many studies report but assays poor. N ~ 200 *Summary:* Most studies report LH and TT in normal prepubertal range.[10,91] With improved assays, TT is reported in the bottom quartile in majority[85], LH to TT ratio is elevated[14], possibly a low TT peak following stimulation.[92] INSL3 is reported as normal (n = 9)[93] *Conclusion:* Mild defects in Leydig cells may be present but difficult to assess prepubertally	*Quality:* Marginal, few studies, N ~ 125 *Summary:* Small studies report INHB and AMH as normal.[10,88,90] Larger study found low INHB in ~1/3 and abnormal AMH (high in ~25%, low in 13%)[40] *Conclusion:* Sertoli cell dysfunction may be present in a subset of boys
Puberty			
Quality: Adequate to excellent, many studies with various comparisons *Summary:* Enlargement in early puberty to max. range 3–10 mL,[92] size plateaus midpuberty and then decreases to ~3 mL in T4-5 PH.[92] Even in early puberty, testicular size smaller than expected for degree of virilization[150] *Conclusion:* Testes enlarge to pubertal size in most. Peak testicular size is variable but typically no more than ~8 mL before decreasing to 3–5 mL in most by late puberty	*Quality:* Adequate, case reports and cross-sectional studies *Summary:* 2 studies, only 6/15 boys in puberty had germ cells in biopsy; none with spermatids.[90,133] Leydig cell hyperplasia in 9/15, fibrosis of the tubules in 15/15 Sertoli cell degeneration in 6/8[90] *Conclusion:* Spermatogenesis is altered in all boys with KS; testicular support cells seem to become abnormal as puberty is initiated, and fibrosis likely progresses with puberty	*Quality:* Adequate, many cross-sectional and several longitudinal studies. Variability in TT assays *Summary:* Median LH elevates by 13–14 y[10,92] and/or T3 PH.[88] TT increases possibly even faster/higher than controls and then plateaus[92] and can decline. ~25% have low TT.[10] LH to TT ratio nearly always high.[88] INSL3 is similar to controls until age 13, then plateaus rather than increasing (n = 14)[93] *Conclusion:* Most boys with KS will have evidence of Leydig cell insufficiency by mid to late puberty	*Quality:* Marginal, several cross-sectional but rare longitudinal studies. Total N ~ 100. Assay variation *Summary:* Median FSH elevates by 12–13 y[10,93] and/or T2-3 PH.[88,92] FSH correlates with age.[10] INHB does not increase as expected in puberty,[97] then decreases below normal range within a year of pubertal onset.[97] Delayed decline of AMH in early puberty[84,151] *Conclusion:* Most boys with KS will have abnormal Sertoli cell biomarkers by early to midpuberty

Adulthood

Quality: Excellent, N > 1000, consistent	*Quality:* Excellent, however, ascertainment bias may be present	*Quality:* Adequate to excellent	*Quality:* Adequate
Summary: Smaller than controls in all,[10] mean volume 3–3.5 mL, range 1–8 mL[10,14]	*Summary:* Sertoli cell only picture most common, scarce patchy areas of germ cells with active spermatogenesis in some (around 50%).[123] Immature and degenerative Sertoli cells, hyalinization of the tubules and Leydig cell hyperplasia[86]	*Summary:* LH elevated in 83%–96%.[10,14] TT below normal in ~50%, lower half of normal in the rest. TT declines with age.[10] INSL3 is often low	*Summary:* FSH elevated in all[10,84,88]; however, degree of elevation does not predict success or failure of TESE. AMH < −2 SD in 85%.[84] INHB below the lower limit of normal or undetectable in all[97]
Conclusions: Adult men with 47,XXY universally have small testes	*Conclusions:* Germ cells are absent or rare; Sertoli and Leydig cells are abnormal, although normal patches may be present	*Conclusion:* Most will have Leydig cell dysfunction; however may be mild in a subset	*Conclusion:* Biomarkers of Sertoli cell function (and germ cells) are nearly universally low in men with KS

Abbreviations: N, total number of subjects in the combined studies; PH, pubic hair; SDS, standard deviation score; T1-5, Tanner stage 1–5.

axis are present in some or all infant boys with KS.[82,83] The 3 studies that reported lower testosterone levels also reported normal luteinizing hormone (LH) levels, potentially raising the question of whether there is some degree of a central pituitary/hypothalamic defect as well as primary hypogonadism. The most recent of these studies reported INSL-3 levels within the normal range.[80]

Biomarkers of Sertoli cell function, including anti-mullerian hormone (AMH) and inhibin B (INHB), are broadly within normal ranges; however, Sertoli cell dysfunction may be present in some infants with KS.[80,81,84] In a study of 68 boys with KS less than the age of 2 years, INHB was lower than the lower limit of normal in ~20%, whereas AMH was occasionally elevated in others.[80] Follicle stimulating hormone (FSH) levels were elevated in 25%, although these were not the individuals that had low INHB levels. Overall, there is insufficient evidence to determine if hypogonadism occurs in infants with KS.

Prepubertal Childhood

Testicular volumes are small, often 1 mL or less, in prepubertal boys with KS.[46,71,73,85] Histologically, germ cell hypoplasia is appreciated, whereas Leydig and Sertoli cells typically appear normal.[76,86,87] Childhood is typically considered the quiescent period of the hypothalamic-pituitary-gonadal axis development.[83] Baseline gonadotropin concentrations as well as stimulation testing with gonadotropin-releasing hormone are described as normal in most studies of prepubertal boys with KS.[79,85,88] The authors have found a small but potentially significant number of boys with elevated gonadotropins for age (LH elevated in 7%, FSH elevated in 10%) in a large sample of 86 boys with KS, 4 to 11 years of age.[40] Serum testosterone concentrations in prepubertal boys with KS are within the normal range for age; however, the majority are in the bottom quartile.[72,85] It is also imperative to note that normal prepubertal hormone concentrations can be lower than the detection limit for many assays, and testosterone radioimmunoassays in particular will overestimate the testosterone concentrations in children.[68] Sertoli cells make up most of the volume of the testes at this age, producing AMH and INHB even during this quiescent period.[89] In KS, small studies have found these biomarkers of Sertoli cell function to be within the normal limits for age most often; however, a few boys with either low INHB or high AMH have been reported.[85,88,90] In a much larger sample of nearly 90 boys with KS, the authors have found a subset who have very low concentrations of AMH or low INHB (~30%), whereas a quarter of subjects had rather elevated levels of AMH.[40] This finding raises the suspicion for Sertoli cell dysfunction and, in addition to germ cell depletion, starting before external signs of puberty in boys with KS. However, it is difficult to conclude whether Leydig cell dysfunction, in particular, defective testosterone production, is present in childhood.

Puberty

Boys with KS in early puberty often have initial enlargement of testes to 6 to 8 mL, an increase in gonadotropins and testosterone to a pubertal range, and development of primary and secondary sex characteristics.[10,14,79,88,91,92] In midpuberty, FSH increases and Sertoli cell biomarkers decline—often to undetectable levels—and testicular volumes decrease. In mid to late puberty, LH typically increases to greater than the normal range, and testosterone declines to low or low-normal for pubertal stage. In one study of 6 subjects followed longitudinally, INSL3 increased to low adult concentrations by a bone age of 12 to 13 years and then plateaued for the next 2 years, although the ratio of INSL3 to LH was much lower than healthy male subjects.[93] Histologic evidence reveals near-absence of germ cells even in early puberty, and structurally abnormal support cells in half.[90] Clinical symptoms of hypogonadism at this age can include incomplete pubertal maturation, persistent pubertal (physiologic) gynecomastia, and relatively tall stature.[14]

There is some evidence to suggest AMH declines more slowly during the peripubertal period in KS compared with XY male subjects.[84] AMH is inversely related to intratesticular testosterone concentration as AMH gene transcription is downregulated in the presence of testosterone binding the androgen receptor on the Sertoli cell.[94] An elevated AMH would therefore be consistent with lower intratesticular testosterone concentration, although intratesticular hormone concentrations in adolescents have not been reported. More studies on serum testicular function biomarkers in boys in early puberty may help to clarify this because it is possible these markers could predict the timing of gonadal failure or future fertility potential. Overall, there is strong evidence to support hypogonadism with germ cells, Sertoli cells, and Leydig cells all being dysfunctional in most boys with KS from midpuberty onward.

Adulthood

Unequivocal testicular dysfunction is observed in adults with KS. Testes are often even smaller than during puberty, and testicular histology typically reveals the absence of germ cells (often a Sertoli-cell only picture), fibrosis and hyalinization of the seminiferous tubules, and Leydig cell hyperplasia.[14,71,95,96] FSH is universally elevated; LH is elevated in the great majority.[10] INHB is usually less than the normal range, whereas AMH is often undetectable.[84,97] Testosterone concentration may be low or low-normal.[10] INSL3, another product of Leydig cells critical for testicular descent and likely germ cell maturation and bone health, is also low.[98]

Intratesticular hormone concentrations have not been thoroughly investigated. Although low intratesticular testosterone would be suspected, a recent study found normal to elevated intratesticular testosterone in biopsies in men with KS.[99] These investigators postulate an abnormal intratesticular vascular bed leading to inadequate secretion of testosterone systemically. Better understanding of the intratesticular hormonal milieu during the critical time of puberty may permit the development of targeted treatments to prevent the degeneration of germ cells, androgen deficiency, and infertility.

MEDICAL MANAGEMENT

Management of patients with KS will involve routine physical examinations, ongoing evaluation for known clinical conditions associated with KS including developmental assessments, and potential androgen supplementation initiated in adolescence. If the diagnosis was made prenatally, a postnatal confirmation of the karyotype should be obtained. For this purpose and for any suspected KS diagnosis, routine chromosome analysis is sufficient, although high-resolution chromosome analysis, fluorescence in situ hybridization for X and Y chromosomes, and comparative genomic hybridization microarray would also reveal the diagnosis.

Infancy

Initial consultation with a pediatric endocrinologist is very important in this interval for reviewing testicular function and the role of androgen replacement with the family. Despite very little published data of prepubertal androgen treatment in infants with KS, the authors have found up to 1 in 5 boys with KS receive androgen treatment in infancy or early childhood.[40] Some of these infants will receive a short course of either intramuscular or topical testosterone for the indication of micropenis. Other clinicians have suggested testosterone treatment should be considered standard of care in infancy,[100] although no therapeutic benefits have been clearly delineated aside from penile growth. There is minimal published data exploring benefits of testosterone in infancy. A recent retrospective study reported higher scores on standardized developmental assessments in multiple cognitive domains at 3 and 6 years of age in boys who had received a short course of testosterone.[101] The retrospective study design, which lacked blinding, randomization, or a delineated protocol, significantly limits generalizability of these findings. A randomized trial of intramuscular testosterone during the mini-puberty period has just started enrollment at Children's Hospital Colorado (NCT#02408445, Principle Investigator (PI): SD).

Some clinicians recommend measuring testosterone, LH, and FSH during the neonatal surge; however, the clinical utility of this information has not been established. Even among 46,XY male subjects, the mini-puberty period is variable with regard to peak hormone concentrations and timing; therefore, these data are not useful in providing evidence-based management decisions or prognostic assessments at this time.[82,102,103] It is quite possible a normal surge may have favorable prognostic implications, such as a milder phenotype, less hypogonadism, or improved fertility potential; however, this has never been reported.

Childhood

The focus during the childhood years should be on educational and psychosocial development needs. There are no published randomized controlled trials of androgen supplementation in prepubertal boys with KS to date. A randomized controlled trial of oral oxandrolone administration in boys 4 to 12 years (NCT#00348946, PI: JR) was recently completed, and published results are anticipated shortly. At this time, there is no clinical indication for androgen treatment in prepubertal boys with KS.

Puberty

At the first sign of puberty or around the age of 10 to 12, boys warrant evaluation by a pediatric endocrinologist. Pubertal progression and growth should be monitored closely, and gonadotropin and testosterone concentrations should be obtained at least annually during this time. Elevated gonadotropin concentrations or plateau of serum testosterone can be seen as puberty progresses and are important in determining when supplemental testosterone is warranted. Signs of relative hypogonadism, such as poor muscle mass, persistent gynecomastia, and stalled virilization, should be assessed. If the patient is obese or on antipsychotic medications, routine laboratory tests to screen for comorbidities should be performed every 2 years according to expert guidelines, including cholesterol levels, hemoglobin A1C (or fasting glucose), and liver function tests.[104,105] The authors recommend these screening tests also be performed in boys with KS and a normal body mass index (BMI) as well, because studies report greater visceral adiposity and a higher risk of these dysmetabolic conditions in all children and adolescents with KS.[15,16] Specifically, elevated low-density lipoprotein cholesterol was observed in 37% and insulin resistance in 24% of prepubertal boys with KS, despite BMI not differing from controls.[15] Although these abnormalities did not reach a threshold necessitating pharmacologic therapy, lifestyle modification, particularly with increased physical activity, would be beneficial and therefore screening around the time of puberty is reasonable and appropriate. There are no data to support the routine measurement of bone density in children or adolescents because bone mineral density has been described as normal.[16]

Because of a lack of definitive research, initiation of testosterone therapy in young adolescents with KS is predominantly clinician-preference. This decision is often based on progression of pubertal development, evolution of hypergonadotropic hypogonadism, development of physical symptoms of androgen deficiency such as persistent gynecomastia, and family preference. A randomized clinical trial of topical testosterone versus placebo in male subjects with KS in early puberty (NCT#01585831) examining psychosocial outcome measures is currently enrolling. When testosterone therapy is initiated, the favored options include intramuscular injections of a testosterone ester or transdermal testosterone gel.[106] Ongoing growth potential can be assessed with a bone age radiograph. A reasonable approach is to start at low doses (100 mg intramuscular injection every 4 weeks or 1 pump per day of 1% or 1.62% testosterone gel) and titrate up until clinical symptoms of hypogonadism improve and serum testosterone concentration is appropriate for stage of pubertal development. Testosterone formulations that have a prolonged duration of action or higher doses are not recommended in adolescents.

Adults

Recommendations for evaluation in adult men with KS include annual measurement of fasting glucose, lipids, hemoglobin A1c, thyroid function tests, and hematocrit as well as intermittent bone density measurement by dual-energy radiograph absorptiometry.[107,108] An interdisciplinary panel from France also recommended baseline and chest radiographs every 2 years, testes and breast ultrasonography, and echocardiography.[107] Research on the cost-effectiveness of these consensus recommendations has been limited.

Untreated adults with KS often will meet criteria for male hypogonadism, defined as a serum testosterone less than 300 ng/dL with clinical symptoms. The Endocrine Society Clinical Practice Guidelines advises on the treatment of male hypogonadism, including KS.[109] Multiple formulations of testosterone are available and outlined in **Table 2**.

Exogenous testosterone can suppress LH, thereby reducing spermatogenesis and potentially decreasing fertility potential.[110] Although high-dose testosterone has the capability to be used as a male birth control method, the antispermatogenic effects are assumed to be temporary.[111,112] Some studies have found less successful sperm retrieval rates in men with KS who have previously been on testosterone treatment, whereas other, more recent studies have found no such association.[113–115] Although there is a lack of randomized controlled trials, the probable benefits of testosterone therapy include positive effects on body composition, bone health, and psychological well-being.[116–119] Overall, these treatment advantages are more convincing than the theoretic risk of fertility decline, particularly with advances in reproductive endocrinology and assisted reproductive technology (ART).

FERTILITY AND REPRODUCTION

The most common reproductive abnormality in KS is nonobstructive azoospermia (NOA), and approximately 11% of men with NOA will have KS.[10,120] In select populations, the ejaculate may contain motile sperm in up to 10% of men with KS; therefore, birth control is advised if fertility is not desired.[35,90,121] However, spontaneous pregnancies are rare and, without ART, men with KS are nearly always infertile.[95] With recent advances of reproductive medicine, sperm can be retrieved via surgical testicular sperm extraction (TESE) in around 50% of men seeking biological fertility.[113,114,122–125] These success rates are similar to men with NOA from other causes.[95,125] Retrieved sperm, either from ejaculate or from TESE, are either used to fertilize an oocyte via intracytoplasmic sperm injection (ICSI) or cryopreserved for

Table 2
Testosterone formulations

Formulation	Adult Regimen	Pharmacokinetic Profile	Advantages	Disadvantages	Adolescent Use
T Cypionate or enanthate 200 mg/mL	150–200 mg intramuscularly (IM) every 2 wk or 75–100 mg/wk	Serum T peaks after the injection, then gradually declines by the end of the dosing interval	Inexpensive, flexibility in dosing	Requires IM injection; peaks and valleys in serum T	Yes, preferred method when small doses are desired
T Gel (1%, 1.62%, 2%)	5–10 g daily	Stable levels of serum T can be attained in the range desired. Transdermal absorption may vary	Ease of application, minimizes variability in serum T	Potential skin-to-skin transfer; skin irritation; daily application	Yes, typically start at 1 pump/d and titrate
Transdermal T patch	5–10 mg Daily (1–2 patches)	Stable levels of serum T can be attained in the range desired. Transdermal absorption may vary	Ease of application	Skin irritation (more frequent), daily application	Possibly. Lowest dose may be too high for many. Not well tolerated
Buccal bioadhesive T tablets	30 mg Controlled release, twice daily	Stable levels of serum T can be attained in the range desired. Absorbed from the buccal mucosa	More rapid metabolism, no transfer	Twice daily administration; buccal irritation	No
T Pellets	3–6 subcutaneous implanted pellets	Serum T peaks at 1 mo, then sustained for 3–6 mo	Eliminates daily administration, stable levels	Requires surgical incision; pellets may extrude; dose cannot be titrated	No
T Nasal gel	11 mg Nasally 3 times daily	Very quick peak and then trough	Ease of application and no transfer to others	Three times daily administration	No
T Undecanoate	750 mg IM every 10 wk	Very stable levels after loading doses	Stable long-term levels avoiding peaks and troughs	Large (3 mL) volume injection; fat pulmonary emboli	No

Adapted from Bhasin S, Cunningham GR, Hayes FJ, et al. Testosterone therapy in men with androgen deficiency syndromes: an Endocrine Society clinical practice guideline. J Clin Endocrinol Metab 2010;95(6):2547.

future ICSI.[124,126] This technology has significantly expanded the options for parenthood for men with KS beyond sperm donation and adoption; however, it is often limited to those with access to large referral centers and monetary resources.

The sperm retrieval success may be increased with the use of micro-TESE, a technique that uses 20 to 25 times magnification to identify larger seminiferous tubules that are more likely to contain active spermatogenesis.[127,128] It is hypothesized that these active spermatogenic foci represent germ cell mosaicism with 46,XY karyotype, potentially representing trisomy rescue during meiosis.[96,123] Micro-TESE may have fewer complications than standard TESE including risk for hematoma and postsurgical hypoandrogenism.[129]

Efforts to identify a consistent predictor for successful sperm extraction have not been fruitful. Testes size, serum hormone concentrations, physical signs of androgenization, age, and history of exogenous testosterone treatment have all been proposed, but have largely failed to differentiate the ~50% of men who will have successful sperm retrieval with TESE.[130,131] Several studies have found greater success rates in sperm retrieval for younger men with KS, which conceptually makes sense, given the progressive decline in spermatogonia number described with age in men with KS.[114,132] Therefore, sperm cryopreservation as early as adolescence has been advocated, potentially even in early puberty before decline in INHB and increase in FSH.[122,133] However, spermatozoa were not found in the ejaculate of 13 adolescent boys with KS,[134] and testicular biopsies in adolescent male subjects have found similar number of spermatogonia to those found in adults with even fewer spermatids.[90,133] Furthermore, several studies have not found age to be a factor in sperm retrieval from TESE, including a recent study where adult men aged 25 to 36 had the same rates of success with TESE as men aged 15 to 24 years.[113] Younger men are also not seeking immediate fertility, therefore requiring cryopreservation, which may yield lower fertilization and pregnancy rates compared with using fresh sperm.[135] Given these findings, along with the high cost of sperm cryopreservation and ethical issues involved in using invasive means to obtain sperm in a minor, it seems most reasonable to wait until the individual with KS is at an age where he can evaluate his options available for fertility, if desired, and provide his own consent to undergo ART.

Although most specialists recommend discontinuation of exogenous testosterone, the use of other pharmacologic agents to enhance sperm retrieval success rates for men with KS is investigational.[110,136–138] The 3 most commonly used medications all attempt to increase endogenous testosterone production, with the premise that higher intratesticular concentration will stimulate spermatogenesis.[137] The first, human chorionic gonadotropin, stimulates Leydig cells by binding to the LH receptor, thereby increasing testosterone production if the Leydig cell is at least partially functional.[137,139] This medication is currently the only US Food and Drug Association-approved medication for male infertility; however, no studies specifically in KS-related infertility have been done. Clomiphene citrate is a selective estrogen receptor modulator that blocks the negative feedback at the level of the hypothalamus and pituitary, thus increasing both LH and FSH secretion.[137,140] Reports of its use in KS date back to the 1970s, although the efficacy of clomiphene has not been proven in KS or men with Sertoli-cell-only morphology.[138,141] Finally, aromatase inhibitors increase the testosterone to estradiol (T/E2) ratio by inhibiting the conversion of testosterone to estrogen, thereby improving spermatogenesis by decreasing the negative inhibition of estrogen and stimulating FSH secretion as well as increasing testosterone levels.[137] Aromatase inhibitors increase sperm volume, sperm concentration, and motility index in men with subfertility and a low T/E2 ratio (<10:1) in a nonrandomized uncontrolled study; however, results were less impressive in a KS subanalysis.[142–144] One study of male subjects with KS and NOA who were treated with one of the above pharmacologic agents when baseline serum testosterone was less than 300 ng/dL found response to treatment (increase in serum testosterone) to be predictive of successful micro-TESE.[114] Others have shown comparable success rates without pretreatment with these pharmacologic agents.[113] Algorithms have been proposed to help aid in determining which pharmacologic agents, if any, should be used before TESE; however, the evidence base is largely limited to a single institution.[114,145]

Most offspring of men with KS are born with a normal karyotype[95]; however, research has demonstrated high rates of aneuploidy from 7% to 46% in spermatids of men with KS.[123,146,147] One hypothesis for this increased risk of aneuploidy is 47,XXY spermatogonia progress through meiosis, yielding hyperhaploid spermatozoa (24,XX and 24,XY).[123] Another potentially more probable hypothesis is that the germ cells that successfully progress through spermatogenesis are predominantly 46,XY; however, the surrounding testicular environment remains unfavorable and increases susceptibility of meiotic abnormalities.[96,148] This finding is consistent with findings of increased risk of autosomal aneuploidy (trisomy 21 and 18) as well as sex chromosome aneuploidy.[147] The routine use of preimplantation genetic diagnosis of embryos fertilized by sperm from men with KS has been proposed; however, this remains an area of debate.[146,147]

In summary, men with KS seeking biological paternity today are no longer considered universally infertile. Various successful approaches for obtaining sperm have been described, including first morning urine (rarely successful),[79,149] ejaculation (up to 10%),[35,121] and TESE (around 50%).[95,114] Typically, the least invasive approaches are attempted first followed by surgical options. Mature sperm can either be used immediately for ICSI or alternatively cryopreserved for future use. Presently, cryopreservation of immature germ cells for the future hope of in vitro differentiation is experimental.

FUTURE CONSIDERATIONS/SUMMARY

A great deal has been learned in the past 70 years since the initial recognition of KS; however, the understanding of the underlying pathophysiology as well as prevention or treatment of manifestations associated with the XXY karyotype is still remarkably limited. The greatest advances for men with KS have arguably been in reproductive endocrinology and ART. Less than 2 decades ago, men with KS were nearly invariably infertile, and now assisted fertility may be successful in half of men seeking to have a biological child. This technology will likely continue to advance rapidly, and it is difficult to predict the possibilities that will exist when the infants born today seek assisted fertility two to three decades from now. If future advances continue to require germ cells for fertilization, it will be prudent to understand the molecular mechanisms involved in germ cell apoptosis in general and in specific for men with KS permitting the exploration and implementation of preventative interventions. Research advances may make it possible to derive sperm from somatic cells; therefore, preservation of germ cells may be unnecessary.

A less distant future consideration is the increased diagnosis rate of KS. There is currently active discussion to make noninvasive prenatal testing part of routine prenatal care independent of maternal age or risk factors.[4] Presuming positive screens for sex chromosome aneuploidy will be followed up with a diagnostic test via amniocentesis or postnatal karyotype, this change in practice would likely increase the number of infants diagnosed with KS by 10-fold. Thousands of parents and health care providers alike will be seeking evidence-based information on sex chromosome aneuploidies, both natural history and intervention to prevent common manifestations. As a research community, we need to focus efforts on patient-centered research outcomes, including predicting phenotypic variation and developing interventions to prevent the unwanted manifestations of KS, with the ultimate goal of helping millions of boys and men with KS worldwide live healthy, normal lives.

REFERENCES

1. Gudeman SR, Townsend B, Fischer K, et al. Etiology of azoospermia in a military population. J Urol 2015;193:1318–21.
2. Nakamura Y, Kitamura M, Nishimura K, et al. Chromosomal variants among 1790 infertile men. Int J Urol 2001;8(2):49–52.
3. Klinefelter HF, Reifenstein EC, Albright F. Syndrome characterized by gynecomastia, aspermatogenesis without aleydigism, and increased excretion of follicle-stimulating hormone. J Clin Endocrinol 1942;2:615–27.
4. Lo JO, Cori DF, Norton ME, et al. Noninvasive prenatal testing. Obstet Gynecol Surv 2014;69(2):89–99.
5. Bojesen A, Juul S, Gravholt CH. Prenatal and postnatal prevalence of Klinefelter syndrome: a national registry study. J Clin Endocrinol Metab 2003;88(2):622–6.
6. Coffee B, Keith K, Albizua I, et al. Incidence of fragile X syndrome by newborn screening for methylated FMR1 DNA. Am J Hum Genet 2009;85(4):503–14.
7. Nielsen J, Wohlert M. Sex chromosome abnormalities found among 34,910 newborn children: results from a 13-year incidence study in Arhus, Denmark. Birth Defects Orig Artic Ser 1990;26(4):209–23.
8. Martin J, Hamilton B, Osterman M, et al. Births: final data for 2013. Natl Vital Stat Rep 2015;64(1):1–65.
9. Abramsky L, Chapple J. 47,XXY (Klinefelter syndrome) and 47,XYY: estimated rates of and indication for postnatal diagnosis with implications for prenatal counselling. Prenat Diagn 1997;17(4):363–8.
10. Pacenza N, Pasqualini T, Gottlieb S, et al. Clinical presentation of Klinefelter's syndrome: differences according to age. Int J Endocrinol 2012;2012:324835.
11. Ferguson-Smith MA, Yates JR. Maternal age specific rates for chromosome aberrations and factors influencing them: report of a collaborative european study on 52 965 amniocenteses. Prenat Diagn 1984;4(Spec No):5–44.
12. Carothers AD, Filippi G. Klinefelter's syndrome in Sardinia and Scotland. Comparative studies of parental age and other aetiological factors in 47,XXY. Hum Genet 1988;81(1):71–5.
13. Herlihy AS, Halliday JL, Cock ML, et al. The prevalence and diagnosis rates of Klinefelter syndrome: an Australian comparison. Med J Aust 2011;194(1):24–8.
14. Aksglaede L, Skakkebaek NE, Almstrup K, et al. Clinical and biological parameters in 166 boys, adolescents and adults with nonmosaic Klinefelter syndrome: a Copenhagen experience. Acta Paediatr 2011;100(6):793–806.
15. Bardsley MZ, Falkner B, Kowal K, et al. Insulin resistance and metabolic syndrome in prepubertal boys with Klinefelter syndrome. Acta Paediatr 2011; 100(6):866–70.
16. Aksglaede L, Molgaard C, Skakkebaek NE, et al. Normal bone mineral content but unfavourable muscle/fat ratio in Klinefelter syndrome. Arch Dis Child 2008; 93(1):30–4.

17. Jiang-Feng M, Hong-Li X, Xue-Yan W, et al. Prevalence and risk factors of diabetes in patients with Klinefelter syndrome: a longitudinal observational study. Fertil Steril 2012;98(5):1331–5.

18. Gravholt CH, Jensen AS, Host C, et al. Body composition, metabolic syndrome and type 2 diabetes in Klinefelter syndrome. Acta Paediatr 2011;100(6):871–7.

19. Bojesen A, Host C, Gravholt CH. Klinefelter's syndrome, type 2 diabetes and the metabolic syndrome: the impact of body composition. Mol Hum Reprod 2010; 16(6):396–401.

20. Swerdlow AJ, Higgins CD, Schoemaker MJ, et al, United Kingdom Clinical Cytogenetics Group. Mortality in patients with Klinefelter syndrome in Britain: a cohort study. J Clin Endocrinol Metab 2005;90(12):6516–22.

21. Ross JL, Roeltgen DP, Stefanatos G, et al. Cognitive and motor development during childhood in boys with Klinefelter syndrome. Am J Med Genet A 2008; 146A(6):708–19.

22. Salbenblatt JA, Meyers DC, Bender BG, et al. Gross and fine motor development in 47,XXY and 47,XYY males. Pediatrics 1987;80(2):240–4.

23. Netley C, Rovet J. Verbal deficits in children with 47,XXY and 47,XXX karyotypes: a descriptive and experimental study. Brain Lang 1982;17(1):58–72.

24. Walzer S, Bashir AS, Silbert AR. Cognitive and behavioral factors in the learning disabilities of 47,XXY and 47,XYY boys. Birth Defects Orig Artic Ser 1990;26(4): 45–58.

25. Tartaglia N, Cordeiro L, Howell S, et al. The spectrum of the behavioral phenotype in boys and adolescents 47,XXY (Klinefelter syndrome). Pediatr Endocrinol Rev 2010;8(Suppl 1):151–9.

26. Boone KB, Swerdloff RS, Miller BL, et al. Neuropsychological profiles of adults with Klinefelter syndrome. J Int Neuropsychol Soc 2001;7(4):446–56.

27. Ratcliffe SG, Masera N, Pan H, et al. Head circumference and IQ of children with sex chromosome abnormalities. Dev Med Child Neurol 1994;36(6):533–44.

28. Rovet J, Netley C, Keenan M, et al. The psychoeducational profile of boys with Klinefelter syndrome. J Learn Disabil 1996;29(2):180–96.

29. Bender BG, Linden MG, Robinson A. Verbal and spatial processing efficiency in 32 children with sex chromosome abnormalities. Pediatr Res 1989;25(6):577–9.

30. Ross JL, Zeger MP, Kushner H, et al. An extra X or Y chromosome: contrasting the cognitive and motor phenotypes in childhood in boys with 47,XYY syndrome or 47,XXY Klinefelter syndrome. Dev Disabil Res Rev 2009;15(4):309–17.

31. Boada R, Janusz J, Hutaff-Lee C, et al. The cognitive phenotype in Klinefelter syndrome: a review of the literature including genetic and hormonal factors. Dev Disabil Res Rev 2009;15(4):284–94.

32. Fruhmesser A, Kotzot D. Chromosomal variants in klinefelter syndrome. Sex Dev 2011;5(3):109–23.

33. Tartaglia N, Ayari N, Howell S, et al. 48,XXYY, 48,XXXY and 49,XXXXY syndromes: not just variants of Klinefelter syndrome. Acta Paediatr 2011;100(6): 851–60.

34. Tartaglia N, Davis S, Hench A, et al. A new look at XXYY syndrome: medical and psychological features. Am J Med Genet A 2008;146A(12):1509–22.

35. Samplaski MK, Lo KC, Grober ED, et al. Phenotypic differences in mosaic Klinefelter patients as compared with non-mosaic Klinefelter patients. Fertil Steril 2014;101(4):950–5.

36. Chang S, Skakkebaek A, Trolle C, et al. Anthropometry in Klinefelter syndrome—multifactorial influences due to CAG length, testosterone treatment and possibly intrauterine hypogonadism. J Clin Endocrinol Metab 2015;100(3):E508–17.

37. Bojesen A, Kristensen K, Birkebaek NH, et al. The metabolic syndrome is frequent in Klinefelter's syndrome and is associated with abdominal obesity and hypogonadism. Diabetes Care 2006;29(7):1591–8.
38. Patwardhan AJ, Eliez S, Bender B, et al. Brain morphology in Klinefelter syndrome: extra X chromosome and testosterone supplementation. Neurology 2000;54(12):2218–23.
39. Bizzarro A, Valentini G, Di Martino G, et al. Influence of testosterone therapy on clinical and immunological features of autoimmune diseases associated with Klinefelter's syndrome. J Clin Endocrinol Metab 1987;64(1):32–6.
40. Davis S, Lahlou N, Bardsley MZ, et al. Longitudinal study of boys with Klinefelter syndrome gives evidence of prepubertal testis defect. San Diego (CA): The Endocrine Society; 2015.
41. Davis S, Lahlou N, Bardsley MZ, et al. Longitudinal gonadal function biomarkers of puberty onset in Klinefelter syndrome. San Diego (CA): Pediatric Academic Society; 2015.
42. Bardsley MZ, Kowal K, Gamber R, et al. Androgen replacement in boys with 47,XXY Klinefelter syndrome: influence on the testicular phenotype. Chicago: Endocrine Society; 2014.
43. Chen X, Williams-Burris SM, McClusky R, et al. The sex chromosome trisomy mouse model of XXY and XYY: metabolism and motor performance. Biol Sex Differ 2013;4(1):15.
44. Lue YH, Wang C, Liu PY, et al. Insights into the pathogenesis of XXY phenotype from comparison of the clinical syndrome with an experimental XXY mouse model. Pediatr Endocrinol Rev 2010;8(Suppl 1):140–4.
45. Bojesen A, Hertz JM, Gravholt CH. Genotype and phenotype in Klinefelter syndrome—impact of androgen receptor polymorphism and skewed X inactivation. Int J Androl 2011;34(6 Pt 2):e642–8.
46. Zinn AR, Ramos P, Elder FF, et al. Androgen receptor CAGn repeat length influences phenotype of 47,XXY (Klinefelter) syndrome. J Clin Endocrinol Metab 2005;90(9):5041–6.
47. Zitzmann M, Depenbusch M, Gromoll J, et al. X-chromosome inactivation patterns and androgen receptor functionality influence phenotype and social characteristics as well as pharmacogenetics of testosterone therapy in Klinefelter patients. J Clin Endocrinol Metab 2004;89(12):6208–17.
48. Huang J, Zhang L, Deng H, et al. Global transcriptome analysis of peripheral blood identifies the most significantly down-regulated genes associated with metabolism regulation in Klinefelter syndrome. Mol Reprod Dev 2015;82(1):17–25.
49. D'Aurora M, Ferlin A, Di Nicola M, et al. Deregulation of sertoli and leydig cells function in patients with klinefelter syndrome as evidenced by testis transcriptome analysis. BMC Genomics 2015;16:1356.
50. Liu N, Qiao Y, Cai C, et al. A sperm component, HSD-3.8 (SPAG1), interacts with G-protein beta 1 subunit and activates extracellular signal-regulated kinases (ERK). Front Biosci 2006;11:1679–89.
51. Viana J, Pidsley R, Troakes C, et al. Epigenomic and transcriptomic signatures of a Klinefelter syndrome (47,XXY) karyotype in the brain. Epigenetics 2014; 9(4):587–99.
52. Zitzmann M, Bongers R, Werler S, et al. Gene expression patterns in relation to the clinical phenotype in Klinefelter syndrome. J Clin Endocrinol Metab 2015; 100(3):E518–23.
53. Fennoy I. Testosterone and the child (0-12 years) with Klinefelter syndrome (47XXY): a review. Acta Paediatr 2011;100(6):846–50.

54. Lahlou N, Fennoy I, Ross JL, et al. Clinical and hormonal status of infants with nonmosaic XXY karyotype. Acta Paediatr 2011;100(6):824–9.

55. Coerdt W, Rehder H, Gausmann I, et al. Quantitative histology of human fetal testes in chromosomal disease. Pediatr Pathol 1985;3(2–4):245–59.

56. Murken JD, Stengel-Rutkowski S, Walther JU, et al. Letter: Klinefelter's syndrome in a fetus. Lancet 1974;2(7873):171.

57. Flannery DB, Brown JA, Redwine FO, et al. Antenatally detected Klinefelter's syndrome in twins. Acta Genet Med Gemellol (Roma) 1984;33(1):51–6.

58. Gustavson KH, Kjessler B, Thoren S. Prenatal diagnosis of an XXY foetal karyotype in a woman with a previous 21-trisomic child. Clin Genet 1978;13(6):477–80.

59. Autio-Harmainen H, Rapola J, Aula P. Fetal gonadal histology in XXXXY, XYY and XXX syndromes. Clin Genet 1980;18(1):1–5.

60. Citoler P, Aechter J. Histology of the testis in XXY fetuses. In: Murken JD, Stengel-Rutdowski S, Schwinger E, editors. Prenatal Diagnosis: Proceedings of the Third European Conference on Prenatal Diagnosis of Genetic Disorders. Stuttgart: Ferdinand Enke; 1979. p. 336–7.

61. Jequier AM, Bullimore NJ. Testicular and epididymal histology in a fetus with Klinefelter's syndrome at 22 weeks' gestation. Br J Urol 1989;63(2):214–5.

62. Ratcliffe SG, Read G, Pan H, et al. Prenatal testosterone levels in XXY and XYY males. Horm Res 1994;42(3):106–9.

63. Kunzig HJ, Meyer U, Schmitz-Roeckerath B, et al. Influence of fetal sex on the concentration of amniotic fluid testosterone: antenatal sex determination? Arch Gynakol 1977;223(2):75–84.

64. Carson DJ, Okuno A, Lee PA, et al. Amniotic fluid steroid levels. Fetuses with adrenal hyperplasia, 46,XXY fetuses, and normal fetuses. Am J Dis Child 1982;136(3):218–22.

65. Abeliovich D, Leiberman JR, Teuerstein I, et al. Prenatal sex diagnosis: testosterone and FSH levels in mid-trimester amniotic fluids. Prenat Diagn 1984; 4(5):347–53.

66. Mean F, Pescia G, Vajda D, et al. Amniotic fluid testosterone in prenatal sex determination. J Genet Hum 1981;29(4):441–7.

67. Sorensen K, Nielsen J, Wohlert M, et al. Serum testosterone of boys with karyotype 47,XXY (Klinefelter's syndrome) at birth. Lancet 1981;2(8255):1112–3.

68. Moal V, Mathieu E, Reynier P, et al. Low serum testosterone assayed by liquid chromatography-tandem mass spectrometry. Comparison with five immunoassay techniques. Clin Chim Acta 2007;386(1–2):12–9.

69. Ivell R, Heng K, Anand-Ivell R. Insulin-like factor 3 and the HPG axis in the male. Front Endocrinol (Lausanne) 2014;5:6.

70. Boas M, Boisen KA, Virtanen HE, et al. Postnatal penile length and growth rate correlate to serum testosterone levels: a longitudinal study of 1962 normal boys. Eur J Endocrinol 2006;154(1):125–9.

71. Ratcliffe SG, Murray L, Teague P. Edinburgh study of growth and development of children with sex chromosome abnormalities. III. Birth Defects Orig Artic Ser 1986;22(3):73–118.

72. Stewart DA, Bailey JD, Netley CT, et al. Growth and development of children with X and Y chromosome aneuploidy from infancy to pubertal age: the Toronto study. Birth Defects Orig Artic Ser 1982;18(4):99–154.

73. Ross JL, Samango-Sprouse C, Lahlou N, et al. Early androgen deficiency in infants and young boys with 47,XXY Klinefelter syndrome. Horm Res 2005;64(1):39–45.

74. Ratcliffe SH. Development of children with sex chromosome abnormalities. Proc R Soc Med 1976;69(3):189–91.

75. Aksglaede L, Petersen JH, Main KM, et al. High normal testosterone levels in infants with non-mosaic Klinefelter's syndrome. Eur J Endocrinol 2007;157(3): 345–50.
76. Muller J, Skakkebaek NE, Ratcliffe SG. Quantified testicular histology in boys with sex chromosome abnormalities. Int J Androl 1995;18(2):57–62.
77. Edlow JB, Shapiro LR, Hsu LY, et al. Neonatal Klinefelter's syndrome. Am J Dis Child 1969;118(5):788–91.
78. Mikamo K, Aguercif M, Hazeghi P, et al. Chromatin-positive Klinefelter's syndrome. A quantitative analysis of spermatogonial deficiency at 3, 4, and 12 months of age. Fertil Steril 1968;19(5):731–9.
79. Ratcliffe SG. The sexual development of boys with the chromosome constitution 47,XXY (Klinefelter's syndrome). Clin Endocrinol Metab 1982;11(3):703–16.
80. Cabrol S, Ross JL, Fennoy I, et al. Assessment of Leydig and Sertoli cell functions in infants with nonmosaic Klinefelter syndrome: insulin-like peptide 3 levels are normal and positively correlated with LH levels. J Clin Endocrinol Metab 2011;96(4):E746–53.
81. Lahlou N, Fennoy I, Carel JC, et al. Inhibin B and anti-Mullerian hormone, but not testosterone levels, are normal in infants with nonmosaic Klinefelter syndrome. J Clin Endocrinol Metab 2004;89(4):1864–8.
82. Forest MG, Sizonenko PC, Cathiard AM, et al. Hypophyso-gonadal function in humans during the first year of life. 1. Evidence for testicular activity in early infancy. J Clin Invest 1974;53(3):819–28.
83. Rey RA. Mini-puberty and true puberty: differences in testicular function. Ann Endocrinol (Paris) 2014;75(2):58–63.
84. Aksglaede L, Christiansen P, Sorensen K, et al. Serum concentrations of Anti-Mullerian Hormone (AMH) in 95 patients with Klinefelter syndrome with or without cryptorchidism. Acta Paediatr 2011;100(6):839–45.
85. Zeger MP, Zinn AR, Lahlou N, et al. Effect of ascertainment and genetic features on the phenotype of Klinefelter syndrome. J Pediatr 2008;152(5):716–22.
86. Aksglaede L, Wikstrom AM, Rajpert-De Meyts E, et al. Natural history of seminiferous tubule degeneration in Klinefelter syndrome. Hum Reprod Update 2006; 12(1):39–48.
87. Ferguson-Smith MA. The prepubertal testicular lesion in chromatin-positive Klinefelter's syndrome (primary micro-orchidism) as seen in mentally handicapped children. Lancet 1959;1(7066):219–22.
88. Bastida MG, Rey RA, Bergada I, et al. Establishment of testicular endocrine function impairment during childhood and puberty in boys with Klinefelter syndrome. Clin Endocrinol 2007;67(6):863–70.
89. Grinspon RP, Loreti N, Braslavsky D, et al. Sertoli cell markers in the diagnosis of paediatric male hypogonadism. J Pediatr Endocrinol Metab 2012;25(1–2): 3–11.
90. Wikstrom AM, Raivio T, Hadziselimovic F, et al. Klinefelter syndrome in adolescence: onset of puberty is associated with accelerated germ cell depletion. J Clin Endocrinol Metab 2004;89(5):2263–70.
91. Topper E, Dickerman Z, Prager-Lewin R, et al. Puberty in 24 patients with Klinefelter syndrome. Eur J Pediatr 1982;139(1):8–12.
92. Salbenblatt JA, Bender BG, Puck MH, et al. Pituitary-gonadal function in Klinefelter syndrome before and during puberty. Pediatr Res 1985;19(1):82–6.
93. Wikstrom AM, Bay K, Hero M, et al. Serum insulin-like factor 3 levels during puberty in healthy boys and boys with Klinefelter syndrome. J Clin Endocrinol Metab 2006;91(11):4705–8.

94. Aksglaede L, Sorensen K, Boas M, et al. Changes in anti-Mullerian hormone (AMH) throughout the life span: a population-based study of 1027 healthy males from birth (cord blood) to the age of 69 years. J Clin Endocrinol Metab 2010;95(12):5357–64.

95. Fullerton G, Hamilton M, Maheshwari A. Should non-mosaic Klinefelter syndrome men be labelled as infertile in 2009? Hum Reprod 2010;25(3):588–97.

96. Sciurano RB, Luna Hisano CV, Rahn MI, et al. Focal spermatogenesis originates in euploid germ cells in classical Klinefelter patients. Hum Reprod 2009;24(9): 2353–60.

97. Christiansen P, Andersson AM, Skakkebaek NE. Longitudinal studies of inhibin B levels in boys and young adults with Klinefelter syndrome. J Clin Endocrinol Metab 2003;88(2):888–91.

98. Overvad S, Bay K, Bojesen A, et al. Low INSL3 in Klinefelter syndrome is related to osteocalcin, testosterone treatment and body composition, as well as measures of the hypothalamic-pituitary-gonadal axis. Andrology 2014; 2(3):421–7.

99. Tuttelmann F, Damm OS, Luetjens CM, et al. Intratesticular testosterone is increased in men with Klinefelter syndrome and may not be released into the bloodstream owing to altered testicular vascularization- a preliminary report. Andrology 2014;2(2):275–81.

100. Wosnitzer MS, Paduch DA. Endocrinological issues and hormonal manipulation in children and men with Klinefelter syndrome. Am J Med Genet C Semin Med Genet 2013;163C(1):16–26.

101. Samango-Sprouse CA, Sadeghin T, Mitchell FL, et al. Positive effects of short course androgen therapy on the neurodevelopmental outcome in boys with 47,XXY syndrome at 36 and 72 months of age. Am J Med Genet A 2013; 161A(3):501–8.

102. Winter JS, Faiman C, Hobson WC, et al. Pituitary-gonadal relations in infancy. I. Patterns of serum gonadotropin concentrations from birth to four years of age in man and chimpanzee. J Clin Endocrinol Metab 1975;40(4):545–51.

103. Chada M, Prusa R, Bronsky J, et al. Inhibin B, follicle stimulating hormone, luteinizing hormone and testosterone during childhood and puberty in males: changes in serum concentrations in relation to age and stage of puberty. Physiol Res 2003;52(1):45–51.

104. American Diabetes Association, American Psychiatric Association, American Association of Clinical Endocrinologists, North American Association for the Study of Obesity. Consensus development conference on antipsychotic drugs and obesity and diabetes. J Clin Psychiatry 2004;65(2):267–72.

105. Barlow SE, Expert C. Expert committee recommendations regarding the prevention, assessment, and treatment of child and adolescent overweight and obesity: summary report. Pediatrics 2007;120(Suppl 4):S164–92.

106. Rogol AD, Tartaglia N. Considerations for androgen therapy in children and adolescents with Klinefelter syndrome (47, XXY). Pediatr Endocrinol Rev 2010;8(Suppl 1):145–50.

107. Radicioni AF, Ferlin A, Balercia G, et al. Consensus statement on diagnosis and clinical management of Klinefelter syndrome. J Endocrinol Invest 2010;33(11): 839–50.

108. Groth KA, Skakkebaek A, Host C, et al. Clinical review: Klinefelter syndrome–a clinical update. J Clin Endocrinol Metab 2013;98(1):20–30.

109. Bhasin S, Cunningham GR, Hayes FJ, et al. Testosterone therapy in men with androgen deficiency syndromes: an Endocrine Society clinical practice guideline. J Clin Endocrinol Metab 2010;95(6):2536–59.

110. Samplaski MK, Loai Y, Wong K, et al. Testosterone use in the male infertility population: prescribing patterns and effects on semen and hormonal parameters. Fertil Steril 2014;101(1):64–9.

111. Forti G, Vannucchi PL, Borghi A, et al. Effects of pharmacological doses of testosterone and dihydrotestosterone on the hypothalamic-pituitary axis function of Klinefelter patients. J Endocrinol Invest 1983;6(4):297–300.

112. Liu PY, Swerdloff RS, Christenson PD, et al, Hormonal Male Contraception Summit Group. Rate, extent, and modifiers of spermatogenic recovery after hormonal male contraception: an integrated analysis. Lancet 2006;367(9520):1412–20.

113. Plotton I, d'Estaing SG, Cuzin B, et al. Preliminary results of a prospective study of testicular sperm extraction in young versus adult patients with nonmosaic 47,XXY Klinefelter syndrome. J Clin Endocrinol Metab 2015;100(3):961–7.

114. Ramasamy R, Ricci JA, Palermo GD, et al. Successful fertility treatment for Klinefelter's syndrome. J Urol 2009;182(3):1108–13.

115. Schiff JD, Palermo GD, Veeck LL, et al. Success of testicular sperm extraction [corrected] and intracytoplasmic sperm injection in men with Klinefelter syndrome. J Clin Endocrinol Metab 2005;90(11):6263–7.

116. Wang C, Cunningham G, Dobs A, et al. Long-term testosterone gel (AndroGel) treatment maintains beneficial effects on sexual function and mood, lean and fat mass, and bone mineral density in hypogonadal men. J Clin Endocrinol Metab 2004;89(5):2085–98.

117. Nielsen J, Pelsen B, Sorensen K. Follow-up of 30 Klinefelter males treated with testosterone. Clin Genet 1988;33(4):262–9.

118. Wang C, Eyre DR, Clark R, et al. Sublingual testosterone replacement improves muscle mass and strength, decreases bone resorption, and increases bone formation markers in hypogonadal men–a clinical research center study. J Clin Endocrinol Metab 1996;81(10):3654–62.

119. Wang C, Swerdloff RS, Iranmanesh A, et al. Transdermal testosterone gel improves sexual function, mood, muscle strength, and body composition parameters in hypogonadal men. J Clin Endocrinol Metab 2000;85(8):2839–53.

120. Van Assche E, Bonduelle M, Tournaye H, et al. Cytogenetics of infertile men. Hum Reprod 1996;11(Suppl 4):1–24 [discussion: 25–6].

121. Lanfranco F, Kamischke A, Zitzmann M, et al. Klinefelter's syndrome. Lancet 2004;364(9430):273–83.

122. Mehta A, Bolyakov A, Roosma J, et al. Successful testicular sperm retrieval in adolescents with Klinefelter syndrome treated with at least 1 year of topical testosterone and aromatase inhibitor. Fertil Steril 2013;100(4):970–4.

123. Yamamoto Y, Sofikitis N, Mio Y, et al. Morphometric and cytogenetic characteristics of testicular germ cells and Sertoli cell secretory function in men with non-mosaic Klinefelter's syndrome. Hum Reprod 2002;17(4):886–96.

124. Friedler S, Raziel A, Strassburger D, et al. Outcome of ICSI using fresh and cryopreserved-thawed testicular spermatozoa in patients with non-mosaic Klinefelter's syndrome. Hum Reprod 2001;16(12):2616–20.

125. Bakircioglu ME, Ulug U, Erden HF, et al. Klinefelter syndrome: does it confer a bad prognosis in treatment of nonobstructive azoospermia? Fertil Steril 2011;95(5):1696–9.

126. Plotton I, Brosse A, Cuzin B, et al. Klinefelter syndrome and TESE-ICSI. Ann Endocrinol (Paris) 2014;75(2):118–25.

127. Deruyver Y, Vanderschueren D, Van der Aa F. Outcome of microdissection TESE compared with conventional TESE in non-obstructive azoospermia: a systematic review. Andrology 2014;2(1):20–4.

128. Schlegel PN. Testicular sperm extraction: microdissection improves sperm yield with minimal tissue excision. Hum Reprod 1999;14(1):131–5.
129. Okada H, Dobashi M, Yamazaki T, et al. Conventional versus microdissection testicular sperm extraction for nonobstructive azoospermia. J Urol 2002; 168(3):1063–7.
130. Vernaeve V, Staessen C, Verheyen G, et al. Can biological or clinical parameters predict testicular sperm recovery in 47,XXY Klinefelter's syndrome patients? Hum Reprod 2004;19(5):1135–9.
131. Gies I, De Schepper J, Van Saen D, et al. Failure of a combined clinical- and hormonal-based strategy to detect early spermatogenesis and retrieve spermatogonial stem cells in 47,XXY boys by single testicular biopsy. Hum Reprod 2012;27(4):998–1004.
132. Sabbaghian M, Modarresi T, Hosseinifar H, et al. Comparison of sperm retrieval and intracytoplasmic sperm injection outcome in patients with and without Klinefelter syndrome. Urology 2014;83(1):107–10.
133. Van Saen D, Gies I, De Schepper J, et al. Can pubertal boys with Klinefelter syndrome benefit from spermatogonial stem cell banking? Hum Reprod 2012;27(2): 323–30.
134. Aksglaede L, Jorgensen N, Skakkebaek NE, et al. Low semen volume in 47 adolescents and adults with 47,XXY Klinefelter or 46,XX male syndrome. Int J Androl 2009;32(4):376–84.
135. Madureira C, Cunha M, Sousa M, et al. Treatment by testicular sperm extraction and intracytoplasmic sperm injection of 65 azoospermic patients with non-mosaic Klinefelter syndrome with birth of 17 healthy children. Andrology 2014; 2(4):623–31.
136. Ramasamy R, Ricci JA, Leung RA, et al. Successful repeat microdissection testicular sperm extraction in men with nonobstructive azoospermia. J Urol 2011;185(3):1027–31.
137. Chehab M, Madala A, Trussell JC. On-label and off-label drugs used in the treatment of male infertility. Fertil Steril 2015;103(3):595–604.
138. Hussein A, Ozgok Y, Ross L, et al. Optimization of spermatogenesis-regulating hormones in patients with non-obstructive azoospermia and its impact on sperm retrieval: a multicentre study. BJU Int 2013;111(3 Pt B):E110–4.
139. Shiraishi K, Ohmi C, Shimabukuro T, et al. Human chorionic gonadotrophin treatment prior to microdissection testicular sperm extraction in non-obstructive azoospermia. Hum Reprod 2012;27(2):331–9.
140. Hussein A, Ozgok Y, Ross L, et al. Clomiphene administration for cases of non-obstructive azoospermia: a multicenter study. J Androl 2005;26(6):787–91 [discussion: 792–3].
141. Adamopoulos DA, Loraine JA, Ismail AA, et al. Endocrinological studies in patients with Klinefelter's syndrome treated with clomiphene. J Reprod Fertil 1971;25(3):409–16.
142. Raman JD, Schlegel PN. Aromatase inhibitors for male infertility. J Urol 2002; 167(2 Pt 1):624–9.
143. Schlegel PN. Aromatase inhibitors for male infertility. Fertil Steril 2012;98(6): 1359–62.
144. Patry G, Jarvi K, Grober ED, et al. Use of the aromatase inhibitor letrozole to treat male infertility. Fertil Steril 2009;92(2):829.e1–2.
145. Reifsnyder JE, Ramasamy R, Husseini J, et al. Role of optimizing testosterone before microdissection testicular sperm extraction in men with nonobstructive azoospermia. J Urol 2012;188(2):532–6.

146. Ferlin A, Garolla A, Foresta C. Chromosome abnormalities in sperm of individuals with constitutional sex chromosomal abnormalities. Cytogenet Genome Res 2005;111(3–4):310–6.
147. Staessen C, Tournaye H, Van Assche E, et al. PGD in 47,XXY Klinefelter's syndrome patients. Hum Reprod Update 2003;9(4):319–30.
148. Mroz K, Hassold TJ, Hunt PA. Meiotic aneuploidy in the XXY mouse: evidence that a compromised testicular environment increases the incidence of meiotic errors. Hum Reprod 1999;14(5):1151–6.
149. Gies I, De Schepper J, Goossens E, et al. Spermatogonial stem cell preservation in boys with Klinefelter syndrome: to bank or not to bank, that's the question. Fertil Steril 2012;98(2):284–9.
150. Wikstrom AM, Dunkel L, Wickman S, et al. Are adolescent boys with Klinefelter syndrome androgen deficient? A longitudinal study of Finnish 47,XXY boys. Pediatr Res 2006;59(6):854–9.
151. Wikstrom AM, Hoei-Hansen CE, Dunkel L, et al. Immunoexpression of androgen receptor and nine markers of maturation in the testes of adolescent boys with Klinefelter syndrome: evidence for degeneration of germ cells at the onset of meiosis. J Clin Endocrinol Metab 2007;92(2):714–9.

Fertility Issues in Disorders of Sex Development

Gabriela Guercio, MD, PhD[a], Mariana Costanzo, MD[a], Romina P. Grinspon, MD, PhD[b], Rodolfo A. Rey, MD, PhD[b,c],*

KEYWORDS

- Aromatase • Gonadal dysgenesis • Ovotestis • Hypospadias • Müllerian remnants
- Ambiguous genitalia • Androgens • AMH

KEY POINTS

- Fertility potential in patients with disorders of sex development is influenced by specific factors related to the causal disorder, and general functional and anatomic features, irrespective of the etiology.
- In patients with testicular dysgenesis, severe forms are raised as females, and motherhood might be possible with hormone replacement and oocyte donation.
- In patients with specific defects of androgen synthesis or action, the absence of uterus and Fallopian tubes hampers motherhood.
- In some virilized 46,XX patients raised as females, fertility is possible after adequate hormonal and surgical treatments.
- Patients raised as males are most frequently oligospermic or azoospermic, with the exception for milder forms, where full spermatogenesis can be achieved spontaneously or after hormonal treatment.

INTRODUCTION

Fertility potential should be considered by the multidisciplinary team when addressing gender assignment, surgical management, and patient and family counseling of individuals with disorders of sex development (DSD) (**Box 1**).

DSD refers to all congenital conditions in which the development of chromosomal, gonadal, or genital sex is atypical.[1] Here we address fertility issues in DSD conditions

Disclosure Statement: The authors have nothing to disclose.
[a] Servicio de Endocrinología, Hospital de Pediatría "Prof. Dr. Juan P. Garrahan", Combate de los Pozos 1881, Buenos Aires C1245AAM, Argentina; [b] CONICET – FEI – División de Endocrinología, Centro de Investigaciones Endocrinológicas "Dr. César Bergadá" (CEDIE), Hospital de Niños Ricardo Gutiérrez, Gallo 1330, Buenos Aires C1425EFD, Argentina; [c] Departamento de Histología, Biología Celular, Embriología y Genética, Facultad de Medicina, Universidad de Buenos Aires, Paraguay 2155, Buenos Aires C1121ABG, Argentina
* Corresponding author. Centro de Investigaciones Endocrinológicas "Dr. César Bergadá" (CEDIE), CONICET – FEI – División de Endocrinología, Hospital de Niños Ricardo Gutiérrez, Gallo 1330, C1425EFD Buenos Aires, Argentina.
E-mail address: rodolforey@cedie.org.ar

Endocrinol Metab Clin N Am 44 (2015) 867–881
http://dx.doi.org/10.1016/j.ecl.2015.07.012   **endo.theclinics.com**

Box 1
Factors that might influence fertility potential in patients with disorders of sex development (DSD)

- Specific factors related to the etiology
- Factors found in most DSD, irrespective of the etiology:
  - Functional and/or anatomic features
  - Features related to the management and/or the surgical corrections

---

affecting the normal pathway of gonadal and/or genital sex differentiation during intra-uterine life (**Fig. 1**). Not discussed are reproductive outcomes in Klinefelter syndrome, Turner syndrome, and congenital adrenal hyperplasia due to 21-hydroxylase deficiency, which are discussed elsewhere in this issue.

46,XY DISORDERS OF SEX DEVELOPMENT

In 46,XY individuals, defects of gonadal differentiation (dysgenetic DSD) or in androgen or anti-Müllerian hormone (AMH) synthesis or action result in incomplete or absent masculinization (see **Fig. 1**). According to the severity of the defect, patients might present with female, ambiguous, or minimally undervirilized external genitalia (micropenis and cryptorchidism).[2] Fertility potential in these patients should be analyzed considering clinical form (or severity of the condition) and sex assignment.

Complete Forms of 46,XY Disorders of Sex Development

Severe gonadal dysgenesis or absent androgen synthesis or action result in female external genitalia. Affected individuals always reared as girls have no possibility for spontaneous fertility because of the lack of oocytes, but pregnancy might be achieved in dysgenetic DSD, owing to the persistence of Müllerian remnants (**Fig. 2**A), with the use of allogenic oocytes (**Table 1**).[3,4]

In defects of androgen synthesis or action, Müllerian structures are generally absent (see **Fig. 2**B). Sporadic cases with presence of minimal Müllerian remnants have been reported,[5,6] but their functionality for embryo implantation has not been reported at present. Nonetheless, the first case of a live birth following uterine allograft transplantation has recently been reported in a patient with congenital absence of the uterus (Rokitansky syndrome),[7] thus opening a promising alternative.

Partial forms of 46,XY Disorders of Sex Development

Partial forms result in a broad phenotypic spectrum, from genital ambiguity to complete virilization in individuals presenting with infertility (see **Table 1**). Depending on the degree of undervirilization of the genitalia, female or male sex of rearing might be possible. For affected patients assigned female, considerations regarding fertility are similar to those discussed for the complete forms.

Fertility in patients raised males might be affected by impaired spermatogenesis secondary to gonadal dysgenesis and/or androgen deficiency, cryptorchidism, anatomic defects of the male reproductive tract (eg, perineoscrotal hypospadias, defects of the epididymis or vas deferens), or complications of genitourinary surgery. Unfortunately, for most patients with DSD reported in infancy or childhood, information regarding pubertal development and/or fertility is not available.

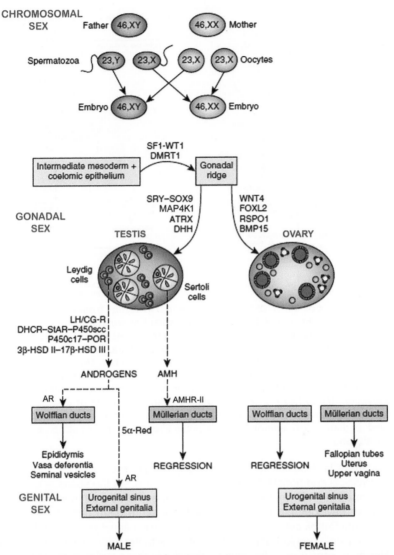

Fig. 1. The 3 stages in normal sexual differentiation. (1) Chromosomal sex is determined by the sex chromosome (X or Y) present in the spermatozoon at fertilization. (2) Gonadal sex differentiation occurs after the sixth week of embryonic life, when the indifferent gonadal ridge takes the testicular or the ovarian pathway, according to the gene expression pattern. (3) Sex of the internal and external genitalia depends on the secretion and action of 2 testicular hormones: testosterone, by Leydig cells, and AMH, by Sertoli cells. Male genital differentiation occurs when androgens (testosterone and DHT) and AMH are present and act through their respective receptors, the AR and AMH type II receptor (AMHR-II). Female differentiation takes place in their absence. (*From* Rey RA, Josso N. Diagnosis and treatment of disorders of sexual development. In: Jameson JL, De Groot LJ, de Kretser D, et al, editors. Endocrinology: adult and pediatric. 7th edition. Philadelphia: Elsevier Saunders; 2015. p. 2086–118; with permission.)

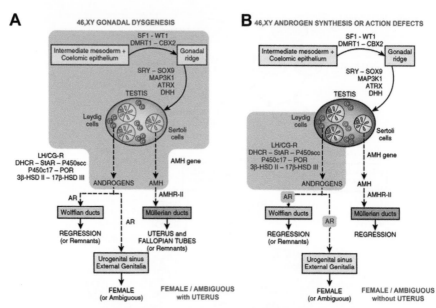

Fig. 2. Pathogenesis of 46,XY DSD. (*A*) Dysgenetic DSD results from defects in testicular differentiation from the gonadal ridge. Both testicular hormones are defective: androgen deficiency results in underdevelopment or complete regression of Wolffian ducts and feminization of the urogenital sinus and external genitalia, whereas AMH deficiency results in the development of the uterus and Fallopian tubes. (*B*) Androgen synthesis defects results from Leydig cell specific dysfunction, whereas androgen action defects results from AR mutations. AMH action is present in both conditions, resulting in Müllerian duct regression. (*From* Rey RA, Josso N. Diagnosis and treatment of disorders of sexual development. In: Jameson JL, De Groot LJ, de Kretser D, et al, editors. Endocrinology: adult and pediatric. 7th edition. Philadelphia: Elsevier Saunders; 2015. p. 2086–118; with permission.)

Testosterone is essential to maintain spermatogenesis and male fertility acting through classical and nonclassical signaling pathways.[8] In the absence of androgen synthesis or action, spermatogenesis rarely progresses beyond meiosis, the blood–testis barrier development is compromised, immature germ cells are prematurely detached from Sertoli cells, and full spermatogenesis cannot be achieved.[8]

Persistently cryptorchid testes might contribute to the decrease in germ cell number.[9] However, considering the primary disorder in these patients, the management of the position of the gonads does not appear to change the reproductive outcome.

Male genitoplasty usually includes chordee correction and penile straightening, urethroplasty, glanuloplasty, correction of scrotal deformities, and orchiopexy. Ejaculation disorders have been reported in adulthood.[10] However, very few studies have evaluated the long-term outcomes,[11–13] and progressive changes in surgical techniques warrant the performance of new studies.

Despite the considerations listed previously, fertility and fatherhood have been reported in a few patients with 46,XY DSD raised as males with milder forms of gonadal dysgenesis or defects in androgen synthesis or action (see **Table 1**).

Partial gonadal dysgenesis

In testicular dysgenesis, germ cells are the most affected cell population, usually leading to incomplete spermatogenesis and increased risk of germ cell tumors.[14] Pubertal

Table 1
Fertility issues in patients with 46,XY disorders of sex development (DSD)

DSD Etiology	Fertility
1. Gonadal dysgenesis • Yp deletions, Xp duplications (DSS), 9p deletions (involving *DMRT1/DMRT2*) • Mutations of genes involved in testicular differentiation: *SRY, SOX9, SF1, WT1, ATRX, DHH, MAP3K1*.	*Severe forms:* raised as females, motherhood possible with hormone replacement and oocyte donation *Milder forms:* raised as males, azoospermia/oligospermia, very rarely spontaneous fatherhood
2. Defects of androgen production • LHCG receptor mutations • Inborn errors of testosterone Biosynthesis: Mutations of StAR, P450scc, P450c17, POR, 3β-HSD, 17β-HSD	*Severe forms:* raised as females, motherhood impossible due to absence of uterus *Milder forms:* raised as males, azoospermia, more rarely fatherhood spontaneous or after hormonal treatment
3. Defects in androgen target organs	
DHT deficiency	*Severe forms:* raised as females, motherhood impossible due to absence of uterus *Milder forms:* raised as males, or changing from female to male gender at puberty, fatherhood possible spontaneously or after hormonal treatment
Androgen insensitivity	*Complete:* Raised as females, motherhood impossible due to absence of uterus *Partial/Mild:* azoospermia/oligospermia, fatherhood possible in rare cases after hormonal treatment
4. Persistent Müllerian duct syndrome • AMH mutations • AMH Receptor mutations	Azoospermia, probably due to long-standing cryptorchidism, or damage of epididymis, vas deferens or testicular blood supply at surgery

Abbreviations: AMH, anti-Müllerian hormone; DHT, dihydrotestosterone; DSS, dosage sensitive sex reversal; HSD, hydroxysteroid dehydrogenase; LHCG, luteinizing hormone/chorionic gonadotropin; POR, P450 oxidoreductase; P450scc, cholesterol side-chain cleavage enzyme; StAR, steroidogenic acute regulatory protein.

development among these patients may be partial, requiring testosterone replacement, but there are also reports on complete pubertal development.[15–17] Most patients are infertile, but there is a huge variability even within the same family. One example is a kindred of four 46,XY individuals with a mutation in *NR5A1*, encoding SF1: all presented with hypospadias at birth; although only one of them also had micropenis and cryptorchidism, the other 3 developed normally, and one fathered 5 children.[16] Another example is related to a mutation in *MAP3K1*, involved in the testicular differentiation pathway: a man with hypospadias and chordee was fertile and fathered 2 children. The father and both children had different degrees of 46,XY gonadal dysgenesis.[18]

Partial androgen synthesis defects

Luteinizing hormone receptor Leydig cell hypoplasia is a rare condition that results from inactivating homozygous or compound heterozygous mutations of the luteinizing hormone–chorionic gonadotropin receptor (LHCGR) in 46,XY subjects. Mild phenotypes have predominantly male external genitalia with micropenis and/or hypospadias or hypergonadotropic hypogonadism without genital ambiguity. Generally these patients are oligospermic and infertile.[12] Successful testicular sperm recovery and fertility have been reported in 2 males (see **Table 1**).[19,20]

Steroidogenic acute regulatory protein and cholesterol side-chain cleavage Defects in the early steps of steroidogenesis include mutations in the steroidogenic acute regulatory protein (StAR) or the cholesterol side-chain cleavage (P450scc) enzyme.[21–23] In late-onset "nonclassical" forms, secondary to mutations that retain partial activity, affected individuals show a broad phenotypic spectrum including normal pubertal development and adult sexual function.[22,24,25] Even though the adult phenotype is indicative of potentially compromised reproductive outcome in many patients, fertility has been reported.[26]

Cytochrome P450c17 Cytochrome P450c17, through its 17α-hydroxylase/17,20-lyase activities, is needed for cortisol and testosterone synthesis. Most of the patients with P450c17 deficiency have been reared as female, and data of patients raised as male are lacking.[21,23] In isolated 17,20-lyase deficiency individuals with 46,XY DSD raised as males usually showed primary hypogonadism requiring testosterone replacement.[27] Fertility has not been reported.

P450 oxidoreductase Mutations in P450 oxidoreductase (POR) cause a complex steroidogenic spectrum including partial P450c17, aromatase (P450C19), and 21-hydroxilase (P450c21) deficiencies.[22,23] The clinical phenotype is remarkably variable and may include skeletal malformations evocative of the Antler–Bixler syndrome.[22,23,28,29] POR deficiency affects genital differentiation in both sexes. Mildly affected male individuals may present with normal or delayed pubertal progression and biochemical signs of compensated hypogonadism. Even though fertility has not been reported, the capacity for spontaneous pubertal development in affected boys justifies a primarily watchful-waiting approach to the evaluation of reproductive outcome.[30] Furthermore, because a 46,XX patient with POR deficiency has been described as a phenotypically normal woman with infertility,[31] it is possible that many XX and XY patients with mild forms of POR deficiency may remain undiagnosed.

3β-hydroxysteroid dehydrogenase type 2 Deficiency of 3β-hydroxysteroid dehydrogenase type 2 (3β-HSD2) impairs steroidogenesis in the adrenals and gonads, leading to glucocorticoid and mineralocorticoid deficiency and ambiguous genitalia. Spontaneous pubertal development has been reported[21–23,32] and it has been suggested that pubertal levels of gonadotropins may increase the expression and activity of type I 3β-HSD in the gonad.[33] Whereas spermatogenic arrest[34] and azoospermia[32] have been observed, a 34-year-old man with adequate spermatogenesis has fathered 2 children.[35] Testicular adrenal rests might compromise fertility in this condition.

17β-hydroxysteroid dehydrogenase type 3 Deficiency of 17β-hydroxysteroid dehydrogenase type 3 (17β-HSD3) is a male-limited disorder affecting testicular conversion of androstenedione to testosterone. Patients with 46,XY with mild forms of 17β-HSD3 deficiency may virilize on their own at puberty.[36] High LH levels enforce testosterone synthesis and the activity of other peripheral 17β-HSD enzymes may also contribute to pubertal virilization. Nevertheless, in adulthood insufficient intratesticular testosterone levels lead to impaired spermatogenesis and azoospermia.[21–23]

5α-reductase type 2 Dihydrotestosterone (DHT) is the main androgen driving the masculinization of the urogenital sinus and external genitalia; however, DHT appears not to play a major role in spermatogenesis. The classical pathway of DHT synthesis involves the action of 5α-reductase type 2 (5α-RD2) in genital skin.[37,38] Affected patients show ambiguous genitalia with hypospadias and cryptorchidism. At puberty, spontaneous virilization occurs. Adult patients report male libido and sexual activity; however, small penis size may impair normal intercourse. Semen analysis is characterized by extremely low volume, increased viscosity, and poor liquefaction, attributed to rudimentary prostate glands and small seminal vesicles.[39,40] Most of the affected individuals are infertile, although spontaneous proven fertility was reported in 2 brothers born with ambiguous genitalia from a Swedish family.[41] In other cases, in vitro fertilization using the patients' sperm cells resulted in successful pregnancies,[38,40] providing support for raising these individuals as males.

AKR1C2/AKR1C4 The alternative pathway of DHT synthesis, found in the human fetal testis and needed for normal male sexual differentiation, involves the AKR1C2 and AKR1C4 enzymes.[23] Recently, compound heterozygous mutations in both genes have been found in families with 46,XY DSD. Even though data regarding age and pubertal status are unknown, one of the patients reported appears to be fertile.[42]

Androgen receptor Androgen receptor (AR) mutations causing partial forms of androgen insensitivity (PAIS) result in a variable phenotypic spectrum, ranging from genital ambiguity to male infertility, a condition known as mild AIS (MAIS).[43] In addition to its effects on gametogenesis, some patients have defects in Wolffian duct derivatives, such as absence or hypoplasia of the vas deferens that might affect reproduction. At present, although challenging, fertility is possible for individuals with PAIS who are raised male.[44–48] In some cases, fertility was spontaneous,[46,47] whereas in others, oligospermia was corrected and the sperm count was restored following high-dose androgen treatment (see **Table 1**).[45]

Anti-Müllerian hormone/anti-Müllerian hormone receptor 2 Defects in testicular AMH production, as well as AMH receptor defects, drive to the same form of internal genital defects in otherwise normally virilized male individuals: the persistent Müllerian duct syndrome (PMDS). The existence of a uterus and Fallopian tubes is an unpredicted finding in boys undergoing surgery for cryptorchidism associated or not with inguinal hernia. Leydig cell androgen production is normal, but azoospermia is common due to the long-standing abnormal position of the gonads or to damage of testicular blood supply during surgical procedures.[49]

46,XX DISORDERS OF SEX DEVELOPMENT

In 46,XX fetuses (**Fig. 3**), virilization along with normal ovarian organogenesis is caused by excessive exposure to androgens of fetal and/or maternal origin (**Table 2**). Virilization can also reflect the existence of testicular tissue: ovotesticular and testicular DSD, which are discussed separately (**Table 3**).

Congenital Adrenal Hyperplasia

Congenital adrenal hyperplasia due to mutations in the *CYP21A2* gene causing 21-hydroxylase deficiency (21OHD) is the most common cause of DSD in 46,XX infants, and is discussed elsewhere in this issue.

With the exception of 21OHD, information on postpubertal gonadal function and adult reproductive outcome and fertility in 46,XX DSD with normal ovarian organogenesis is scarce.

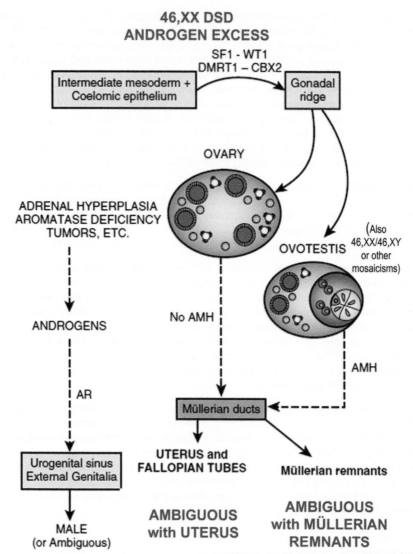

Fig. 3. Pathogenesis of 46,XX DSD. Androgen excess may derive from abnormal adrenal function (congenital adrenal hyperplasia), aromatase deficiency or androgen-secreting tumors in 46,XX fetuses with normal ovarian development. Alternatively, ovotestes can develop in 46,XX individuals with or without SRY, and also in individuals with 46,XX/ 46,XY or other mosaicisms carrying a Y chromosome. In patients with ovotesticular DSD, the presence or absence of Müllerian remnants depends on the amount of testicular tissue secreting AMH. (*From* Rey RA, Josso N. Diagnosis and treatment of disorders of sexual development. In: Jameson JL, De Groot LJ, de Kretser D, et al, editors. Endocrinology: adult and pediatric. 7th edition. Philadelphia: Elsevier Saunders; 2015. p. 2086–118; with permission.)

Table 2
Fertility issues in 46,XX disorders of sex development (DSD) due to exposure to excessive androgens

DSD Etiology	Fertility
Congenital adrenal hyperplasia • 21-hydroxylase deficiency • 11β-hydroxylase deficiency • 3β-HSD deficiency • POR deficiency	*Classic forms:* raised as females: fertility possible if adequate hormonal and surgical treatments
Aromatase deficiency	Unknown

Abbreviations: HSD, hydroxysteroid dehydrogenase; POR, P450 oxidoreductase.

11β-hydroxylase

11β-hydroxylase deficiency (11OHD) due to mutations in the *CYP11B1* gene is a rare form of congenital adrenal hyperplasia. In classic forms, newborns are virilized like in 21OHD, but mineralocorticoid activity is not deficient due to the accumulation of 11-deoxycortisol and 11-deoxycorticosterone. Despite multiple publications on 11OHD, data about fertility are scarce. Only one successful pregnancy in one properly treated woman has been reported.[50] Caution should be taken for sexually active women who attempt pregnancy because spironolactone, used for hypertension management, is potentially teratogenic.[51]

3β-HSD2

Like 21OHD and 11OHD, 3β-HSD2 deficiency virilizes the 46,XX fetus; however, the androgen excess is less severe, and genital surgery is rarely required.[51] As the girl grows, however, the main problems are due to androgen excess and hypogonadism. Deficiency of 3β-HSD2 might variably affect normal ovarian estrogen synthesis. Regular menses and evidence of progesterone secretion have been described in one female individual with the classic form of the disease; however, there is no information on fertility.[52]

P450 oxidoreductase

Subjects with 46,XX and POR deficiency present with partial in utero virilization without postnatal progression. This is the result of at least 2 mechanisms: partial placental aromatase deficiency and androgen biosynthesis through the fetal alternative steroidogenic pathway.[22,29,30,51] The relative contribution of each mechanism varies with the different POR mutations involved. Affected patients generally present with complete absence of puberty, but partial and even complete pubertal development have been reported.[30,31] The disruptive impact of mutant POR on sterol synthesis and metabolism might contribute to ovarian cyst development in addition to high gonadotropin levels resulting from estrogen deficiency. CYP51A1 requires electron transfer from POR for catalytic activity and catalyzes the conversion of lanosterol to meiosis-activating sterols (MAS). Follicular fluid MAS has been shown to be crucial for the resumption of oocyte meiosis at puberty and also support oocyte maturation.[30] Fertility has never been reported.

Aromatase Deficiency

Aromatase (P450arom) deficiency is a rare form of 46,XX DSD due to fetoplacental androgen excess. Aromatase catalyzes the synthesis of estrogens from androgens.

In postnatal life, the effect of excessive androgens and insufficient estrogens is responsible for a variable clinical picture. In complete forms, affected female individuals are born with ambiguous genitalia and progress to hypergonadotropic hypogonadism with pubertal delay, primary amenorrhea, and hyperandrogenism. Some patients develop enlarged ovaries and large ovarian cysts, sometimes requiring surgical removal for torsion, pain, or bleeding. Those factors, along with surgical consequences of genital reconstruction, might affect reproduction in these women. Variable phenotypes have been described and some affected female individuals have spontaneous breast development and uterine growth despite androgen excess and virilization.[53–55] However, information about the course of the disease in adulthood and long-term consequences on fertility is unknown. Data on the long-term follow-up of these patients might clarify our understanding of the reproductive outcomes.

Management of Fertility Issues

In 46,XX DSD due to exposure to excessive androgens, the focus and goals of treatment change as the patient grows and becomes an adult when reproduction may become a concern.

Assisted reproduction might be an alternative to offer to women who cannot spontaneously conceive. In some conditions, adequate clinical and surgical management during infancy and childhood might anticipate the long-term complications, as seen in 21OHD and 11OHD CAH.

OVOTESTICULAR AND TESTICULAR DISORDERS OF SEX DEVELOPMENT

Ovarian differentiation is the normal pathway in 46,XX fetuses (see **Fig. 1**). However, testicular tissue may differentiate in fetuses with 46,XX/46,XY or other Y-bearing mosaicisms or in 46,XX individuals with translocations of Yp carrying the SRY gene; interestingly, testicular tissue can also develop in 46,XX fetuses devoid of SRY.[56] Testicular tissue can exist together with ovarian tissue, a condition known as ovotesticular DSD (previously called true hermaphroditism, see Ref.[1], or as the only gonadal tissue, a condition known as 46,XX testicular DSD, previously named XX male, see Ref.[1]). In patients carrying SRY, the underlying pathophysiology is easily understood (see **Fig. 1**), whereas in 46,XX SRY-negative patients, recent studies have unveiled defects in potentially antitesticular genes, like RSPO1,[57] and overexpression of protesticular genes, like SOX9[58] and SOX3.[59]

Table 3		
Fertility issues in 46,XX testicular disorders of sex development (DSD) and in ovotesticular DSD independently of the karyotype		
DSD Etiology	**Fertility**	
46,XX Testicular DSD	Raised as males: azoospermia due to the existence of 2 X chromosomes and absence of Y chromosome	
Ovotesticular DSD	Raised as females: pregnancy possible spontaneously or following the use of ART with the patient's own oocytes. Raised as males: azoospermia/oligospermia, very rarely fatherhood spontaneously or after ART (TESE + ICSI)	

Abbreviations: ART, assisted reproductive technology; ICSI, intracytoplasmic sperm injection; TESE, testicular sperm extraction.

Ovotesticular Disorders of Sex Development

The diagnosis of ovotesticular DSD is histologic and requires the existence of seminiferous cords and ovarian follicles with oocytes. The most prevalent karyotype is 46,XX, but 46,XX/46,XY or other mosaicisms also can occur (see **Fig. 3**). The degree of virilization depends on the amount of functional testicular tissue. The ovarian tissue usually develops more normally than the testicular portion. Therefore, the preservation of ovarian tissue at surgery in patients raised as females may be of major importance for the achievement of pregnancy, either spontaneous or following the use of assisted reproductive techniques with the patient's own oocytes. To date, there are fewer than 15 cases of pregnancy reported in patients with ovotesticular DSD raised as females; most of them have had complications, for example, preterm labor or morbidity related to the delivery process, due to the female reproductive tract defects.[60] For patients raised as males, the considerations are similar to those previously described for 46,XY partial dysgenesis. A successful intracytoplasmic sperm injection (ICSI) procedure with subsequent live birth has been reported after testicular sperm extraction from a 46,XX/46,XY azoospermic male patient.[61]

46,XX Testicular Disorders of Sex Development

Most patients with this condition have normal male genitalia, but cases with genital ambiguity also have been reported. Like patients with Klinefelter syndrome, XX males have normal testicular function until midpuberty, with spontaneous progression of secondary sex characteristics.[62] However, the existence of 2 X chromosomes and the absence of a Y chromosome drive to germ cell degeneration, small testes, and azoospermia.[63]

SUMMARY

As patients with DSD grow and become adults, reproduction arises as an important issue. The establishment of a multidisciplinary team facilitating close interaction among the pediatrician, adult endocrinologist, gynecologic/urologic surgeon, fertility specialist, and clinical psychologist with experience in these conditions is mandatory for the long-term follow-up and the achievement of an integrated approach to the patient.

A better characterization of the more recently described conditions and detailed information about the long-term follow-up of patients with DSD reported in infancy or childhood is important to address the lifelong consequences, as in other chronic medical conditions.

Assisted reproduction might be an alternative to offer to those who cannot spontaneously conceive.

REFERENCES

1. Lee PA, Houk CP, Ahmed SF, et al. Consensus statement on management of intersex disorders. Pediatrics 2006;118:e488–500.
2. Rey RA, Grinspon RP. Normal male sexual differentiation and aetiology of disorders of sex development. Best Pract Res Clin Endocrinol Metab 2011;25:221–38.
3. Jorgensen PB, Kjartansdottir KR, Fedder J. Care of women with XY karyotype: a clinical practice guideline. Fertil Steril 2010;94:105–13.
4. Creatsas G, Deligeoroglou E, Tsimaris P, et al. Successful pregnancy in a Swyer syndrome patient with preexisting hypertension. Fertil Steril 2011;96:e83–5.

5. Nichols JL, Bieber EJ, Gell JS. Case of sisters with complete androgen insensitivity syndrome and discordant Mullerian remnants. Fertil Steril 2009;91:932.e15–8.

6. Corbetta S, Muzza M, Avagliano L, et al. Gonadal structures in a fetus with complete androgen insensitivity syndrome and persistent Mullerian derivatives: comparison with normal fetal development. Fertil Steril 2011;95:1119.e9–14.

7. Brännström M, Johannesson L, Bokström H, et al. Livebirth after uterus transplantation. Lancet 2015;385:607–16.

8. Walker WH. Non-classical actions of testosterone and spermatogenesis. Philosophical Trans R Soc Lond B Biol Sci 2010;365:1557–69.

9. Rey RA. Early orchiopexy to prevent germ cell loss during infancy in congenital cryptorchidism. J Clin Endocrinol Metab 2012;97:4358–61.

10. Rynja SP, de Kort LM, de Jong TP. Urinary, sexual, and cosmetic results after puberty in hypospadias repair: current results and trends. Curr Opin Urol 2012;22: 453–6.

11. Migeon CJ, Wisniewski AB, Gearhart JP, et al. Ambiguous genitalia with perineoscrotal hypospadias in 46,XY individuals: long-term medical, surgical, and psychosexual outcome. Pediatrics 2002;110:e31.

12. Sircili MHP, de Queiroz e Silva FA, Costa EMF, et al. Long-term surgical outcome of masculinizing genitoplasty in large cohort of patients with disorders of sex development. J Urol 2010;184:1122–7.

13. Tourchi A, Hoebeke P. Long-term outcome of male genital reconstruction in childhood. J Pediatr Urol 2013;9:980–9.

14. Chemes HE, Venara M, Del Rey G, et al. Is a CIS phenotype apparent in children with disorders of sex development? Milder testicular dysgenesis is associated with a higher risk of malignancy. Andrology 2015;3:59–69.

15. Warman DM, Costanzo M, Marino R, et al. Three new SF-1 (NR5A1) gene mutations in two unrelated families with multiple affected members: within-family variability in 46,XY subjects and low ovarian reserve in fertile 46,XX subjects. Horm Res Paediatr 2011;75:70–7.

16. Ciaccio M, Costanzo M, Guercio G, et al. Preserved fertility in a patient with a 46,XY disorder of sex development due to a new heterozygous mutation in the NR5A1/SF-1 gene: evidence of 46,XY and 46,XX gonadal dysgenesis phenotype variability in multiple members of an affected kindred. Horm Res Paediatr 2012; 78:119–26.

17. Guercio G, Rey RA. Fertility issues in the management of patients with disorders of sex development. Endocr Dev 2014;27:87–98.

18. Pearlman A, Loke J, Le CC, et al. Mutations in MAP3K1 cause 46,XY disorders of sex development and implicate a common signal transduction pathway in human testis determination. Am J Hum Genet 2010;87:898–904.

19. Martens JW, Verhoef-Post M, Abelin N, et al. A homozygous mutation in the luteinizing hormone receptor causes partial Leydig cell hypoplasia: correlation between receptor activity and phenotype. Mol Endocrinol 1998;12:775–84.

20. Bakircioglu ME, Tulay P, Findikli N, et al. Successful testicular sperm recovery and IVF treatment in a man with Leydig cell hypoplasia. J Assist Reprod Genet 2014; 31:817–21.

21. Mendonça BB, Costa EM, Belgorosky A, et al. 46,XY DSD due to impaired androgen production. Best Pract Res Clin Endocrinol Metab 2010;24:243–62.

22. Miller WL, Auchus RJ. The molecular biology, biochemistry, and physiology of human steroidogenesis and its disorders. Endocr Rev 2011;32:81–151.

23. Auchus RJ, Miller WL. Defects in androgen biosynthesis causing 46,XY disorders of sexual development. Semin Reprod Med 2012;30:417–26.

24. Parajes S, Kamrath C, Rose IT, et al. A novel entity of clinically isolated adrenal insufficiency caused by a partially inactivating mutation of the gene encoding for P450 side chain cleavage enzyme (CYP11A1). J Clin Endocrinol Metab 2011;96:E1798–806.
25. Tee MK, Abramsohn M, Loewenthal N, et al. Varied clinical presentations of seven patients with mutations in CYP11A1 encoding the cholesterol side-chain cleavage enzyme, P450scc. J Clin Endocrinol Metab 2013;98:713–20.
26. Metherell LA, Naville D, Halaby G, et al. Nonclassic lipoid congenital adrenal hyperplasia masquerading as familial glucocorticoid deficiency. J Clin Endocrinol Metab 2009;94:3865–71.
27. Miller WL. The syndrome of 17,20 lyase deficiency. J Clin Endocrinol Metab 2012; 97:59–67.
28. Fukami M, Nishimura G, Homma K, et al. Cytochrome P450 oxidoreductase deficiency: identification and characterization of biallelic mutations and genotype-phenotype correlations in 35 Japanese patients. J Clin Endocrinol Metab 2009; 94:1723–31.
29. Krone N, Reisch N, Idkowiak J, et al. Genotype-phenotype analysis in congenital adrenal hyperplasia due to P450 oxidoreductase deficiency. J Clin Endocrinol Metab 2012;97:E257–67.
30. Idkowiak J, O'Riordan S, Reisch N, et al. Pubertal presentation in seven patients with congenital adrenal hyperplasia due to P450 oxidoreductase deficiency. J Clin Endocrinol Metab 2011;96:E453–62.
31. Sahakitrungruang T, Huang N, Tee MK, et al. Clinical, genetic, and enzymatic characterization of P450 oxidoreductase deficiency in four patients. J Clin Endocrinol Metab 2009;94:4992–5000.
32. Alos N, Moisan AM, Ward L, et al. A novel A10E homozygous mutation in the HSD3B2 gene causing severe salt-wasting 3{beta}-hydroxysteroid dehydrogenase deficiency in 46,XX and 46,XY French-Canadians: evaluation of gonadal function after puberty. J Clin Endocrinol Metab 2000;85:1968–74.
33. Yoshimoto M, Kawaguchi T, Mori R, et al. Pubertal changes in testicular 3 beta-hydroxysteroid dehydrogenase activity in a male with classical 3 beta-hydroxysteroid dehydrogenase deficiency showing spontaneous secondary sexual maturation. Horm Res 1997;48:83–7.
34. Schneider G, Genel M, Bongiovanni AM, et al. Persistent testicular delta5-isomerase-3beta-hydroxysteroid dehydrogenase (delta5-3beta-HSD) deficiency in the delta5-3beta-HSD form of congenital adrenal hyperplasia. J Clin Invest 1975;55:681–90.
35. Rhéaume E, Simard J, Morel Y, et al. Congenital adrenal hyperplasia due to point mutations in the type II 3 beta-hydroxysteroid dehydrogenase gene. Nat Genet 1992;1:239–45.
36. George MM, New MI, Ten S, et al. The clinical and molecular heterogeneity of 17betaHSD-3 enzyme deficiency. Horm Res Paediatr 2010;74:229–40.
37. Thigpen AE, Davis DL, Milatovich A, et al. Molecular genetics of steroid 5 alpha-reductase 2 deficiency. J Clin Invest 1992;90:799–809.
38. Costa EM, Domenice S, Sircili MH, et al. DSD due to 5alpha-reductase 2 deficiency—from diagnosis to long term outcome. Semin Reprod Med 2012;30:427–31.
39. Cai LQ, Fratianni CM, Gautier T, et al. Dihydrotestosterone regulation of semen in male pseudohermaphrodites with 5 alpha-reductase-2 deficiency. J Clin Endocrinol Metab 1994;79:409–14.
40. Katz MD, Kligman I, Cai LQ, et al. Paternity by intrauterine insemination with sperm from a man with 5{alpha}-reductase-2 deficiency. N Engl J Med 1997;336:994–8.

41. Nordenskjold A, Ivarsson SA. Molecular characterization of 5 alpha-reductase type 2 deficiency and fertility in a Swedish family. J Clinendocrinol Metab 1998; 83:3236–8.

42. Flück CE, Meyer-Boni M, Pandey AV, et al. Why boys will be boys: two pathways of fetal testicular androgen biosynthesis are needed for male sexual differentiation. Am J Hum Genet 2011;89:201–18.

43. Hughes IA, Davies JD, Bunch TI, et al. Androgen insensitivity syndrome. Lancet 2012;380:1419–28.

44. Grino PB, Griffin JE, Cushard WG Jr, et al. A mutation of the androgen receptor associated with partial androgen resistance, familial gynecomastia, and fertility. J Clin Endocrinol Metab 1988;66:754–61.

45. Yong EL, Ng SC, Roy AC, et al. Pregnancy after hormonal correction of severe spermatogenic defect due to mutation in androgen receptor gene. Lancet 1994;344:826–7.

46. Giwercman A, Kledal T, Schwartz M, et al. Preserved male fertility despite decreased androgen sensitivity caused by a mutation in the ligand-binding domain of the androgen receptor gene. J Clinendocrinol Metab 2000;85: 2253–9.

47. Chu J, Zhang R, Zhao Z, et al. Male fertility is compatible with an Arg(840)Cys substitution in the AR in a large Chinese family affected with divergent phenotypes of AR insensitivity syndrome. J Clin Endocrinol Metab 2002;87:347–51.

48. Wisniewski AB, Mazur T. 2009 46,XY DSD with female or ambiguous external genitalia at birth due to androgen insensitivity syndrome, 5alpha-reductase-2 deficiency, or 17beta-hydroxysteroid dehydrogenase deficiency: a review of quality of life outcomes. Int J Pediatr Endocrinol 2009;2009:567430.

49. Josso N, Rey R, Picard JY. Testicular anti-Mullerian hormone: clinical applications in DSD. Semin Reprod Med 2012;30:364–73.

50. Simm PJ, Zacharin MR. Successful pregnancy in a patient with severe 11-beta-hydroxylase deficiency and novel mutations in CYP11B1 gene. Horm Res 2007;68:294–7.

51. Auchus RJ, Chang AY. 46,XX DSD: the masculinised female. Best Pract Res Clin Endocrinol Metab 2010;24:219–42.

52. Zachmann M, Vollmin JA, Murset G, et al. Unusual type of congenital adrenal hyperplasia probably due to deficiency of 3-beta-hydroxysteroid dehydrogenase. Case report of a surviving girl and steroid studies. J Clin Endocrinol Metab 1970;30:719–26.

53. Lin L, Ercan O, Raza J, et al. Variable phenotypes associated with aromatase (CYP19) insufficiency in humans. J Clin Endocrinol Metab 2007;92:982–90.

54. Belgorosky A, Guercio G, Pepe C, et al. Genetic and clinical spectrum of aromatase deficiency in infancy, childhood and adolescence. Horm Res 2009;72: 321–30.

55. Marino R, Perez Garrido N, Costanzo M, et al. Five new cases of 46,XX aromatase deficiency: clinical follow-up from birth to puberty, a novel mutation, and a founder effect. J Clin Endocrinol Metab 2015;100:E301–7.

56. Berkovitz GD, Fechner PY, Marcantonio SM, et al. The role of the sex-determining region of the Y chromosome (SRY) in the etiology of 46,XX true hermaphroditism. Hum Genet 1992;88:411–6.

57. Parma P, Radi O, Vidal V, et al. R-spondin1 is essential in sex determination, skin differentiation and malignancy. Nat Genet 2006;38:1304–9.

58. Cox JJ, Willatt L, Homfray T, et al. A SOX9 duplication and familial 46,XX developmental testicular disorder. N Engl J Med 2011;364:91–3.

59. Moalem S, Babul-Hirji R, Stavropolous DJ, et al. XX male sex reversal with genital abnormalities associated with a de novo SOX3 gene duplication. Am J Med Genet A 2012;158A:1759–64.
60. Schultz BA, Roberts S, Rodgers A, et al. Pregnancy in true hermaphrodites and all male offspring to date. Obstet Gynecol 2009;113:534–6.
61. Sugawara N, Kimura Y, Araki Y. Successful second delivery outcome using refrozen thawed testicular sperm from an infertile male true hermaphrodite with a 46, XX/46, XY karyotype: case report. Hum Cell 2012;25:96–9.
62. Aksglaede L, Jorgensen N, Skakkebæk NE, et al. Low semen volume in 47 adolescents and adults with 47,XXY Klinefelter or 46,XX male syndrome. Int J Androl 2009;32:376–84.
63. Vorona E, Zitzmann M, Gromoll J, et al. Clinical, endocrinological, and epigenetic features of the 46,XX male syndrome, compared with 47,XXY Klinefelter patients. J Clin Endocrinol Metab 2007;92:3458–65.

Index

Note: Page numbers of article titles are in **boldface** type.

A

Adrenal hyperplasia, congenital, 873–875
 3ß-HSDA deficiency in, 875
 11ß-hydroxylase deficiency in, 875
 defective steroidogenesis in, 705–706
 fertility treatments in, 709
 forms of, 706–707
  and effects on fertility, 706–707
 glucocorticoid replacement in, 709
 infertility and reproductive function in, **705–722**
 men with, diagnosis and evaluation of, 713
  due to glucocorticoid overtreatment, 713
  fertility and fecundity rates in, 710–711
  fertility in, 710–715
  fertility treatments in, 713–715
  Legdig cell dysfunction in, 712
  psychological factors and, 713
  Sertoli cell dysfunction in, 712
  testicular adrenal rest tumors in, 711–712, 713–715
 P450 oxidoreductase deficiency in, 875
 pregnancy and fertility rates in, 707
 pregnancy in, management and outcomes of, 709–710
 reduced fertility in, factors contributing to, 707–709
 women with, fertility in, 707–709
Androgen insensitivity, androgen receptor mutations and, 873
Aromatase deficiency, 875–876
 fertility issues in, management of, 876

C

Cancer, adolescent, types of, 800–801
 childhood, in females, antimüllerian hormone and, 744
  chemotherapy in, gonadal damage due to, 743–744
   stem cell transplantation with, 744
  Childhood Cancer Survival Study of, 744, 746
  fertility and alkylating agents in, 744
  long-term survivors of, fertility in, 742–743
  radiation therapy and, 745–746
  in males, chemotherapy in, gonadal damage due to, 740
   stem cell transplantation in, 740–741
  Childhood Cancer Survival Study of, 741, 743
  fertility and alkylating agents in, 741

Endocrinol Metab Clin N Am 44 (2015) 883–888
http://dx.doi.org/10.1016/S0889-8529(15)00135-8
0889-8529/15/$ – see front matter © 2015 Elsevier Inc. All rights reserved.

Cancer (*continued*)
      fertility rates after stem cell transplantation in, 741–742
      long-term survivors of, fertility in, 740–743
      radiation therapy and, 742–743
    survival rates for, 739
    survivors of, gonadal function and fertility among, **739–749**
    types of, 800
  fertility preservation in, 799–800
Childhood, cancer in. See *Cancer, childhood*
Cholesterol side-chain cleavage mutations, 872
Cryopreservation, gamete, 802–812
Cryptorchidism, acquired, and fertility, 755–756
  and fertility, **751–759**
  sperm concentration and adult testicular size after, 753–755
  treatment of, paternity rates following, 752–753

D

Dihydrotestosterone synthesis, 5α-reductase type 2 action and, 872–873
  AKR1C2/AKP1C4 and, 873

E

Embryo, cryopreservation of, 810–811
Estrogens, in treatment of gender dysphoria, 777–778, 782

F

Fertility, cryptorchidism and, **751–759**
  in disorders of sex development, **867–881**
  male, factors influencing, 765
  potential for, evaluation of, 803–804
  preservation of, counseling for, 804–806
    ethical and psychosocial considerations for, 803
    in children and adolescents, **799–820**
    in oncologic conditions, 799–800
    in postpubertal boys, 807–808
    in postpubertal girls, 809–812
    in prepubertal boys, 806
    in prepubertal girls, 808–809
    indications for, 800–802
    informed consent for, 804, 805
    process of, 799
    treatment options for, 806, 807
  prognostic factors for, in idiopathic hypogonadotropic hypogonadism, 828–829
Fertility treatments, in men with congenital adrenal hyperplasia, 713–715

G

Gamete cryopreservation, 802–812
Gender dysphoria, and ambiguous genitalia, 799

completely reversible interventions in, 775–776, 777
diagnosis of, 775, 776
epidemiology of, 774
etiology of, 774–775
irreversible interventions in, 779
partially reversible interventions in, 777–779
reproductive desires and, 782
treatment of, 775–779
    psychological outcomes of, 779–781
    reproductive and fertility outcomes of, 781–782
Gender dysphoric individuals, psychological outcomes and reproductive issues among, **773–785**
Genitalia, ambiguous, gender dysphoria and, 799
Germ cell loss, in cryptorchidism, 752
Germ cell proliferation, during childhood, 751
Germ cells, effect of treatment with chorionic gonadotropin or gonadotropin-releasing hormone on, 752
Glucocorticoid overtreatment, men with congenital adrenal hyperplasia due to, 713
Gonadal suppression, medical, 811
Gonodal dysgenesis, partial, sex development and, 870–871

H

Hypogonadism, hypergonadotropic, in Klinefelter syndrome, 844
    hypogonadotropic, 822
        functional, 824
            and hypothalamic amenorrhea, 826, 827
            pregnancy in, 826
            resumption of menses in, 824–826
        idiopathic, 827–829
            in men, 828
            in women, 828
            prognostic factors for fertility in, 828–829
    varicoceles and, 837

I

Infertility, adolescent varicoceles and, **835–842**
    adult male, varicoceles and, 837

K

Klinefelter syndrome, aneuploidy in offspring of men with, 856
    clinical features of, 844–845
    definition of, 843–844
    diagnosis of, 844
    epidemiology of, 844
    fertility and reproductive abnormalities in, 853–856
        management of, 855
    future considerations in, 856–857
    hypergonadotropic hypogonadism in, 844

Klinefelter (*continued*)
  medical management of, in adults, 853, 854
    in childhood, 852
    in infancy, 851–852
    in puberty, 852–853
  pathophysiology of, 845
  testicular development in, fetal, 846
    function, and pathology in, 845–851
    in adulthood, 851
    in infancy, 846–850
    in prepubertal childhood, 850
    in puberty, 850–851
    primary literature in, 847–849
  testis development and fertility potential in, **843–865**

L

Leydig cell dysfunction, in men with congenital adrenal hyperplasia, 712
Leydig cell hypoplasia, 871–872

M

Male obesity. See *Obesity, male*.
Müllerian duct syndrome, persistent, 873

O

Obesity, male, **761–772**
    affecting sexual maturation and fertility, 762
    and pubertal development, 769
    earlier onset of, pubertal changes in, 762–763, 764
    earlier trend toward puberty and maturation in, 762
    effects of puberty on, 766
    effects on reproduction, 767–768
    in childhood and adolescence, 763–764
    influence on timing of puberty, 766–767
    sexual development in, 764–765
Oocyte(s), human, cryopreservation of, 802–803
  immature, in vitro maturation of, 809–810
  mature, cryopreservation of, 809
Ovarian injury, in long-term survivors of childhood cancer, 743
Ovarian tissue cryopreservation, 808
Ovarian transposition/oophoropexy, 808–809

P

Polycystic ovarian syndrome, anovulation in, mechanisms of, 788–790
  dehydroepiandrosterone sulfate changes in women with, 791, 792
  fertility improvement in, during late reproductive age, 790–792
    testosterone changes in women with, 791
  infertility treatment in, rational approach to, 793–794

menopausal age in women with, 792–793
pathophysiology of, 789–790
reproductive outcome in, in anovulatory and ovulatory patients, 787–788
reproductive system outcome among patients with, **787–797**
testosterone changes in women with, 791
Puberty, and maturation, earlier trend toward, in obesity, 762
  delayed, adult height and, 823
    bone mineral density and fracture and, 823–824
    definition of, 821
    hypogonadotropic causes of, fertility issues in, **821–834**
    self-limited, 822, 824
  male, and reproduction, adipose tissue modulation of, 768–770
    childhood growth and fat development influencing, 765

S

Sertoli cell dysfunction, in men with congenital adrenal hyperplasia, 712
Sex development, disorders of, fertility issues in, **867–881**
    fertility potential in, factors influencing, 868
  ovotesticular and testicular disorders of, 876–877
  partial androgen synthesis defects in, 871–873
    3ß-Hydroxysteroid dehydrogenase type 2, 872
    17ß-Hydroxysteroid dehydrogenase type 3, 872
    cytochrome P450c17 deficiency, 872
    P450 oxidoreductase mutations, 872
  partial gonadal dysgenesis and, 870–871
  46,XX disorders of, 873–876
    fertility issues in, 876
    pathogenesis of, 874
  46,XY disorders of, 868–873
    complete forms of, 868, 870, 871
    fertility issues in, 868, 871
    partial forms of, 868–873
Sexual differentiation, normal, three stages in, 868, 869
Sperm, human, cryopreservation of, 802, 807–808
  in vitro maturation of, 806
Sperm concentration, and adult testicular size, after cryptorchidism, 753–755
Spermatogonial stem cell transplantation, 806
Stem cell transplantation, in childhood cancer, 740–741, 741–742, 744
  spermatogonial, 806
Steroidogenegis, defective, in congenital adrenal hyperplasia, 705–706
Steroidogenic acute regulatory protein mutations, 872

T

Testicular adrenal rest tumors, in men with congenital adrenal hyperplasia, 711–712, 713–715
Testicular tissue freezing, 806
Testosterone, in gender dysphoria, 778–779, 782
Testosterone formulations, in hypogonadism in Klinefelter syndrome, 853, 854
Trachelectomy, radical, 811

Transsexualism, 774
Turner syndrome, assisted reproductive technology in, 728–729
    gonadotropins and ovarian hormone production in, 727
    menstrual function in, 727–728
    ovarian and uterine growth in, 727
    phenotypic features of, 725
    pregnancy in, cardiovascular disease and, 730–731
        cesarean section delivery in, 732
        diabetes and glucose metabolism in, 731–732
        hepatic disease and, 731
        outcomes of, 729–730
        professional society recommendations in, 732–734
        risks and complications of, 730–732
        thyroid disease and, 731
    prepregnancy counseling in, 732, 734
    pubertal maturation in, 727–728
    women with, features of, 723–724
        ovarian development in, 724–727
        reproductive issues in, **723–737**

U

Uterine transplantation, 812

V

Varicocele(s), adolescent, 838–839
        and infertility, **835–842**
    and adult male infertility, 837
    conditions associated with, 836, 837
    definition of, 835
    hypogonadism and, 837
    painful, 837
    pathophysiology of, 836–837
    physical examination to identify, 836
    repair of, approach to, 839–840
        effect of, 839
    treatment of, indications for, 837–839

X

Xenotransplantation, 806

United States Postal Service

Statement of Ownership, Management, and Circulation
(All Periodicals Publications Except Requester Publications)

1. Publication Title	2. Publication Number	3. Filing Date
Endocrinology and Metabolism Clinics of North America	0 0 0 - 2 7 5	9/18/15

4. Issue Frequency	5. Number of Issues Published Annually	6. Annual Subscription Price
Mar, Jun, Sep, Dec	4	$330.00

7. Complete Mailing Address of Known Office of Publication (Not printer) (Street, city, county, state, and ZIP+4®)

Elsevier Inc.
360 Park Avenue South
New York, NY 10010-1710

Contact Person
Stephen R. Bushing
Telephone (Include area code)
215-239-3688

8. Complete Mailing Address of Headquarters or General Business Office of Publisher (Not printer)

Elsevier Inc., 360 Park Avenue South, New York, NY 10010-1710

9. Full Names and Complete Mailing Addresses of Publisher, Editor, and Managing Editor (Do not leave blank)

Publisher (Name and complete mailing address)

Linda Belfus, Elsevier Inc., 1600 John F. Kennedy Blvd., Suite 1800, Philadelphia, PA 19103

Editor (Name and complete mailing address)

Lauren Boyle, Elsevier Inc., 1600 John F. Kennedy Blvd., Suite 1800, Philadelphia, PA 19103-2899

Managing Editor (Name and complete mailing address)

Adrianne Brigido, Elsevier Inc., 1600 John F. Kennedy Blvd., Suite 1800, Philadelphia, PA 19103-2899

10. Owner (Do not leave blank. If the publication is owned by a corporation, give the name and address of the corporation immediately followed by the names and addresses of all stockholders owning or holding 1 percent or more of the total amount of stock. If not owned by a corporation, give the names and addresses of the individual owners. If owned by a partnership or other unincorporated firm, give its name and address as well as those of each individual owner. If the publication is published by a nonprofit organization, give its name and address.)

Full Name	Complete Mailing Address
Wholly owned subsidiary of	1600 John F. Kennedy Blvd, Ste. 1800
Reed/Elsevier, US holdings	Philadelphia, PA 19103-2899

11. Known Bondholders, Mortgagees, and Other Security Holders Owning or Holding 1 Percent or More of Total Amount of Bonds, Mortgages, or Other Securities. If none, check box ☐ None

Full Name	Complete Mailing Address
N/A	

12. Tax Status (For completion by nonprofit organizations authorized to mail at nonprofit rates) (Check one)
The purpose, function, and nonprofit status of this organization and the exempt status for federal income tax purposes:
☐ Has Not Changed During Preceding 12 Months
☐ Has Changed During Preceding 12 Months (Publisher must submit explanation of change with this statement)

13. Publication Title	14. Issue Date for Circulation Data Below
Endocrinology and Metabolism Clinics of North America	September 2015

15. Extent and Nature of Circulation			Average No. Copies Each Issue During Preceding 12 Months	No. Copies of Single Issue Published Nearest to Filing Date
a. Total Number of Copies (Net press run)			787	614
b. Legitimate Paid and/ Or Requested Distribution (By Mail and Outside the Mail)	(1)	Mailed Outside County Paid/Requested Mail Subscriptions stated on PS Form 3541. (Include paid distribution above nominal rate, advertiser's proof copies and exchange copies)	338	254
	(2)	Mailed In-County Paid/Requested Mail Subscriptions stated on PS Form 3541. (Include paid distribution above nominal rate, advertiser's proof copies and exchange copies)		
	(3)	Paid Distribution Outside the Mails Including Sales Through Dealers And Carriers, Street Vendors, Counter Sales, and Other Paid Distribution Outside USPS®	177	191
	(4)	Paid Distribution by Other Classes of Mail Through the USPS (e.g. First-Class Mail®)		
c. Total Paid and or Requested Circulation (Sum of 15b (1), (2), (3), and (4))			515	445
d. Free or Nominal Rate Distribution (By Mail and Outside the Mail)	(1)	Free or Nominal Rate Outside-County Copies included on PS Form 3541	38	37
	(2)	Free or Nominal Rate In-County Copies included on PS Form 3541		
	(3)	Free or Nominal Rate Copies mailed at Other classes Through the USPS (e.g. First-Class Mail®)		
	(4)	Free or Nominal Rate Distribution Outside the Mail (Carriers or Other means)	38	37
e. Total Nonrequested Distribution (Sum of 15d (1), (2), (3) and (4))			38	37
f. Total Distribution (Sum of 15c and 15e)			553	482
g. Copies not Distributed (See instructions to publishers #4 (page #3))			234	132
h. Total (Sum of 15f and g)			787	614
i. Percent Paid and/or Requested Circulation (15c divided by 15f times 100)			93.13%	92.32%

* If you are claiming electronic copies go to line 16 on page 3. If you are not claiming Electronic copies, skip to line 17 on page 3.

16. Electronic Copy Circulation	Average No. Copies Each Issue During Preceding 12 Months	No. Copies of Single Issue Published Nearest to Filing Date
a. Paid Electronic Copies		
b. Total paid Print Copies (Line 15c) + Paid Electronic copies (Line 16a)		
c. Total Print Distribution (Line 15f) + Paid Electronic Copies (Line 16a)		
d. Percent Paid (Both Print & Electronic copies) (16b divided by 16c X 100)		

☐ I certify that 50% of all my distributed copies (electronic and print) are paid above a nominal price

17. Publication of Statement of Ownership
If the publication is a general publication, publication of this statement is required. Will be printed in the **December 2015** issue of this publication.

☐ Publication not required.

18. Signature and Title of Editor, Publisher, Business Manager, or Owner	Date
Stephen R. Bushing	September 18, 2015
Stephen R. Bushing – Inventory Distribution Coordinator	

I certify that all information furnished on this form is true and complete. I understand that anyone who furnishes false or misleading information on this form or who omits material or information requested on the form may be subject to criminal sanctions (including fines and imprisonment) and/or civil sanctions (including civil penalties).

PS Form 3526, July 2014 (Page 3 of 3)

Moving?

Make sure your subscription moves with you!

To notify us of your new address, find your **Clinics Account Number** (located on your mailing label above your name), and contact customer service at:

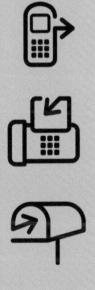

Email: journalscustomerservice-usa@elsevier.com

800-654-2452 (subscribers in the U.S. & Canada)
314-447-8871 (subscribers outside of the U.S. & Canada)

Fax number: 314-447-8029

Elsevier Health Sciences Division
Subscription Customer Service
3251 Riverport Lane
Maryland Heights, MO 63043

*To ensure uninterrupted delivery of your subscription, please notify us at least 4 weeks in advance of move.

ELSEVIER

Printed and bound by CPI Group (UK) Ltd, Croydon, CR0 4YY

07/10/2024

01040499-0020